LEGAL ISSUES IN MENTAL HEALTH CARE

LEGAL ISSUES IN MENTAL HEALTH CARE

Barbara A. Weiner, J.D.
Weiner and Eglit, Ltd.
Highland Park, Illinois

and

Robert M. Wettstein, M.D.
Western Psychiatric Institute and Clinic
University of Pittsburgh School of Medicine
Pittsburgh, Pennsylvania

Springer Science+Business Media, LLC

Library of Congress Cataloging-in-Publication Data

Weiner, Barbara A.
Legal issues in mental health care / Barbara A. Weiner and Robert M. Wettstein.
p. cm.
Includes bibliographical references and index.

1. Mental health laws--United States. 2. Mental health personnel--United States--Handbooks, manuals, etc. I. Wettstein, Robert M. II. Title.
[DNLM: 1. Forensic Psychiatry--United States. 2. Mental Health Services--United States--legislation. WM 33 AA1 W4L]
KF3828.W45 1993
344.73'044--dc20
[347.30444]
DNLM/DLC
for Library of Congress 92-49114
CIP

10 9 8 7 6 5 4 3 2

DOI 10.1007/978-1-4899-1654-9

To all the mental health professionals
with whom we have worked,
and who have taught us
much of what we know

Preface

I. OVERVIEW

Legal Issues in Mental Health Care is aimed at the mental health clinician who provides services on either an inpatient or an outpatient basis. It is written for psychiatrists, psychologists, social workers, nurses, and other therapists to help them understand and manage legal issues in their daily practice. The issues covered apply to therapists who work for an agency or hospital as well as those who work independently.

The book is meant to serve as a handbook, but it also provides a quick resource as legal questions arise which are related to the obligations of the therapist. It addresses the legal issues that confront the clinician. It is not aimed at the clinician who specializes in forensic mental health issues, because the information provided does not reach that level of detail or sophistication. Nor is it aimed at the scholar, because our goal is to provide practical information in a clear and concise format. We have not addressed the wide array of laws protecting the mentally disabled from discrimination—most notably, the Americans with Disabilities Act (1990) and the Fair Housing Act. Most states also have laws that prohibit discrimination in employment, services, and housing. These issues are beyond the scope of this book because we are addressing the legal issues that arise in providing care, rather than the rights of mentally disabled persons.

II. ORGANIZATION OF THE BOOK

The book consists of eleven chapters and a Glossary of Legal Terms. The Glossary provides a quick reference to legal terms that readers are likely to encounter in their practice. The first two chapters are designed to introduce clinicians to the legal system and the attorney's role. Chapter 1, "Introduction to the Legal System," provides an overview of the American legal system and will familiarize the reader with the state and federal court systems, and how to find legal citations. Chapter 2, "The Role of the Attorney in the Mental Health System," discusses the attorney's perspective and the various positions attorneys may represent. There is also discussion of attorneys' fees and how to hire a competent attorney.

Chapters 3–11 discuss legal issues in the clinical context. Specific advice is offered regarding how to respond when a legal issue arises within the clinical context. Although Chapter 6 specifically addresses professional liability, the other clinical chapters also discuss avoiding charges of malpractice when specific issues are raised.

Near the end of each of the clinical chapters is a section entitled "Commonly Asked Questions," which is designed to provide specific advice to the reader about many of the most frequent queries that arise on the topic. In a few instances, the questions and answers will repeat what is in the text. Most, however, introduce new material. If an answer is needed to a specific question, this section is the first place the reader should look. Further information on the topic will then be found in the text of the chapter. We view this section as one of the most valuable features of the book.

At the end of each chapter is a bibliography, in which we have included recent legal cases as well as articles and books. The legal cases chosen are those that have had a major impact on the law in the area, are representative of a trend in the law, or are particularly interesting for other reasons. If readers are interested in reviewing the legal cases, they should first identify those cases in their own jurisdiction, whether federal or state. The selected articles and books are those we believe are worth reading on a particular topic. The bibliography provides readers with a resource if they wish additional information; it is not necessarily comprehensive, but only a supplementary resource.

III. THE AUTHORS' PERSPECTIVE

This book reflects our perspective that there is a need for a practical volume on how the law affects the clinician. It grew out of our combined experience that knowledge of mental health law not only can protect the clinician but, more important, can be made to serve the therapeutic needs of patients. Both authors have worked in this field for more than a decade, and each has been involved in delivering mental health services, as well as training mental health professionals. For 18 years, Barbara Weiner has been an attorney specializing in mental health law. Her practice has concentrated on representing health care providers, including community mental health agencies, hospitals, nursing homes, and individual mental health professionals. At one point in her career, she was the executive director of a not-for-profit grant-in-aid mental health agency.

Robert M. Wettstein is an academic psychiatrist with subspecialty training and experience in law and psychiatry. Much of his work involves consultation and training mental health clinicians in clinical-legal issues. Additionally, he has been a consultant to mental health and legal professionals regarding both policy issues and specific litigation.

The book was conceived based on the authors' experience that there is a need for this type and level of knowledge. The issues addressed and the "Commonly Asked Questions" that have been included are those repeatedly raised by the mental health professionals who consult us. We hope through this book that our experience will be translated into useful information which will be valuable in the reader's daily practice.

V. LEGAL ADVICE

This book is designed to be a ready resource when a legal issue arises within the clinical context. However, it is not a substitute for individual legal counsel, nor does it attempt to answer all questions about situations that may be encountered. Mental health law is continuously in a state of flux, and the laws of each state vary significantly. When there is concern about a legal issue, advice from an attorney experienced in mental health law should be sought as appropriate. The authors do not accept responsibility for any misapplication or misinterpretation of the information contained in this book.

V. NOMENCLATURE

We need to add a few words about nomenclature. We recognize that some mental health professionals view the people they see as "clients" and that others view them as "patients." These terms are largely interchangeable from our perspective. In the text, we have often used the term *client* for those receiving outpatient care and *patient* for those who are hospitalized, but the nature of the material is such that this cannot be done uniformly, so there is some deliberate randomness in usage. We have also found it easier to use the male form of pronouns, although these words should be thought of as referring equally to women and men unless the context specifically calls for the male description.

VI. ACKNOWLEDGMENTS

This publication was supported in part by National Institutes of Health grant LM 04437 from the National Library of Medicine. We gratefully acknowledge their support for our work.

We also wish to acknowledge the contribution of Kathleen M. Quinn, M.D., who not only served as the primary author of Chapter 10 but also assisted with Chapters 7 and 11.

We would like to thank Richard Elliott, M.D., Linda Grossman, Ph.D., Sue Liles, R.N., and Karen Meyer, M.S.W., for serving as valuable commentators as we wrote each chapter. Additional thanks are due to Elizabeth B. Manning, J.D., for her consultation and to Diane Dip for her research assistance. We are also grateful to Nancy Fisher, who assisted with the manuscript.

We would also like to express our gratitude to Loren Roth, M.D., M.P.H., David Kupfer, M.D., and Thomas Detre, M.D. and the staff at Western Psychiatric Institute and Clinic in Pittsburgh for providing the resources to complete this work.

Contents

1. Introduction to the Legal System **1**

I. The Law in Our Society 1
II. Sources of Law 3
A. Constitutional Law 3
B. Statutory Law 4
C. Regulatory Law 5
D. Case Law 5
III. The Court System 5
A. The Federal Court System 6
B. The State Courts 9
C. The Juvenile Justice System 11
IV. The Lawsuit 12
A. The Criminal Case 12
B. The Civil Case 12
C. Rights of Parties Involved in Litigation 13
D. Rights of Parties during a Trial 14
V. The Legal System of Citation 16
A. The Law Library 16
B. Citation of Cases 16
C. Statutory Citations 18
D. Regulatory Citations 20
E. Law Review Articles 20
F. The Mental and Physical Disability Law Reporter 21
G. Updating Legal References 21
VI. Conclusion 22
VII. Bibliography 22

2. The Role of the Attorney in the Mental Health System **23**

I. The Adversarial Process 23
II. The Attorney's Perspective 24
III. Points of Attorney Involvement 26

A. Representing the Mentally Disabled 26
B. Representing the State 28
C. Representing the Family 28
D. Representing the Treatment Facility 29
E. Representing the Treatment Provider 29
F. Representing Children in Juvenile Proceedings 30
IV. Problems in Representing the Mentally Disabled 30
V. When to Contact an Attorney 31
VI. Hiring an Attorney 33
VII. Attorneys' Fees 35
A. Flat Fee 35
B. Range Fee 36
C. Hourly Fee 36
D. Percentage Fee 36
E. Contingent Fee 36
VIII. The Attorney's Impact on the Mental Health System 37
IX. Bibliography 38

3. Involuntary Hospitalization 41

I. Historical Perspective 41
II. Admission Status 43
A. Voluntary Admission 44
B. Informal Admission 45
C. Emergency Admission 45
D. Observational Commitment 46
E. Civil Commitment 46
III. The State's Power to Civilly Commit 47
A. *Parens Patriae* 47
B. Police Power 47
IV. The Civil Commitment Standard 47
V. Determining When Someone Merits Commitment 48
A. Mental Illness 48
B. Danger to Others 49
C. Danger to Self 51
D. Inability to Care for Self: Grave Disability 52
E. Other Commitment Criteria 52
VI. Initiating the Civil Commitment Process 53
A. Recommendations for Completing Commitment Papers 54
VII. The Civil Commitment Hearing 55
A. Rights of the Patient 55
B. The Role of the Prosecutor 58
C. Expectations of the Mental Health Professional at Trial 58
VIII. Outpatient Commitment 59
IX. Duration of Commitment 60
A. Clinical Indications for Discharge or Recommitment 61
X. Financial Responsibility for the Costs of Institutional Care 62
XI. Commonly Asked Questions 63

Appendix: State Civil Commitment Procedures 65
XII. Bibliography 76

4. Rights of Hospitalized Patients 81

I. *Wyatt v. Stickney* 81
II. Communication 82
A. Mail 82
B. Visitation 83
C. Telephone 84
III. Access to an Attorney 85
IV. Presumption of Competency 86
V. Humane Care and Treatment 87
VI. Least Restrictive Alternative 88
VII. Periodic Review 90
VIII. Patient Employment 91
IX. Right to Manage Funds 92
A. Representative Payee 93
X. Right to Refuse to Participate in Research 95
XI. Personal Possessions 97
XII. Religious Freedom 98
XIII. Voting Rights 98
XIV. Commonly Asked Questions 98
Appendix: Patients' Rights 100
XV. Bibliography 104

5. Legal Issues in Providing Treatment 109

I. Legal Basis for Challenging Treatment or Lack Thereof 110
II. Right to Treatment 110
A. Case Law 111
B. Present Status 112
C. Clinical Implications of a Right to Treatment 112
III. The Right to Habilitation 114
A. Case Law 114
B. Present Status 115
IV. Informed Consent to Treatment 115
A. Competency to Consent to Treatment 116
B. Voluntariness 117
C. Information 118
D. Implications of the Right to Refuse Treatment 118
V. The Right to Refuse Treatment for Mental Illness 119
A. The Right to Refuse Psychotropic Medication 120
B. Legal Regulation of Electroconvulsive Therapy 133
C. Legal Regulation of Restraints and Seclusion 134
D. Legal Regulation of Behavior Modification 136
E. Legal Regulation of Psychosurgery 137
VI. Commonly Asked Questions 138
VII. Bibliography 140

6. Professional Liability **149**

I. Malpractice 150
A. Negligence 150
B. Attorney's Analysis of a Malpractice Case 152
C. Proving Professional Negligence 154
II. Potential Areas of Malpractice Liability 158
A. Suicide and Attempted Suicide 158
B. Failure to Diagnose 160
C. Negligent Release 161
D. Sexual Activity with a Patient 161
E. Improper Psychotherapy 163
F. Abandonment 164
G. Negligent Administration of Medication 165
H. Electroconvulsive Therapy 166
I. Negligent Psychological Evaluation 167
J. Social Worker Negligence 167
III. Problems in Proving Liability against Mental Health Professionals 168
IV. Other Causes of Liability 169
A. Lack of Informed Consent 169
B. Breach of Confidentiality 171
C. Duty to Protect Third Parties 171
D. Failure to Report Child Abuse 171
E. Civil Rights Suits 172
V. Hospital or Agency Liability 173
VI. Suits against Supervisory Personnel 174
VII. Suits against State Employees 175
VIII. Malpractice Insurance 176
IX. Record Keeping 177
A. Record Keeping Functions 177
B. Contents of Records 178
X. Malpractice Prevention 181
A. Communication 181
B. Empathy 181
C. Limitations 181
D. Informed Consent 182
E. Fees 182
F. Comprehensive Evaluation 182
G. Consultation 182
H. Continuity of Care 182
I. Knowing the Relevant Law and Institutional Policies 183
XI. Responding to a Malpractice Lawsuit 183
XII. Coping with a Malpractice Lawsuit 185
XIII. Conclusion 186
XIV. Commonly Asked Questions 187
XV. Bibliography 191

7. Confidentiality **201**

I. The Importance of Confidentiality 201
II. What is Considered Confidential 202
III. Breach of Confidentiality 203
A. When the Therapist Can Breach Confidentiality 203
B. Advising Clients about Confidentiality 206
C. Waiver of Confidentiality by the Client 207
D. Disclosure to Investigative Agencies 208
E. Clinical and Social Erosions of Confidentiality 208
IV. Privileged Communications 210
A. Physician–Patient Privilege 211
B. Psychologist–Patient Privilege 211
C. Psychotherapist–Patient Privilege 211
D. To Whom the Privilege Belongs 212
V. Exceptions to the Therapist–Patient Privilege 212
A. Court-Ordered Examinations 213
B. Patient-Litigant Exception 213
VI. Nonstatutory Protection of Confidentiality 217
A. The Ethics of the Mental Health Professional 217
B. The Common Law 218
C. The Constitutional Right of Privacy 218
VII. Minors' Confidentiality 219
VIII. Confidentiality of Drug Abuse and Alcoholism Treatment Records . 219
IX. Acquired Immunodeficiency Syndrome 221
X. Group and Family Therapy 222
XI. Disclosure of Records 222
A. Patient Access 223
B. Statutory Access by Others 223
C. The Records of Minors 224
D. Obligation to Patient 224
E. Disclosure in Publications 224
XII. Responding to a Subpoena 225
XIII. Commonly Asked Questions 225
XIV. Bibliography 230

8. The Duty to Protect Third Parties and Negligent Release **237**

I. The Duty to Protect Third Parties 238
A. Legal Theory 238
B. The *Tarasoff* Decisions 239
C. Post-*Tarasoff* Decisions 240
D. Meaning of *Tarasoff* for Mental Health Professionals 242
E. When There Is a Duty to Protect Third Parties 242
F. Methods of Discharging the Duty to Protect 243
G. Problems Presented by the Duty to Protect 245
H. Avoiding Liability 246

I. Duty-to-Protect Statutes 247
J. Conclusion 249
II. Negligent Release 249
A. Negligent Release Cases: Plaintiff Verdict 250
B. Negligent Release Cases: Defense Verdict 252
C. When Liability Is Likely 253
D. Avoiding Liability 253
E. Conclusion 255
III. Liability for Motor Vehicle Accidents 256
IV. Managed Care 257
V. Commonly Asked Questions 258
Appendix: American Psychiatric Association's Model Statute on the Physician's Duty to Take Precaution Against Patient Violence 262
VI. Bibliography 263

9. Competency and Guardianship 273

I. Types of Competency 274
II. Impact of Competency in the Treatment Setting 276
A. Competence to Consent to Health Care 276
B. Competency Evaluations 276
C. Competency Standards 280
D. When the Person Is Decisionally Incapacitated 281
III. Court Proceedings for Adjudicating Incompetence 282
A. Definition of Incompetence 282
B. Initiation Proceedings 282
C. Rights at the Hearing 282
D. Role of the Mental Health Professional 283
E. Finding of Incompetency 284
IV. Rights Affected by Being Declared Incompetent 284
A. Incompetent as to the Estate 285
B. Incompetent as to the Person 285
V. Appointment of a Guardian 287
A. Selection of a Guardian 287
B. The Guardian's Authority 287
C. Surrogate Decision Making: Principles and Practices 290
VI. Dealing with the Guardian in the Treatment Setting 292
VII. Restoration to Competency 293
VIII. Other Protective Devices 293
A. Representative Payee 293
B. Adult-Protective Services 294
C. Elder Abuse Reporting 294
D. Public Guardian 295
E. Advance Directives 296
F. Surrogate Consent Law 299
IX. Conclusion 299

X. Commonly Asked Questions 300
XI. Bibliography 303

10. Legal Rights of Children 309
Kathleen M. Quinn and Barbara A. Weiner

I. Competency 310
A. Emancipated Minor 311
B. Mature Minor 311
II. The Child Witness 312
III. Access to Medical Care 314
A. Emergency Care 314
B. Parents' Refusal of Treatment 315
C. Handicapped Infants 315
D. Parental Consent 316
E. Child's Role in Treatment Decisions 317
F. Consent by Nonparents 318
IV. Reproductive Rights 318
A. Access to Contraceptives 319
B. Venereal Disease Counseling 319
C. Abortion 319
D. Sterilization 320
V. Access to Outpatient Counseling 320
A. Substance Abuse 320
B. Mental Health Services 321
VI. Psychiatric Hospitalization of Minors 322
VII. Confidentiality of Records 324
VIII. Participation in Research 325
IX. Child Abuse and Neglect 326
A. Reporting Abuse and Neglect 326
B. Investigation of Abuse and Neglect 327
C. Actions to Protect the Child 328
D. Liability of the Caseworker 329
X. Divorce and Child Custody 329
A. Legal Definitions 330
B. Evaluating the Child's Best Interests 331
C. Recommending Joint Custody 332
D. Mediating Custody Disputes 333
E. Acting as Therapist to One of the Parties 333
F. Confidentiality Issues 334
XI. Access of Disabled Children to an Education 334
XII. Juvenile Justice System 336
A. Role of the Mental Health Professional 337
B. Charging the Child as an Adult 337
C. The Future 338
XIII. Commonly Asked Questions 338
XIV. Bibliography 341

11. Involvement with Litigation **349**
I. Why Attorneys Need Expert Witnesses 350
II. Mental Health Professionals in the Courtroom 351
A. Civil Commitment 351
B. Proceedings Related to Children 351
C. Guardianship and Incompetency Proceedings 352
D. Personal Injury Cases 352
E. Workers' Compensation and Disability Claims 353
F. Criminal Cases 353
III. Why the Professional Should Serve as an Expert Witness 355
IV. What to Expect from an Attorney 356
A. Background of the Case 356
B. Clarification of the Legal Issue 356
C. Clarification of What the Attorney Wants 357
D. Access to All Records 357
E. The Evaluator's Setting the Terms of the Evaluation 357
F. Fees 358
G. Conferences 358
V. When a Case Should Be Declined 359
VI. Preparing Reports 360
A. Preparation for Writing the Report 360
B. Format for the Report 360
C. Content of the Report 362
VII. Consulting with the Attorney before Trial 363
VIII. Depositions 364
IX. Testifying at Trial 366
A. Preparation 366
B. Testifying 367
C. Cross-Examination 370
X. Commonly Asked Questions 371
XI. Bibliography 374

Glossary of Legal Terms **377**

About the Authors **387**

Index **389**

1

Introduction to the Legal System

I. The Law in Our Society • **II. Sources of Law** • A. Constitutional Law • B. Statutory Law • C. Regulatory Law • D. Case Law • **III. The Court System** • A. The Federal Court System • B. The State Courts • C. The Juvenile Justice System • **IV. The Lawsuit** • A. The Criminal Case • B. The Civil Case • C. Rights of Parties Involved in Litigation • D. Rights of Parties during a Trial • **V. The Legal System of Citation** • A. The Law Library • B. Citation of Cases • C. Statutory Citations • D. Regulatory Citations • E. Law Review Articles • F. *The Mental and Physical Disability Law Reporter* • G. Updating Legal References • **VI. Conclusion** • **VII. Bibliography**

An overall understanding of the legal system is important for placing in context the system's specific impact on the mental health professional. This chapter introduces the legal system, beginning with a brief history of its development. The chapter sets forth the sources of law in the United States and describes the federal and state court systems. We explain the mechanics of filing a lawsuit, including the rights of the parties. The chapter concludes with a description of the legal system of citation, with examples which should facilitate the reader's use and understanding of legal references.

I. THE LAW IN OUR SOCIETY

The law is a body of rules by which we govern ourselves. It is a reflection of society's history, aspirations, and values and provides a framework within which disagreement and confrontations can be either averted or resolved in a manner short of physical violence. The law seeks to reconcile society's competing demands for continuity and change in a way that encourages social growth yet preserves those principles basic to our democratic ideals. The notion behind the need for laws is the need to find ways to settle disputes. Rules are the heart of the law.

Every society has had a system of laws, whether formal or informal. The earliest formal set of laws which has been preserved is the Code of Hammurabi, which was developed about 2000 B.C. This code set down the kinds of punishment to be used for a variety of offenses and established amounts of payment for various services rendered. About 1200 B.C., Moses presented the Ten Commandments to the Hebrews. This listing of what have come to be fundamental normative values in Judeo-Christian societies have had a profound influence on every subsequent body of Western law.

The ancient Greeks were the first to introduce the concept that laws are made by humans, not gods, and can be changed by them to meet their changing needs. In 450 B.C., the Romans produced the Law of the Twelve Tables, which governed their daily lives. This formed the basis for the civil laws. The legal profession began in Rome at this time. During the Middle Ages, Roman law was rediscovered and revived. Today, most nations in Western Europe, hearkening back to Roman law, are civil law countries; that is, they follow the Roman tradition of codifying rules. This civil law system is a collection of basic principles to be applied to the individual case. It still exists in Europe, and in the United States it was adopted by Louisiana.

The bulk of the American legal system was adopted from the English, whose common law system is not codified but is based on case law. In this system, the law rests on a body of opinion written and developed by judges in the course of deciding particular cases. The notion is that if similar cases are decided in a similar way, consistency will result and people can fashion their behavior and relationships in reliance upon the predictable legal consequences which the case law doctrine prescribes. Basic to the common law is the concept of *precedent*, which means that the court will seek to adhere to its own previous decisions, or to the intervening decision of a higher court on the same issue.

Today, the American legal system is a combination of the common law and a codified system of laws. Our government is a federal system which is a dual system of government, the state and the federal. The United States Constitution and the constitutions of the various states provide the framework for all of our laws. There is a dual system of legislatures and courts, resulting in different laws in each jurisdiction. We are thus governed by the federal laws as well as those enacted by the various states. These parallel legal systems interlock at the level of the United States Supreme Court, since some state court rulings can be reviewed by the U.S. Supreme Court. When there is a conflict between a state law and a federal law, the federal law overrides the state law. It is also possible for someone to violate both federal and state laws at the same time. For example, if someone kills a person at a Veterans Administration hospital, the person has violated both the federal and the state prohibitions against murder. In such a case, the state and federal authorities will reach a decision between them as to who will prosecute the case.

There are many ways to conceptualize the law. For our immediate purposes, we will divide the law between public and private law. Broadly speaking, the private law has five primary divisions: contracts, property, associations, torts, and family law. Contract law is concerned with agreements between people and the legal effects of such agreements. When a reference is made to commercial litigation, one is usually speaking of problems concerning a contract dispute. Property law relates to problems concerning the ownership and use of real property. The law of associations concerns itself with the way people come together as groups to accomplish things. For example, it would cover corporations or the development of partnerships for the purposes of delivering health services. Tort law is concerned with private civil wrongs. Suits claiming some type of personal injury, such as malpractice claims or suits filed as a result of accident cases, are tort actions. Finally, family law is concerned with issues such as divorce, child custody, guardianship, and adoption proceedings.

Public law deals with the framework of the state, the operations of the state, and the relationship between the state and the individual. It includes not only the regulation of individual conduct through the criminal law but also the regulation of many types of actions through a wide variety of laws which govern most aspects of our daily life.

II. SOURCES OF LAW

There are four primary sources of law in the United States: (1) the United States Constitution and the constitutions of the various states, (2) statutes, (3) regulations, and (4) decisions by courts, referred to as *case law*.

A. Constitutional Law

The United States Constitution is our fundamental legal charter. It sets forth, typically without much embellishment, the powers of the three branches of the federal government: the presidency, the Congress, and the federal court system. The federal government is one of enumerated powers; thus, if a power is not set forth in the Constitution it is deemed beyond the reach of any federal entity to exercise. Since the language of the Constitution typically is vague, there is much room for potential expansion so as to bring within the federal sway powers which do not appear on the face of the document. Moreover, the Necessary and Proper Clause of Article I of the Constitution sets forth the groundwork for the doctrine of implied powers, by empowering the Congress to pass laws necessary and proper for carrying out the specifically enumerated powers lodged in the Constitution.

Of particular relevance to mental health professionals is the Commerce Clause contained in Article I of the Constitution, which gives to the Congress the power to regulate commerce. The Supreme Court has broadly interpreted *commerce*. Thus, virtually any activity which has some effect on commerce, no matter how tenuous, is within the purview of Congress. The commerce power gives Congress the authority over many health-related issues, such as the regulation of prescription medication.

Also contained in Article I of the Constitution is the authority for Congress to spend money for the general welfare. This broad language provides support for Congress' creation of the National Institutes of Health (NIH) and the National Institutes of Mental Health (NIMH) and for statutes providing federal funding for clinical, educational, and research programs in the mental health area.

In addition to setting forth powers of the federal government, the Constitution—through the first 10 amendments, commonly known as the Bill of Rights—sets forth a number of constraints on the federal government. Most of these pertain to persons charged with or convicted of federal crimes. However, the Fifth Amendment's Due Process Clause contains a broad-ranging guarantee of individual liberty in civil settings as well: "no person shall be deprived of life, liberty, or property without due process of law." This provision can, for simplicity, be understood here as constituting a guarantee that the federal government must act fairly. The Supreme Court has read into the Due Process Clause a further protection, that is, an equal protection guarantee that persons who are similarly situated must be treated similarly. The analogue of the Fifth Amendment is the Constitution's Fourteenth Amendment, which likewise contains a due process provision, as well as an explicit guarantee of equal protection. The Fourteenth Amendment's constraints apply to state and local governments.

It is the Due Process and Equal Protection clauses which are the source of the explosion of civil rights and civil liberties decisions that have characterized the last 30 years of Supreme Court and lower federal court jurisprudence. In the mental health area, challenges to civil commitment standards and practices, to the care received within state mental health facilities, and to the services available to the mentally disabled within the community have all been based in part on constitutional claims grounded in these provisions. These class action lawsuits, which began proliferating in the late 1960s, have resulted in a revolution in the care of the mentally disabled.

In addition to the Equal Protection and Due Process clauses, other provisions of the United States Constitution have also been relied upon to challenge mental health treatment conditions. Most notable is the First Amendment's guarantee of freedom of thought and the constitutionally protected right of privacy, which have served as the basis for recognizing the right of an involuntarily hospitalized patient to refuse treatment in a nonemergency setting.

Although many of the legal challenges in the mental health area have been based on the United States Constitution, each state has its own constitution, usually modeled on the federal document. These state constitutions set forth the powers of the state governments and the limitations on their powers. Typically, a state constitution also has its listing of guaranteed rights, which rights are typically the same as those set forth in the federal Constitution, but sometimes they articulate even more extensive protections.

B. Statutory Law

Statutory law is law that has been enacted by elected legislative bodies. The United States Congress creates the federal laws. The state legislatures pass the state laws. Local governing bodies pass ordinances, which are laws that apply within their jurisdiction. Each level of legislative body, the local, the state, and the federal, has certain areas which are within its jurisdiction.

The procedures by which laws are passed by the United States Congress illustrates how ideas become laws. A bill is first introduced into either the House of Representatives or the Senate. The bill is assigned a number and is assigned to the appropriate congressional committee. If the committee is interested in the proposal, it will hold hearings and eventually vote on the bill. A committee report will be issued with a recommendation that the bill be either passed or defeated. About 85% of the bills introduced die in committee. If voted out of committee, the bill is scheduled for a vote in the respective chamber of Congress in which it was introduced. Debate occurs on the proposed legislation and a vote is taken. If the bill passes one house of Congress, it is sent to the other chamber for action, and the same process occurs in the other chamber. If the two versions of the bill differ, it is sent to a conference committee, consisting of members from each chamber who work out the final bill. If the bill then passes both houses of Congress it is sent to the President. It becomes law upon the signing of the act by the President or his not taking action within 10 days of its passage. At that point, the bill becomes part of the federal laws.

A similar system exists within the states, with the governor being the key person to sign the legislation. Thus, statutes are pronouncements by legislatures that are declarations of the law. These same legislative bodies that passed the law also have the ability to amend, repeal, revise, or supersede it. In addition, the courts examine the constitutionality and validity of the law.

C. Regulatory Law

Regulatory law has the same authority as a statute. Rules and regulations (they mean the same thing) passed by administrative agencies have the authority of law. They are adopted as part of the authority given the agency by the legislative body which created it. In the federal system, for example, when an agency proposes to adopt a rule, it must provide the public with notice of the proposed rule. This is done by publication in the *Federal Register*. There is then a period of time during which the public can comment on the effect of the proposed rule. After the commentary period, the agency can decide to withdraw, modify, or adopt the rule. If the rule is adopted, it is published in the Code of Federal Regulations (CFR) so that people can be aware of it. When state agencies adopt a rule, they may have a less formal process, although there is usually a means of providing interested public groups with notice and an opportunity for comment. Few states have a formal system for publishing their rules.

Government agencies are often called upon to interpret their rules through administrative decisions. These decisions are often published for federal agencies but are less likely to be published for state agencies, particularly those which deal with mental health professionals, such as the state mental health department. To learn the rules and their interpretation by a state mental health agency often requires directly inquiring of the agency.

D. Case Law

Case law consists of the holdings of appellate courts, which interpret the law. Appellate decisions are usually published, so that it is possible for attorneys to know how a court has ruled on a particular issue. Since one of the goals of the legal system is to be predictable, knowing the precedents set by the courts allows individuals to know what to expect from the courts when they are confronted with an identical or similar situation. The next section will discuss this subject in some detail.

III. THE COURT SYSTEM

Much of law is fundamentally concerned with the resolution of disputes. This is primarily accomplished through the court system. The judge and/or jury hears the facts and the legal arguments and renders a decision based upon the questions presented to it. That decision may recognize that the plaintiff, the party bringing the suit, has specific rights and is entitled to the relief requested from the court; alternatively, it may find there was not a sufficient basis to find for the plaintiff and thus rules in the defendant's favor. When a case is presented to the court, it can decide only the dispute before it, based on the facts and legal arguments presented by the parties.

In the United States, there are two parallel court systems: the federal and the state. The systems are similar in that there is a trial court (lower court) in which the parties appear before a judge, and there are appellate courts (higher courts).

The judiciary perform a number of functions. Perhaps their primary purpose is to analyze the rules of our society and, when they have been violated, to set the punishment. This is most commonly done in the criminal justice system but also applies when one party sues another and the court enforces the civil law by granting specific statutory relief or monetary damages. The courts also interpret the laws and administrative regulations and apply them in specific circumstances. Finally, the courts are called upon to settle disputes between individuals or organizations, based on their legal rights.

A. The Federal Court System

The federal courts have jurisdiction over only certain matters. Matters which involve the federal government as a party, challenges based on the U.S. Constitution, or the violation of federal laws or regulations are most likely to be filed in federal court. There are certain areas of law which are exclusively heard in the federal courts. These include issues of bankruptcy, maritime law, treaties with foreign governments, and matters relating to patent, copyright, and postal regulation. In addition, cases which involve diversity of citizenship can be filed in federal court. A diversity case is one in which the parties are from different states. For example, ABC Corporation is located in New York, and it entered into a contract with XYZ Corporation, which is located in California, to produce parts at its plant in Indiana. If XYZ failed to comply with the terms of the contract, ABC could bring suit in a federal district court in either New York, California, or Indiana, based on diversity jurisdiction. There are also times when an act is a violation of both federal and state law. A person may be prosecuted under either system in those instances.

The U.S. Constitution provides that federal judges are appointed for life by the President of the United States with the advice and consent of the Senate. Congress determines the number of district courts and courts of appeal and the number of judges assigned to each court. Congress also determines the matters over which the court will have jurisdiction, as limited by Article III of the Constitution. (See Figure 1.1.)

1. *The Federal District Courts*

As of 1993, there were 94 federal district courts in the United States. Each state has at least one district court. In the more populated states, there may be multiple district courts. Illinois, for example, has three federal district courts, one for the Northern District of Illinois, one for the Central District of Illinois, and one for the Southern District of Illinois.

When a case is filed in federal district court, it is randomly assigned to a judge. The federal district court is the federal trial court, and the parties will appear before the judge and have the opportunity to present their view of the facts and their interpretation of the law. After all the evidence has been presented, the judge—or jury, if there is one—will render a decision.

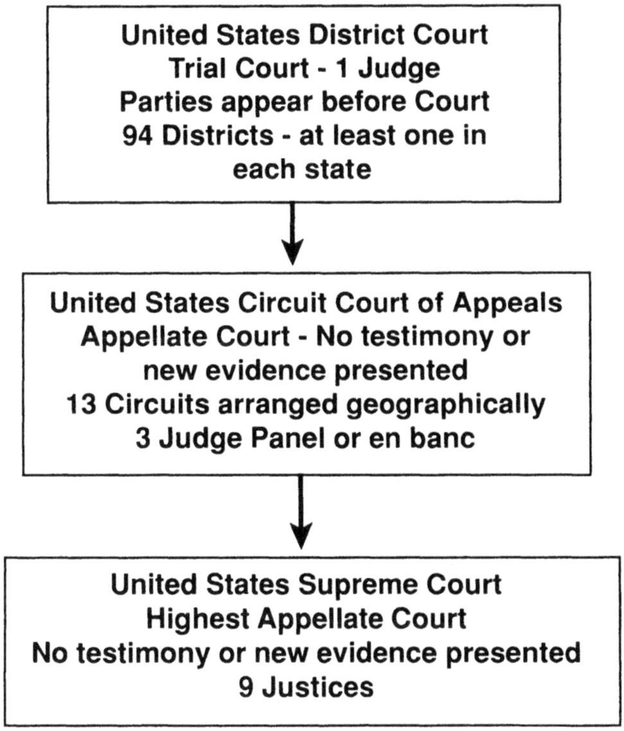

Figure 1.1. The federal court system. Arrows indicate the direction in which appeals are taken.

2. *The Circuit Courts of Appeals*

The United States is geographically divided to form 13 Circuit Courts of Appeals, which are identified by number with two exceptions. The number of judges in each circuit varies and is determined by the Congress. The circuits are numbered 1 to 11, in addition to the Circuit Court for the District of Columbia and the Federal Circuit, which handles copyright and patents. (See Figure 1.2 for the division of the circuits.) As a matter of right, a losing party in the federal district court can appeal to the circuit court of appeals. The appeal is filed in the circuit in which the district court is located.

A hearing in the Circuit Court of Appeals usually consists of three judges reviewing the decision of the district court. In rare instances, when the case is considered unusually important, the full court of appeals may hear the case *en banc*. This means that the case will be heard by all the judges belonging to that circuit court of appeals.

Appellate review can be based on the claim that the district judge either interpreted the law incorrectly or did not apply the law properly to the facts in the case. The arguments are generally articulated through, and based on, the legal briefs and the trial court record. No testimony is given in the appellate process. A brief generally consists of three parts: (1) a statement of the facts, which basically tells the story of the case; (2) questions presented that the appellant wants the court to address;

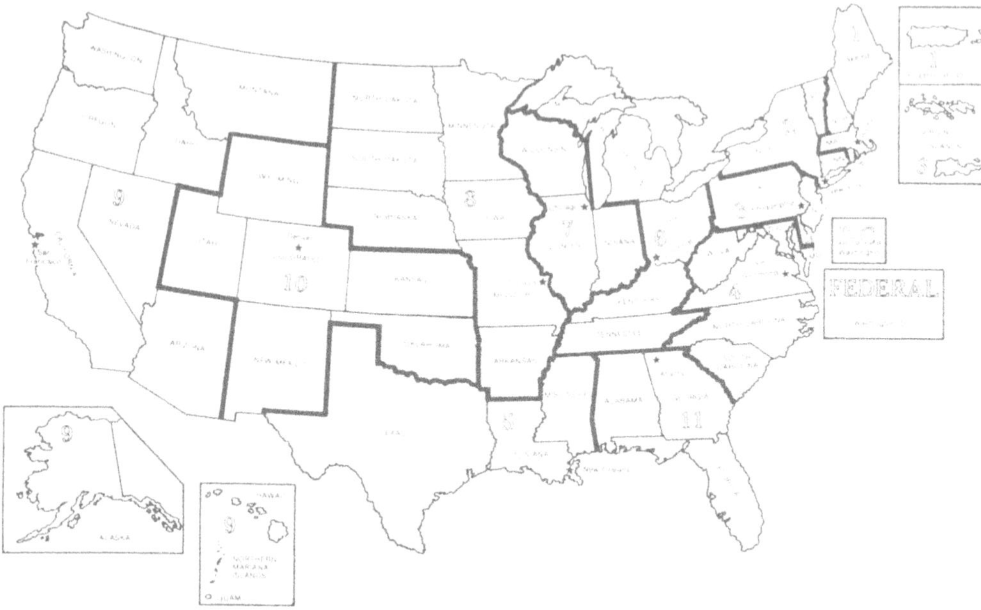

Figure 1.2. The 13 federal judicial circuits.

and (3) the argument, which consists of legal sources to try to convince the court that the trial court ruled correctly or incorrectly, depending on the attorney's position. The attorneys representing the parties are given an opportunity to make short oral arguments after the briefs have been filed. After considering the oral and written arguments, the judges render an opinion. A minimum of two judges forms the majority opinion, which either affirms or reverses the trial court's decision. If an opinion is written, there may be both a majority and a dissenting opinion.

Decisions rendered by the Court of Appeals constitute the law binding precedent in that Circuit. The majority of decisions by the court are published, so that people can be aware of how the court interprets the law on a particular issue within that Circuit.

Although a losing party in the District Court has a right to appeal to the Circuit Court of Appeals, the costs involved in attorneys' fees and the time it takes for a final decision to be rendered makes the losing party think carefully before proceeding further. When the cost and time factors are combined with the recognition that Appellate Courts give a great deal of weight to the findings of the trial court regarding the credibility of witnesses, one can understand the hesitance of those with limited funds to appeal no matter how convinced they are of the merit of their case.

3. The United States Supreme Court

The United States Supreme Court consists of nine justices appointed by the President of the United States to life terms. It is the highest judicial body in the country. A ruling by the Court applies throughout the United States.

The Supreme Court actually hears and decides few cases during its nine-month term each year. Attorneys who wish to have a case heard by the Court present what is known as a petition for a writ of *certiorari*, which calls upon the Court to exercise its discretion and schedule the case for full review. The Court rejects the great majority of petitions for *certiorari*. The Court accepts only those cases which it wishes to hear. Most often the Court will accept a case if it wants to clarify an earlier opinion, or if there is a split of opinion among the various circuits. For example, if the Sixth Circuit Court of Appeals held that a "beyond a reasonable doubt" standard was needed before someone could be civilly committed, and the Seventh Circuit Court of Appeals held that civil commitment required only proof by "clear and convincing evidence," the Supreme Court might accept the case to clarify which single standard should apply throughout the country.

When a case is scheduled for full review before the Supreme Court, a brief is filed setting forth the legal arguments as to why the appealing party believes the Circuit Court of Appeals ruled incorrectly. The opposing party files a response brief setting forth why the court ruled correctly and disputing the arguments made by the petitioner. Often, a group that has an interest in the case but is not a party to the litigation will seek the Court's permission to file an *amicus curiae* (friend of the court) brief, which brings to the Court's attention its position on the matter. The *amicus curiae* briefs are often filed by associations of professionals and set forth data which might not find its way into the briefs of the parties. These briefs will bring to the Court's attention the impact of a decision on the constituency group.

The Court schedules brief oral arguments. Once the Court has considered all the materials before it, including the record from the trial court, the decision from the circuit court of appeals, and the briefs filed in the Supreme Court, including any *amicus* briefs, the justices render a decision. The decision addresses the narrowest legal point, deciding no more than is necessary to settle the controversy. For many attorneys, what the Court does not decide is often as important as what it does decide. Rarely do all the justices agree, and so a decision will have a majority and dissenting opinions, with some justices writing concurring opinions. A concurring opinion means that the justice agrees with the result but wants to clarify, expand upon, or disagree with the reasoning set forth by the majority.

It is rare for a case to be heard by the United States Supreme Court. The appeals process is costly and lengthy. It is not unusual for the Court to render a decision five years or more after the original trial court decision. Since the Court can decide which cases it will choose to hear and will rule on only the narrowest issue, it is only in the exceptional case that an attorney will advise a client to begin the process to seek a review by the United States Supreme Court.

B. The State Courts

Like the federal court system, the state court system consists of at least three levels of courts. The lowest level is the trial court, which has various names, depending on the jurisdiction. It may be known as the court of common pleas, the superior court, or the circuit court. In some states it is known as the supreme court or supreme bench. The higher courts usually consist of two levels of appeals court, usually denominated the Court of Appeals and the Supreme Court. The constitution of the particular state sets forth the powers of the court. (See Figure 1.3.)

The state courts address a much wider variety of issues and hear many more cases than the federal courts. Areas such as divorce, probate, and landlord–tenant

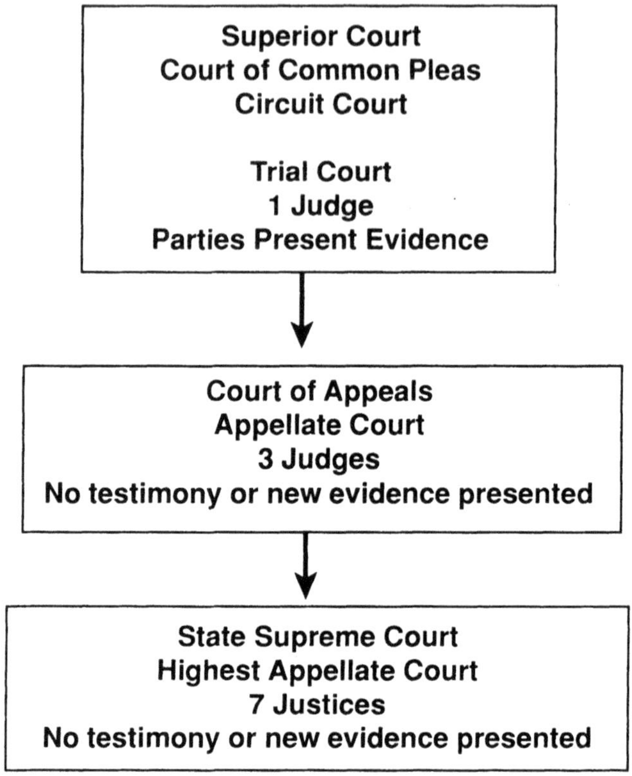

Figure 1.3. The state court system. Arrows indicate the direction in which appeals are taken.

problems are heard only in state courts. Although there is a federal criminal code, the vast majority of criminal matters are heard by state court judges. Except for class action lawsuits which challenge specific aspects of the mental health system on constitutional grounds, the vast majority of litigation which involves mental health professionals occurs in the state court system. This includes civil commitment hearings, guardianship proceedings, and malpractice actions.

Selection of judges to serve within the state court system varies among the states. In many jurisdictions, the judges are elected for specific terms of office. In others, the judges are appointed for a specific term. At the end of the term the judge may have to be reappointed or reelected, depending on the state law. Terms of office for judges vary depending upon the state and on the court to which the judges are appointed or elected.

1. The Trial Court

The trial court is the lowest court in the state system. It has different names in the various states. Depending on the jurisdiction, it may be known as the circuit court, the court of common pleas, the superior court, or the supreme court. Whatever its name, in the trial court the parties appear before one judge (or a jury) and argue their case. After a consideration of the evidence and the legal arguments, a decision is rendered. As a matter of right, the losing party may appeal the decision.

The decision of a trial court has no precedential value and applies only to the parties in that particular case.

2. *The Court of Appeals*

The state court of appeals usually consists of a three-judge panel which reviews the decision of the trial court. The appellate court has before it the record of the proceedings from the trial court. The attorneys for the parties will have filed legal briefs setting forth their arguments either in support of or against the decision of the trial court. The parties will not testify, and the attorneys will be given the opportunity to present brief oral arguments. The basis for the appeal must be that the trial judge either interpreted the law incorrectly or, based on the facts before the court, did not apply the law properly in that situation. Appellate courts give great weight to the decision of the trial court, since the parties were personally present before it and do not appear in the appellate court. Decisions of the appellate court apply to all cases within the geographical area covered by the court. In some states there may be only one appellate court. In larger states there may be numerous appellate courts. Each court of appeals is responsible for a specific geographical area.

3. *The State Supreme Court*

The highest court of the state is usually called the supreme court. For example, the highest court in Illinois is the Illinois Supreme Court, but this is not necessarily the case in all states. In contrast, the highest court in New York is named the New York Court of Appeals. New York also has an intermediate court of appeals. The state's highest courts are the courts of last resort; that is, if a case is lost there, there is no further place to present an appeal. Most state supreme courts consist of seven justices.

Like the U.S. Supreme Court, the state supreme court can decide if it wishes to hear a case. If it chooses to hear a case, it will have the record from the trial court as well as the briefs filed in the appellate court. The attorneys handling the appeal, through legal briefs, try to establish why the appellate court ruled erroneously or correctly, depending upon their perspective. The court usually hears short oral arguments after it has considered the arguments presented in the legal briefs. It will then render an opinion. As in the U.S. Supreme Court, there may be a majority opinion and dissenting opinions with concurring opinions.

C. The Juvenile Justice System

In almost every jurisdiction a special court has been established to handle cases involving children. Juvenile courts usually address issues related to a child's being delinquent in behavior. A juvenile delinquent is a child who has been adjudicated to have committed an act which, if done by an adult, would be considered a crime. Juvenile courts also have authority to address issues of abuse and neglect of the child by his parents or guardians.

The first juvenile court was established in Chicago in 1899. The founders of the juvenile court believed that children who had committed crimes should not be treated as adults and subjected to the harsh environments in which adult offenders were confined. Juvenile court judges are given more latitude in finding a way to "help" the child, rather than punish him. This can include involving social workers in the life of the child, special education programs, probation, or institutionalization in a "reform" or "training" school. These institutions are usually operated by the state department of corrections.

Until the late 1970s, juveniles had few rights in the legal system. As a result of a series of United States Supreme Court decisions, juveniles who are charged with acts of delinquency now have almost the same rights as adults who are charged with crimes. These include representation by an attorney, the ability to examine and cross-examine witnesses, and the right to testify. To protect the child, the names of juveniles are not released when a crime occurs, and their hearings are not open to the public. Judges in juvenile court have much flexibility in designing a punishment which is likely to result in helping the child become rehabilitated. If a child is sent to a correctional institution it cannot be for a period beyond his reaching the age of 21, unless the child has been tried as an adult.

In cases of abuse and neglect the court also has authority to consider a wide variety of alternatives in fashioning a remedy which protects the child. These may include forcing the parents into therapy, making the abusive parent leave the home, or providing homemaker services. The child may also be taken away from the parents, and an abusive parent may be imprisoned.

Since the late 1960s questions have been raised about the value and effectiveness of juvenile courts in addressing the needs of the children who come before them. Although there have been many complaints, obvious solutions are not apparent.

IV. THE LAWSUIT

The filing of a lawsuit is the formal means by which one party, the plaintiff, notifies another party, the defendant, that he is seeking recourse through the court system for some harm he alleges to have occurred to him. Whether the legal action involves a loss of liberty or monetary damages determines the rights that a defendant has during the course of the suit. (See Table 1.1 for a summary of the steps involved in suing someone.)

A. The Criminal Case

Someone who is charged with a crime is prosecuted through the criminal justice system. The case will be entitled something like *People of the State of Michigan v. John Doe*. The state will be represented by a state's attorney or the district attorney, who is called the prosecutor. John Doe is the defendant, since he is defending against the charges the state has placed against him. He will be represented by an attorney. If he can independently afford to hire an attorney, he will be represented by a private attorney; if he does not have sufficient funds to hire an attorney, a private attorney or public defender will be appointed to represent him without charge.

B. The Civil Case

When a civil case is filed, the case is named after the parties involved. If Susan Smith wishes to sue Michael Jones for breach of contract, for example, the case would be referred to as *Smith v. Jones*. In this case, Susan Smith is the plaintiff, meaning she is the person complaining that she has been harmed and her rights have been

Table 1.1. Steps in Bringing a Lawsuit to Trial

1. Drafting a complaint. This states the basis for the lawsuit and sets forth the relief requested.
2. Filing the complaint in the trial court.
3. Serving the defendant with a copy. This gives him notice of the suit.
4. Defendant files an answer and makes a counterclaim if he desires.
5. Discovery. Each party can gain more information about the issues directly related to the lawsuit.
6. Filing pretrial motions. These are usually related to the sufficiency of the complaint or compliance with discovery.
7. The trial. This is the opportunity for the parties to present to the court the evidence which supports their positions.
8. The court's decision and entry of the order.

violated. Michael Jones is the defendant. He is accused by Ms. Smith of having violated her rights, and he must defend against her claims.

C. Rights of Parties Involved in Litigation

In order to ensure fairness in our system, both parties to a lawsuit have specific rights before their case is heard and during the course of the trial. These rights include notice, discovery, answer, and counterclaim.

1. Notice

Notice requires that the person being sued be made aware of the suit. This is accomplished by serving the defendant with a copy of the complaint filed against him. The complaint must be sufficiently specific so that the defendant knows what is the basis of the suit and what remedy is being sought.

2. Discovery

Each party to a suit has a right to learn more from the other party about the issues which are raised in the lawsuit. For example, if Susan Smith is suing Michael Jones for malpractice, she has a right to discover a copy of the records he kept on her as a patient. Michael Smith, in defending the suit, has a right to know on what basis she is claiming that malpractice occurred. If she sought another professional psychiatric opinion and obtained further treatment, he will be entitled to copies of those records. He might also argue that Ms. Smith's problems existed before she consulted him and might thus seek copies of records from treatment providers who saw her before he saw her. What may be discovered is often broad and is within the discretion of the trial court judge. The discovery process is frequently time-consuming and can result in prolonging the case for many months, sometimes years, before it proceeds to trial. Yet, discovery is the chief reason a case will be settled out of court. Often, once both sides are fully informed of the strengths and weaknesses of each side, they can realistically evaluate the situation and reach a reasonable settlement, without incurring the costs of a trial.

3. *Answer*

This is the formal means by which the defendant can respond to the suit. He may deny all the allegations in the complaint. He may admit some allegations and deny others, or he may admit the allegations but set forth a defense for his actions. In a criminal case, the answer is the defendant's response to whether he is guilty or not guilty. In a civil case, there will be a written answer.

4. *Counterclaim*

The counterclaim permits the defendant in a civil case not only to answer the complaint filed, but also to set forth a complaint against the plaintiff. For example, if ABC Corporation sues XYZ Corporation for breach of contract, XYZ may deny that it breached the contract and may set forth a counterclaim against ABC for not paying $50,000 for a shipment of materials.

D. Rights of Parties during a Trial

A party's rights at trial depend upon whether the case is civil or criminal. To complicate matters further, there are some instances in which the case is civil but there is a loss of liberty, such as in a civil commitment proceeding, and the defendant will be entitled to additional rights. (See Table 1.2 for a summary of rights at trial.)

1. *Witnesses*

In both civil and criminal proceedings, the parties have a right to call witnesses to establish or defend their positions. In addition to calling witnesses, each party usually serves as its own primary witness to set forth the facts as it perceives them.

2. *Examination and Cross-Examination*

On direct examination, each party has the opportunity to ask questions of its own witness. On cross-examination, the witness is questioned by the other side. Redirect examination occurs when the witness is again questioned by the attorney for the side originally calling that witness. The purpose of redirect examination, and then recross-examination, is to further clarify points brought out in the witness's earlier testimony.

Table 1.2. Rights of Parties at Trial

1. Notice of proceedings and opportunity to respond.
2. Representation by an attorney if loss of liberty is involved.
3. Admission of evidence in support of the position of each party.
4. Examination and cross-examination of witnesses.
5. Ability to present legal arguments in support of position.
6. Decision by a judge or jury. Basis for decision will be explained if made by a judge.
7. Right to appeal.

3. *Representation by an Attorney*

Individuals have the right to represent themselves in litigation, known as *pro se* representation. They also have the right to hire an attorney to represent them. Only in instances where someone can be deprived of liberty is he automatically entitled to an attorney paid for by public funds if he is indigent. This occurs in all criminal proceedings carrying a penalty of imprisonment and in civil commitment proceedings. Defendants are also guaranteed legal representation for the purpose of appealing their criminal conviction. In other cases, there is no legally guaranteed right to an attorney. However, because of the complicated nature of legal proceedings, most people who seek redress through the court system hire an attorney to represent them.

4. *Jury*

Whether one has a right to a jury trial depends on the type of litigation involved. In all criminal proceedings, the individual is entitled to request a jury trial. Although not mandated by the U.S. Supreme Court, criminal trial juries consist of 12 persons. The jury's decision to convict the defendant must be unanimous. When the jury cannot reach a unanimous decision, there is a hung jury and a new trial may result. There can also be a mistrial when the jurors cannot agree, when newly discovered evidence is brought out at the trial, or when either attorney engages in outrageous conduct before the jury.

In many types of civil proceedings, the parties can also ask for a jury. This may be a smaller jury, such as six persons. There are also many types of litigation in which a jury is not permitted, for example, in contested child custody disputes. In civil cases, depending on the state, there may or may not be the requirement of a unanimous jury verdict. Most cases, both civil and criminal, are tried without a jury.

5. *Standard of Proof*

This is the weight of evidence necessary to determine if the plaintiff has presented his case successfully. There are three standards of proof. The lowest standard is "preponderance of the evidence," which is the standard of proof used in most civil actions. On a scale from zero to 100, it is at 51, meaning that the plaintiff needs to have just more than half of the evidence in his favor to win the suit.

The "clear and convincing evidence" standard is at approximately 75 on the scale. This is the standard used in most jurisdictions for civil commitment proceedings and termination of parental rights. The "beyond a reasonable doubt" standard is used for criminal proceedings. This standard requires that the judge or jury be approximately 95% convinced that the defendant committed the crime with which he is charged.

6. *Right to Appeal*

As a matter of right, the loser in the trial court can appeal the decision to a court of appeals. The appeal will argue that either the trial judge interpreted the law incorrectly or that he misapplied the law based on the facts of the case. An indigent criminal defendant is entitled to a copy of the trial record for appeal purposes. A nonindigent defendant must bear the full cost of his appeal. The appellate court can uphold the decision of the trial court or can reverse it and remand the case for a new trial on the issue on which it has reversed.

V. THE LEGAL SYSTEM OF CITATION

This section will introduce the reader to the law library and the legal system of citation. The law library contains the primary tools of the attorney's profession. Having a rudimentary understanding of the legal system of citation will make it possible for the mental health professional to know which court decided a case, and to research further to determine if there are later statutory or case law developments in the area of concern.

A. The Law Library

A law library is similar to other libraries in that books and periodicals are arranged systematically and a librarian may be available to offer assistance. Like other libraries, law libraries are progressively becoming computerized, and access to a computerized data base may be the best way to identify and locate reference materials. The law library is different from other libraries in that almost all the materials contained within its walls relate to the law. There are basically three categories of law books:

1. Those which contain the statutory or quasi-statutory laws. These are the original laws passed by a body legally authorized to do so, such as the Congress or a state legislature. The most common quasi-statutory laws are rules (the same as regulations), which are written by agencies to enact the laws passed by legislative bodies.
2. Those containing appellate cases, which are published in law reporters (discussed in Section B below).
3. Those books which explain the law, such as periodicals, treatises, or law reviews.

In addition to the law books, there are also numerous resources to help locate the law, such as digests and indexes. For the attorney, the law library is the most important resource in the practice of his profession.

There are now at least two computerized legal research systems. These are Lexis and Westlaw. Through access to a computer, legal research has been revolutionized. These systems are in the process of adding all previously reported cases, statutes, and in some instances citations of law review articles. By entering key words about which the researcher needs information, he can quickly find the pertinent cases, as well as law review articles related to the subject.

Generally the public has access to a law library through the local court system. In addition, many law schools will permit members of the public to use their library, although they will probably not permit the withdrawal of books and other materials.

B. Citation of Cases

Since an appellate decision may have precedential value, it is important for attorneys to be able to find what the courts have held on a particular issue. This is accomplished through reading the case law. Case law consists of the decisions handed down by the courts, usually appellate courts, and it is published in law reporters. Reporters are law books which contain the appellate decisions from the various state and federal courts. There are separate reporter systems for the federal and state courts as well as separate systems for the various levels of courts. Whenever a case is cited, there is a reference to the volume of the reporter in which the case can be found and its page number. For example, in the case *O'Connor v. Donaldson*, 422 U.S. 563 (1975), *422* refers to the volume number of the *United States* reporter where the case can be found, *563* refers to the specific page on which the case begins in the volume, and *1975* is the year the case was decided. (See Figure 1.4.) Each year there are approximately 50,000 cases reported in the various reporter systems.

1. *The Federal District Court*

These decisions of the Federal District Courts are reported in the *Federal Supplement*, referred to as *F.Supp.* For example, in the case *Rogers v. Okin*, 478 F.Supp. 1342 (D. Mass. 1979), which addresses a patient's right to refuse medication, *478* refers to the volume number of the *Federal Supplemental Reporter*, where it is published; *1342* refers to the page number where the case begins; *D. Mass.* means the case was decided in the Massachusetts Federal District Court; and *1979* was the year in which the case was first decided.

2. *Circuit Court of Appeals*

Appellate decisions are reported in the *Federal Reporter*, referred to as *F.* or *F.2d.* When the *Rogers* case was appealed, the decision of the circuit court of appeals was reported as *Rogers v. Okin*, 634 F.2d 650 (1st Cir. 1980). This means that the decision in this case can be found in Volume 634 of the *Federal Reporter*, second edition, and begins on page 650. The case was decided by the First Circuit Court of Appeals in 1980.

3. *The United States Supreme Court*

Decisions of the United States Supreme Court can be found in any of three reporter systems: the *United States Reporter*, or *U.S.*; the *Supreme Court Reporter*, or *S. Ct.*; and the *United States Law Week* reporter, or *U.S.L.W.* (See Table 1.3). Most cases are referred to by the "U.S." citation. The reference to *Law Week* is usually used before the case has been published in either the United States or Supreme Court

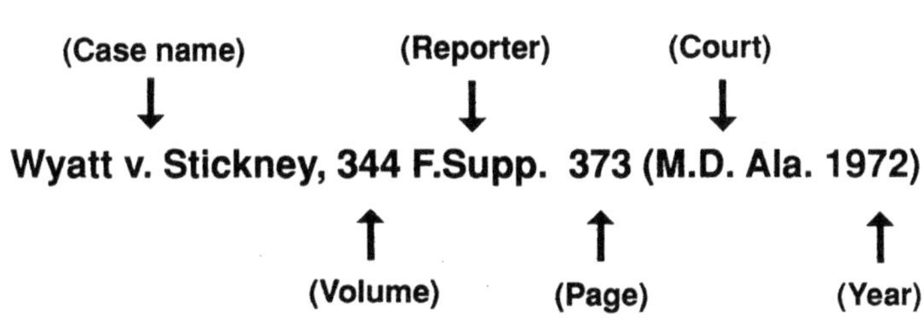

Figure 1.4. Reading a case citation. The case of *Wyatt v. Stickney* is found in Volume 344 of the Federal Supplement (F. Supp.) as shown.

Table 1.3. Citations to Federal Court Opinions

Court	Reporter	Reporter abbreviation
United States District Court	*Federal Supplement*	F. Supp.
United State Circuit Court of Appeals	*Federal Reporter*	F. or F.2d
United States Supreme Court	*United States Reporter*	U.S.
	Supreme Court Reporter	S.Ct.
	United States Law Week	U.S.L.W.

reporters. *Law Week* is a weekly publication that makes available Supreme Court decisions, as well as a synopsis of other important decisions within a short time of the decision's being handed down. In the case of Supreme Court decisions, they are available in *Law Week* within a week of the Court's having rendered its opinion. In addition, Supreme Court decisions are immediately available by computerized access in a limited number of facilities.

As another example, when the *Rogers v. Mills* case was appealed to the United States Supreme Court, the case became *Mills v. Rogers*, 457 U.S. 291 (1982). The reversal of the order of the parties reflects who filed the appeal. This means that the case can be found in Volume 457 of the U.S. Reports beginning at page 291. The reader immediately knows that any decision published in the U.S. Reports is a Supreme Court decision; this one was handed down in 1982. This same decision was also reported at 102 S.Ct. 2442 in the *Supreme Court Reporter*, and 50 LW 4677 in the *Law Week Reporter*.

4. The State Court System

State appellate court decisions can be found as part of the National Reporter System published by West Publishing Company. The National Reporter System divides the United States into seven geographical areas, and the cases from a state are reported in the regional reporter for that area. (See Figure 1.5.)

For each reporter, there is now a second series. For example, *Guardianship of Richard Roe*, 421 N.E.2d 40 (Mass. 1981) can be found in Volume 421 of the second series of the *North Eastern Reporter* at page 40. It was a Massachusetts state court case decided in 1981.

In addition to the *National Reporter System*, 32 of the 50 states publish their own official reporters. Thus, as in the United States Supreme Court cases, a state case may have parallel citations. In the case *State v. Krol*, 68 N.J. 236, 344 A.2d 289 (N.J. 1975), the first citation refers to the 68th volume of the *New Jersey State Reporter* at page 236, and the second cite refers to Volume 344 of the *Atlantic Reporter* (second series) at page 289.

C. Statutory Citations

1. Federal Laws

Laws enacted by the United States Congress are published in the United States Code, referred to as U.S.C. The Code is published by the federal government and

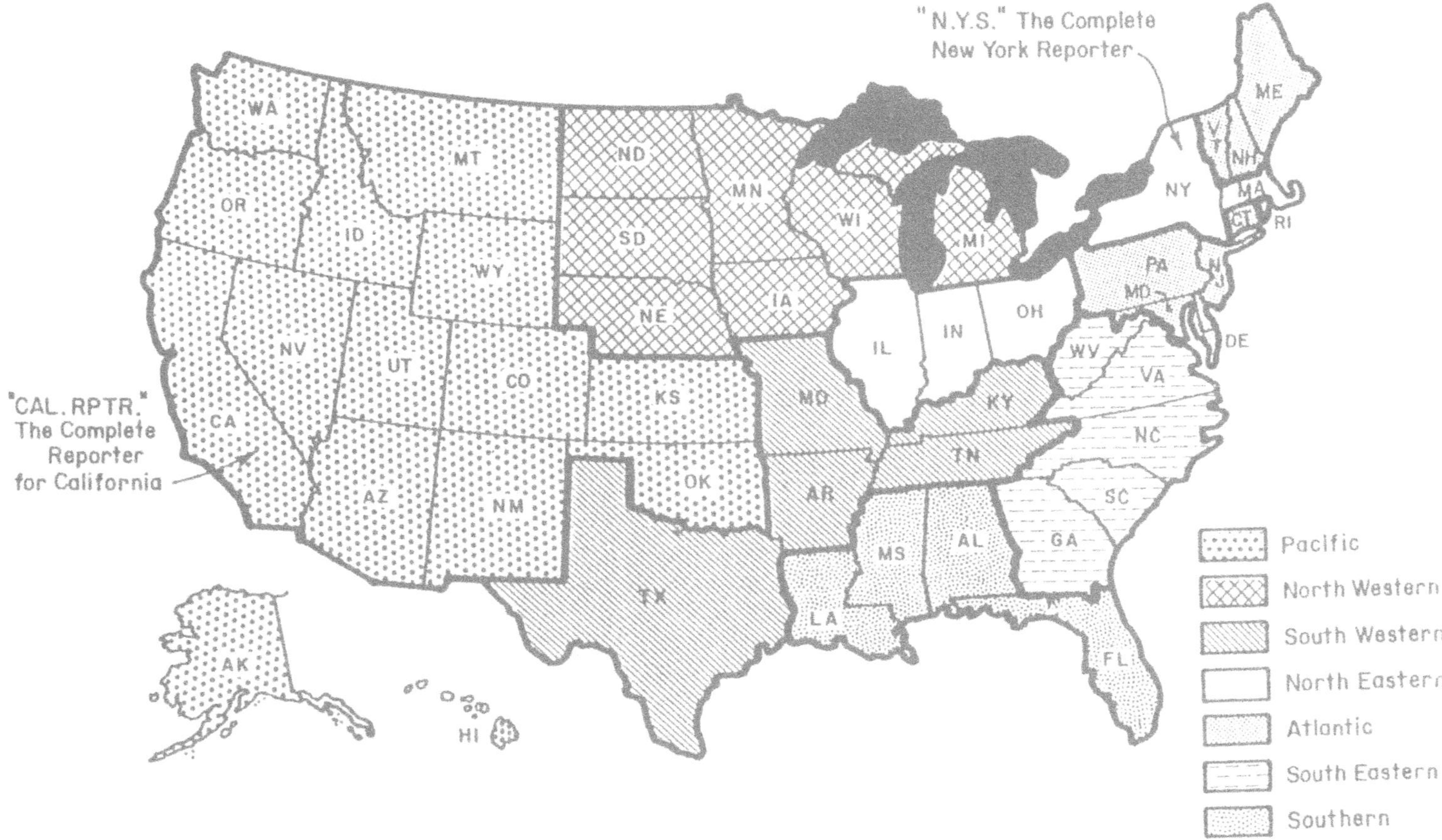

Figure 1.5. The National Reporter System. The seven reporters are abbreviated as: Atlantic (A.), North Eastern (N.E.), North Western (N.W.), Pacific (P.), South Eastern (S.E.), South Western (S.W.), and Southern (So.). The system also includes the *Supreme Court Reporter,* the *Federal Reporter,* the *Federal Supplement, Federal Rules Decisions,* the *New York Supplement,* and *West's California Reporter.* Reprinted with permission, West Publishing Co.

includes the United States Constitution and its amendments, as well as federal laws. These laws are divided into 50 titles with many subdivisions. The U.S.C. has a four-volume index which lists acts by their popular names and provides cross-references for the researcher. For example, the Education for All Handicapped Children Act of 1975 is cited as Pub. L. No. 94-142, 20 U.S.C. Sec. 1400 (1976), meaning that the act is found in Volume 20 of the United States Code at Section 1400. In addition to the U.S.C., the United States Code Annotated (U.S.C.A.) is published by West Publishing and is located in every law library. The primary advantage of the U.S.C.A. over the U.S.C. is that it provides a summary of cases with the citations which have interpreted the statute.

2. *State Laws*

Each state publishes its laws and has its own method of deciding where a law fits in its codification scheme. States also provide a subject index at the end of their codes so the researcher can find the laws on a particular topic. In addition to the official set of statutes, West Publishing Company publishes the laws of 21 of the most populated states in a manner which is similar to the U.S.C.A. For example, the insanity defense standard in Illinois is found at Ch. 38 Ill. Rev. Stat. Sec. 6-1. This means that this law is in Volume 38 of the Illinois Revised Statutes at Section 6-1. In the official statutes, all that appears is the law. In the annotated laws published by West, there are brief descriptions of cases which have interpreted the law, as well as references to law review articles on the topic if applicable.

D. Regulatory Citations

Administrative agencies are created by legislative bodies. Their regulations have as much impact on citizens as statutes, and their decisions have the same authority as case law. There is a specific rule-making process for both federal and state agencies before their rules can be put into effect, the process varying with the jurisdiction.

The regulations of federal agencies can be found in the Code of Federal Regulations (CFR). This is a codification of the general and permanent regulations of the various agencies. The CFR is divided into 50 titles, which represent broad subject areas of regulatory action. The regulations of primary concern to the mental health professional are those of the Department of Health and Human Services (HHS). These are codified in Volume 45 of the Code of Federal Regulations, referred to as 45 CFR. For example, the regulations on the protection of human subjects are contained in 45 CFR 46. At the beginning of Section 46 is a table of contents which lists the subsections for the topic.

State regulations are often harder to locate, since few states publish their rules in a formal manner. The rules that a mental health professional would most likely want to be cognizant of are those of the mental health agency and the state professional licensing agency. In many instances, these rules are not published, and a telephone call to the agency might result in an unhelpful response. It often appears that only when something has been done improperly will the agency have the ability to cite a specific rule which has been violated.

E. Law Review Articles

The mental health professional will frequently see a reference to a law review article. Most law schools publish law reviews, and some even publish several law reviews which address specific topics, such as labor law or civil rights. Law review articles generally give a detailed analysis of the law on a particular topic. Sometimes the article analyzes a case or statute in depth. Law reviews are usually kept alphabetically on the shelves of the law library.

The *Index to Legal Periodicals* provides a researcher with the means of finding law review articles on particular topics. The index is published monthly, and it annually provides a title, author, and subject index. References to law review articles contain many abbreviations. One example is "Plotkin, Limiting the Therapeutic Orgy: Mental Patients' Right to Refuse Treatment, 72 Nw. U.L.Rev. 461 (1978)." This citation provides the author's last name and the title of the article; *72* is the volume number of the *Northwestern University Law Review, 461* is the page number on which the article begins, and *1978* is the year the article was published. Another example is "Rhoden, The Right to Refuse Psychotropic Drugs, 15 Harv. C.R.-C.L.L.Rev. 363 (1980)." This 1980 article by Rhoden is published in Volume 15 of the *Harvard Civil Rights-Civil Liberties Law Review* at page 363.

F. The *Mental and Physical Disability Law Reporter*

The *Mental and Physical Disability Law Reporter* (MPDLR), published six times a year, is a project of the Commission on Mental and Physical Disability Law of the American Bar Association. First published in 1976, it is the most comprehensive source of developments in mental health law. The reporter includes not only reports of cases but also legislative proposals and enactments. Often federal and state regulations will be noted. Topical articles are also included. For those who wish to keep abreast of developments in this field, this reporter is highly recommended. It is perhaps the best source of providing up-to-date information on the broad range of topics in mental health law. Although many clinicians may not be able to afford an individual subscription, it is a worthwhile resource for the library of any facility or agency that delivers mental health services, or for groups of practitioners who share expenses. This reporter is often cited in the mental health law literature. In a legal citation, it will be cited as "MDLR before 1984" or "MPDLR after 1984" when "Physical" was added to the title. Information or subscriptions can be obtained from the American Bar Association, 1800 M Street, N.W., Washington, D.C. 20036-5886.

While the *Mental and Physical Disability Law Reporter* is an excellent source of information on mental health law developments, there are several other publications in the mental health law area which clinicians are likely to find useful in their practice and which may be located in their facility libraries. Several of the best known include *Behavioral Sciences and the Law, Bulletin of the American Academy of Psychiatry and the Law, International Journal of Law and Psychiatry, Journal of Psychiatry and Law,* and *Law and Human Behavior*. These are published four or six times per year, depending upon the journal, and cover clinical, research, and policy issues in the mental health law area. Subscription information can be obtained from an issue of the journal or by contacting the publisher of the journal.

G. Updating Legal References

Finding legal references may be useless unless one understands how to update them. A reference to a law which has subsequently been amended or repealed is meaningless. It is erroneous to cite a case for a proposition when the case has been overruled. Thus the law library provides the resources to keep current on all legal developments.

The Shepard's citation provides a means of locating and evaluating the status of legal cases. (A pamphlet on how to use this service can be obtained by writing Shepard's/McGraw-Hill, P.O. Box 1235, Colorado Springs, Colorado 89001.) Shepard's publishes citators to cover all federal and state court decisions, federal and state laws, and law review articles. For example, if the researcher wanted to know whether *Wyatt v. Stickney*, 344 F.Supp. 373, had been overturned on appeal, he would go to the Shepard's citator for this volume of the *Federal Supplement*. Once the researcher located the references to Volume 344, he would search for page 373; there he will find a list of further numbers which will refer to other cases in which this case was cited or further decisions on this particular case. To further understand what subsequently occurred with the case, the researcher would need to refer to the Shepard's references at the front of the index to see if the various letters mean the case was cited, reversed, and so on. For further clarification, the researcher should examine the relevant cases cited.

The Shepard's citation system can be used for statutes as well as cases. In addition, in the back of each volume of state or federal statutes there is a "pocket part." This provides the latest update on a statute. In instances where the code is annotated, such as the United States Code, the pocket part will also provide brief descriptions of cases which have recently been decided relating to that statute.

Westlaw and Lexis, the two computerized legal research systems, have made it much easier to perform the initial research and then update cases, statutes, or other citations. By correctly citing the case or statute, the computer will update any developments. In addition, by using "key words," the researcher can find related developments on a topic.

VI. CONCLUSION

The information presented in this chapter is only enough to help guide the mental health professional to the appropriate section of the law library. Developing skills in legal research, as in medical and social science research, takes training and practice. Thus, if the reader finds himself in the law library with some idea of what he wants, he should not hesitate to ask the librarian for assistance. Once one begins to use the law library, it becomes easier on each successive visit.

VII. BIBLIOGRAPHY

Coco, A. (1982). *Finding the law: A workbook on legal research for lay persons, prepared for Bureau of Land Management*. Washington, DC: U.S. Government Printing Office.

Elias, S. (1986). *Legal research: How to find and understand the law* (3rd ed.). Berkeley: Nolo Press.

Friedman, L. M. (1984). *American law*. New York: W. W. Norton.

Harnett, B. (1984). *Law, lawyers, and laymen, making sense of the American legal system*. San Diego: Harcourt Brace Jovanovich.

Llewellyn, K. N. (1962). *The bramble bush*. New York: Oceana.

Statsky, W. P. (1986). *Legal research and writing: Some starting points* (2nd ed.). St. Paul: West.

Wren, C., & Wren, J. (1984). *The legal research manual*. Madison, WI: A-R Editions, Inc.

2

The Role of the Attorney in the Mental Health System

I. The Adversarial Process • II. The Attorney's Perspective • III. Points of Attorney Involvement • A. Representing the Mentally Disabled • B. Representing the State • C. Representing the Family • D. Representing the Treatment Facility • E. Representing the Treatment Provider • F. Representing Children in Juvenile Proceedings • **IV. Problems in Representing the Mentally Disabled • V. When to Contact an Attorney • VI. Hiring an Attorney • VII. Attorneys' Fees** • A. Flat Fee • B. Range Fee • C. Hourly Fee • D. Percentage Fee • E. Contingent Fee • **VIII. The Attorney's Impact on the Mental Health System • IX. Bibliography**

This chapter will address the various points of interface between attorneys and the mental health system. Discussion will center on the type of proceedings which relate to the mentally disabled as well as the special problems presented to the attorney by having a mentally disabled person as a client. However, before one can analyze the unique role the attorney has played in relation to the mental health system, it is important to have some understanding of the attorney's perspective. The chapter will also discuss when to contact an attorney, and how to hire an attorney, including fee arrangements. The chapter concludes with a discussion of the attorney's impact on the mental health system.

I. THE ADVERSARIAL PROCESS

The American legal system has developed its own unique process for determining the merits of a legal case. Known as the *adversarial system,* this approach requires a neutral and passive fact finder, reliance on the contesting parties to present the evidence, and a highly structured setting for presenting the case. The fact finder, either a judge or a jury, is expected to refrain from any conclusion until all the evidence has been presented and, to ensure impartiality, must refrain from actively participating in the gathering of the evidence.

The contesting parties are responsible for the production of all the evidence upon which the decision is to be based. This requirement has the dual advantages of insulating the fact finder from involvement in the case and requiring the parties to put forward what they believe to be their most important proof. The litigation is thus focused on the questions of the greatest importance to the litigants, and a decision tailored to their needs is therefore more likely. Because of the complexity of legal questions and the intricacy of our legal system, litigants usually hire attorneys to represent them in their lawsuits. The attorney brings to the process an ability to organize and present the material in a way which comports with the rules of procedure and in a manner acceptable to the court.

There are elaborate rules for conducting the trial, as well as for pretrial and posttrial actions. The rules of procedure set the stage for the confrontation of the parties at the trial. This confrontation leads to the presentation of all the evidence upon which the decision will be based. Rules of evidence protect the fact finder from evidence which is likely to be unreliable or unfairly prejudicial to one of the parties. These rules confine the judge to the role of a manager of the proceedings. Although trials are often likened to battles, attorneys are prevented from winning "at any cost" by rules of procedure and a set of ethical standards which governs their behavior during the representation of a client. Thus, the trial gives the parties whose interests are adverse to each other the opportunity in a structured setting to have an independent fact finder determine which litigant's position is supported by more evidence, and that party becomes the winner in the lawsuit.

Appellate courts have the authority to review the decision of the trial court to determine if the court and the litigants complied with the rules of procedure. This review process, and the authority of the appellate court to redress the errors of the trial court, encourages the attorneys and judges to adhere to the requirements of the law; otherwise they may be reversed on appeal.

Concepts that make up the adversarial system have been around for approximately 700 years, although the actual system as it exists today did not exist until around 1700. For almost 300 years, this approach has provided a system of justice that helped establish the United States as a country where wrongs can be addressed and corrected in a fair and equitable manner. We do not have inquisitions, and each side has the opportunity to state its case during its day in court.

II. THE ATTORNEY'S PERSPECTIVE

Perhaps the most difficult thing for mental health professionals or any layperson to understand about the legal system is the perspective of the attorney. Questions frequently arise: How can an attorney represent someone he knows is guilty? Why does the attorney fight to prevent the civil commitment of someone who the attorney believes needs hospitalization? Obviously, the attorney's perspective is different from that of the mental health professional. The mental health professional has been trained to seek the "medical best interest" of the person, which is measured by the training, experience, and personal values of the individual practitioner. The fundamental ethical consideration is to promote health and maximize life.

In contrast, the ethical obligations of the attorney are more complex than defining the medical best interest of his client. Attorneys function in the adversarial system; they believe that the trial setting affords a fair opportunity for the opposing interests to clash and will result in an equitable solution to the conflict. This requires attorneys to counsel clients about the benefits and costs of each legal alternative, but the ultimate decision of which path to follow is the client's. Thus, while the attorney is the adviser, the client must make the final decision. The attorney may disagree with the client's decision and believe the approach the client has chosen is not in his best interest, yet the attorney has the responsibility to accept the client's decision if he is going to represent the client. Although the attorney may disagree with his client, he must zealously advocate his client's position by asserting and protecting the client's legal claims, rights, and interests. The attorney, for example, may know that his client is guilty of murder, yet he believes that everyone is entitled to representation and the full rights guaranteed by the legal system. He further believes that through the trial process the truth will be determined and justice will be served. If the attorney believes that he cannot provide the client with the proper representation, then he is obligated to decline the case or withdraw at the point when he believes he is not serving the best legal interests of his client.

The attorney has many responsibilities to his client. The first is to be objective and dispassionate in analyzing the client's case. The importance of this responsibility cannot be overemphasized. Often the client is involved in the issue and can see only his side, with no awareness of the legal merits of the case. Perhaps this objectivity is the most important service the attorney can provide. He needs to advise the client about the potential likelihood of success and various legal strategies to be employed in the situation. This can be done only if the attorney is familiar with the law in the area or researches the topic so that he becomes current with legal developments in the area under discussion. The attorney must then share his knowledge with his client and explain the areas where there are questions about how the law can be interpreted. This critical advice will determine whether a suit will be filed or how it will be defended. It might encourage the client to settle the case without going forward with litigation. The initial analysis of the case sets the stage for all the later proceedings.

The attorney and client must have an open and honest relationship in which the client keeps the attorney advised of all the facts and developments, and the attorney advises the client of any actions he is proposing to take. The attorney must keep abreast of the law in the area and advise his client accordingly. The attorney must inform his client when there are developments in the case, and he cannot take any final action without the client's approval. Finally, the attorney must provide the services to which he agreed, and for the fee agreed upon.

An important concept underlying the attorney–client relationship is that of attorney–client privilege. This testimonial principle was adopted in England in 1577 and exempted attorneys from providing evidence on matters their clients had discussed with them. Today, the privilege is recognized in every state. It provides that matters discussed by the client with the attorney which are meant to be kept confidential are privileged and cannot be discovered in legal proceedings. This testimonial privilege provides the client the freedom to be completely open and honest with his attorney. It makes it possible to fully reveal past illegal activity, if any, and allows full discussion of the events leading to the present charges without fear that the attorney will notify the criminal justice authorities. The attorney–client privilege recognizes that individuals often do not seek legal assistance unless they have been involved in questionable or illegal activities. Thus, the privilege is the only way the person can admit his activity to his attorney and receive competent legal advice.

This evidentiary privilege is intended to protect and preserve the privacy of the client's concerns, interests, and affairs and to ensure that the client will be willing to disclose sensitive and personal information to the attorney. Confidentiality is expected not only of the attorney but also of those employed by him who learn about the particular case. The privilege remains in effect indefinitely, unless the client authorizes disclosure or unless one of the exceptions to the privilege arises. There are few exceptions to the attorney–client privilege; the two most notable are if the client sues the attorney for malpractice, or if the client reveals plans to be involved in future criminal activity. In the latter event, the attorney, as an officer of the court, has an obligation to breach confidentiality and come forward with his knowledge.

III. POINTS OF ATTORNEY INVOLVEMENT

An attorney can represent five possible parties involved in mental health issues: (1) the patient/client, (2) the state, (3) the family of the patient/client, (4) the treatment facility, and (5) the treatment provider. This section will briefly discuss the types of cases in which the attorney may be consulted.

A. Representing the Mentally Disabled

The mentally disabled need legal representation on a variety of issues which affect the general public, such as divorce, wills, or real estate; they also need special representation related to disability (see Table 2.1). The most common types of cases in which mental disability is a factor are the following:

1. Civil Commitment Proceedings

The disabled person may be represented by a private attorney but is more commonly represented by a public defender specifically assigned to this task or, in less populated areas, by a court-appointed attorney. In civil commitment proceedings (discussed in Chapter 3), the goal of the attorney for the disabled person is to try to prevent, or at least minimize, hospitalization when the patient has decided he does not wish to enter the hospital voluntarily. Although the attorney may identify the need for hospital-based treatment, he is responsible for representing the expressed wishes of his client, and for using the full force of the legal system to make sure the client's position against hospitalization is represented.

Table 2.1. Attorney Representation of the Mentally Disabled

1. Civil commitment hearings
2. Transfer and discharge hearings
3. Protecting rights within the institution
4. Advocating for rights within the community
5. Defending the disabled in criminal proceedings
6. Incompetency and guardianship proceedings

2. *Rights within the Institution*

Most mental health codes set forth the rights of the disabled person within the institution (see Chapter 4). Sometimes the only way to enforce these rights is with a lawsuit or the threat of a lawsuit. In other instances, a mentally disabled person is entitled to representation at transfer or discharge hearings. Generally, in these proceedings the mentally disabled person will be represented by a public interest attorney. This may be a member of a legal aid organization which is funded by the federal, state, or local government, or it could be a member of an advocacy group which has been specifically funded to represent the mentally disabled. In the past, particularly for the developmentally disabled, there has been funding available for this type of representation. With the cutback in federal funds for legal services, this money has greatly diminished, although there has been a recent resurgence of some federal funds for protection and advocacy services for the mentally disabled. However, a growing number of states have funded their own advocacy systems for the mentally disabled. Governmental funding for these programs is essential to ensure the rights of the disabled, since these cases are not likely to generate fees and therefore would not be acceptable to most attorneys in private practice.

In addition to seeking to enforce individual rights within the institution, "class action" lawsuits have been brought to attempt systematic change. A *class* can be broadly defined. For example, it may include all adults at a facility, or all women on a particular unit, or all persons within the state mental health system. The goal of a class action suit is to bring about specific changes in the system to benefit the identified class. These lawsuits have had a major impact in eliciting widespread changes in the mental health system, thus resulting in improved services to the mentally ill and developmentally disabled. These suits are usually undertaken by legal aid organizations. With the decrease in funding legal services for the mentally disabled, in conjunction with major changes in mental health codes which often reflect court victories in class action litigation, the numbers and scope of these suits in the mental health area have diminished.

3. *Rights within the Community*

In a few states there are specific advocacy programs for the mentally disabled which provide for representation for general legal matters. However, if specific rights are to be enforced, such as providing services for the developmentally disabled within the school system, or providing more community treatment or habilitation programs, these suits are usually brought as class action lawsuits by legal aid or advocacy agency attorneys. These attorneys might also represent the disabled in seeking social security or other entitlement program benefits. Few private attorneys take such cases except on a *pro bono* (without fee) basis because they would not generate sufficient fees.

4. *Representation in Criminal Proceedings*

The fact of mental disability may have an impact on an individual's progress through the criminal justice system. It may determine whether he is charged with a crime or diverted directly into the mental health system for treatment. It may affect whether he is found competent to stand trial or is found to be criminally responsible. Finally, mental disability may influence the sentence the individual receives, including being required to obtain treatment. In these cases, although mental disability may distinguish the defendant from other defendants, he will not be given special representation because of this fact. Like others charged with crimes, he will be represented either by a private attorney if he can afford it, or by a public defender if he cannot. In those cases where the court assumes the cost of representation, the court will also provide funds for the attorney to hire experts to assist him in preparing the defendant's defense. The court will approve each expenditure, though limits may be placed on how much can be spent on experts.

B. Representing the State

Although treatment providers or family members may seek the civil commitment of a particular individual, these proceedings are brought in the name of the state under either its police or its *parens patriae* powers. This is the case because individuals do not have the right to institutionalize someone, but the state does have this power. The attorney acting on behalf of the state will be an official of a governmental agency. Depending upon the state, he will be referred to as an assistant attorney general, an assistant district attorney, or an assistant state's attorney. This attorney presents the evidence which supports commitment for the mentally disabled person. He will call witnesses, including the treatment staff, police, and the family, to testify to help make his case.

In addition to commitment proceedings, the representative of the state will be involved if the mentally disabled person is charged with a crime. This attorney will prosecute the defendant in the hopes of convicting him of the crime with which he is charged. As in commitment proceedings, the state is represented by a prosecutor, who is known as an assistant attorney general, a district attorney, or a state's attorney. His goal is to represent the interests of the community by ensuring that those who commit crimes will be brought to justice for their actions. This attorney will also represent the state when there is an effort to suspend or terminate parental rights.

C. Representing the Family

There will be times when the family of the mentally disabled person will take steps that the disabled person will view as adverse to his interests. This commonly occurs when the family seeks civil commitment, and the disabled person does not believe he needs to be committed. In this instance, the family may hire a private attorney to intervene with the state's attorney to initiate civil commitment proceedings, or to be sure that their position is advocated at the commitment hearing, although the state's attorney will present the bulk of the case for commitment.

In other instances, the family may seek to have the disabled person declared legally incompetent so that he will no longer have the authority to make personal decisions or manage his financial affairs (see Chapter 9, "Competency and Guardianship"). They will hire a private attorney to file the appropriate court documents for this to be accomplished. In many states, the court will appoint an attorney to represent the allegedly disabled person, and thus the family and the respondent may be on opposing sides of the petition for a declaration of legal incompetency.

Attorneys may also become involved in representing families who are seeking to enforce rights on behalf of their disabled relative. This could include suing to guarantee the person's statutory rights, such as access to educational or other entitlement programs. It might also involve filing a wrongful death action, which could include a suit against the facility or treatment provider claiming that malpractice was the cause of death (see Chapter 6, "Professional Liability").

D. Representing the Treatment Facility

Attorneys representing the treatment facility have a wide range of legal responsibilities. They will be responsible for handling the legal matters in which the facility is involved, including patient rights, contracts, labor negotiations and discipline, and other legal matters. If a staff member is sued in his capacity as an employee, the facility attorney becomes involved. Much of the attorney's time is spent advising the facility on a broad range of legal issues and responding to questions of individual staff members.

When the treatment facility is operated by a governmental agency, the attorney will be a government attorney. Few state mental health agencies have their own attorneys for each treatment or habilitation facility. Usually the state mental health agency has attorneys to represent its facilities, or in less populated states, these legal services may be provided by attorneys from the attorney general's staff. In either event, if the attorney has much experience in representing mental health and developmental disability facilities, he will be a good source of answers to specific questions relating to the rights of the disabled.

If the treatment facility is private, a private attorney who works full time at the facility or an outside attorney, usually a member of a law firm, will provide legal advice and consultation. An outside attorney, because of the wide variety of organizations he is likely to represent, may not be as knowledgeable about specific issues relating to the mentally disabled as an attorney who works full time with these issues. However, if he is presented with a mental health law problem, he will research the appropriate law on the issue so he can provide the proper advice.

E. Representing the Treatment Provider

There are occasions when the individual treatment provider seeks legal consultation relating to issues which arise during his professional activities. If the legal issues arise in a treatment facility setting, then the provider can consult the attorney for the facility. However, if the issues arise in a private practice setting, the practitioner will need to consult a private attorney. For legal issues which relate to the rights of the mentally disabled, it may at times be difficult to find attorneys with the requisite experience and knowledge. The best source are attorneys who represent treatment facilities, or those who advise professional organizations.

If the treatment provider receives notice of a lawsuit for actions which arise out of providing mental health services, he should immediately contact his insurance carrier, who will provide him with an attorney. If the provider is uncomfortable with the attorney chosen by the insurance company, he has the option of requesting a different one. If the suit is brought as a result of services provided in the treatment facility, the attorney for the facility should also be notified immediately. It is advisable for mental health professionals to be aware of at least a local attorney whom they can retain when they need consultation on mental health issues. This should be someone who is familiar with this area of the law. Some mental health professionals who are experienced or trained in law and mental health may also be helpful to the treatment provider in these situations.

F. Representing Children in Juvenile Proceedings

When a child is charged as a delinquent, he is entitled to legal representation by an attorney. In urban areas, this is likely to be someone from the public defender's office. In rural areas, it is more likely to be a court-appointed attorney who is paid on a per case basis. In some jurisdictions, the attorney is a strong advocate and approaches the proceeding in a manner similar to the way he would represent an adult charged with a crime. In other jurisdictions, the attorney is likely to be less adversarial and to spend more of his time seeking alternative sentencing solutions, which will avoid institutionalization.

In addition to the attorney's role in delinquency proceedings, attorneys are also involved when child abuse charges are before the court. An attorney for the child, referred to as the GAL, or guardian *ad litem*, is appointed. This attorney is charged with ensuring that the child's interests will be protected. This may mean fighting vigorously to have a child removed from his parents, or to have a parent removed from the home.

IV. PROBLEMS IN REPRESENTING THE MENTALLY DISABLED

The concepts which underlie the attorney's ethical obligations to his client originated from the perspective that the client is a mentally competent individual. Thus, once the attorney explains the law to the client or suggests various alternatives, the client must choose which legal course of action to follow. The attorney is then responsible for advocating that position, although he may disagree with it. In contrast, when the client is mentally disabled, because of either mental retardation or mental illness, perhaps the rules should be different. There are, however, few ethical guidelines for these situations, and mentally disabled clients pose special problems for the attorney who seeks to undertake their representation.

The first issue presented is whether the disabled person is able to hire, rationally communicate with, and pay an attorney. Clearly there are times when disabled people need and are entitled to legal representation. Yet some disabled people are so incapacitated by their mental disorders that they fail to recognize the need for legal representation or are unable to communicate meaningfully with any attorney who might be appointed in their behalf. To compensate for their disability in terms of hiring attorneys, some states have developed specific advocacy programs for the mentally disabled. The underlying assumption of some of these programs is that the advocate will represent the best medical interests of the disabled (in contrast with their expressed wishes, which may be distorted by their illness) and will seek to ensure that they will obtain all the legal rights guaranteed them.

A second conflict may arise when the attorney has a long-standing relationship with both an individual and his family. The family seeks the attorney's representation to take an action which the client perceives as adverse to his interests, such as declaring him legally incompetent to manage financial matters. In this instance, the attorney may be aware of the psychological decompensation of the client, yet the client does not believe he is mentally impaired and wishes to be represented by his attorney. In this case, to avoid any conflict or even the appearance of impropriety by representing both the individual and the family, the attorney would be wise to refer the family elsewhere. This referral, however, would not preclude the attorney from advising his client to agree to have others manage his affairs if he believes this course would be most beneficial to the client. However, until the client is declared legally incompetent or the attorney withdraws from representing him, the attorney must follow the directives of his client.

A third problem situation arises when an attorney is hired by an executive of a company to represent the company as well as handle the executive's personal legal matters. Once the attorney becomes aware of the executive's failing mental abilities, he has a duty to bring them to the attention of the corporation's board of directors. At that point, he must choose whether he will represent the executive or the corporation in the conflict which is likely to arise. He cannot continue to serve the interests of both since their interests are now adverse to each other.

When the client is severely or profoundly retarded, and thus clearly incapacitated to make decisions about any aspect of his life, the attorney can represent the disabled person in a way which would seem to protect his best interests as judged by what a reasonable person would do in similar circumstances. However, when the client is mentally ill, the distinction between rationality and irrationality may be more elusive. Because a client chooses a course which seems irrational to many may not mean that this position should be rejected. After all, each person has a right to make foolish decisions. The issue for the attorney becomes one of whether he should undertake representation of this client, and in what fashion. The attorney is ethically obligated not to file suit or pursue a course of action which seems meritless. Thus, although the attorney is required to follow the wishes of his client, there are limits to this command, particularly when there can be a division of opinion on a course of action. These problems are particularly acute in the area of medical decision making. In these cases, the client may decide to forego a life-saving or life-sustaining treatment that offers a high chance of success because of what appears to be an irrational belief. This type of case poses difficult legal and ethical problems for the attorney, as well as for the treatment provider. In cases where the refusal of treatment seems irrational, the treatment provider or family may seek to have the person declared legally incompetent so as to be able to compel him to accept the necessary treatment (see Chapter 9). The matter then shifts to a court, which will decide how the individual's interests should be served.

Few would argue that the mentally disabled do not need or are not entitled to legal representation. These cases often pose complicated legal and ethical problems for the attorney. Nevertheless legal representation is provided. The mental health professional must be sensitive to the fact that the attorney is often grappling with these issues while trying to accommodate the needs and desires of his client.

V. WHEN TO CONTACT AN ATTORNEY

Many questions of a legal nature are likely to arise during the course of the therapist's practice. These relate to the rights of the patient/client as well as to the therapist's legal obligations. Areas of practice which commonly require legal consultation include confidentiality, protecting members of the public from a dangerous patient, the right of the disabled to refuse treatment, or their right to various entitlement programs. The law in each state is different, and thus what is read in a professional journal or heard at a seminar may not apply in the therapist's state. These issues merit correct legal consultation, which can be offered only by an attorney who is current on the status of the law in the state where the therapist is practicing.

Perhaps the most common circumstance in which the mental health professional should seek legal advice is upon receipt of a subpoena for either records or testimony (see Table 2.2). In the case of a subpoena for records (*subpoena duces tecum*), the therapist should never automatically provide the attorney with a copy of the requested records. The therapist should first contact the patient to whom the records relate and notify that person of the subpoena. The therapist should also inform the patient what the records contain so he can decide if he wishes them to be released. If the therapist is then authorized to release the records, a written consent should be obtained from the patient. If not, and the patient does not want the records released, the patient should contact an attorney who should attempt to quash the subpoena. Until the therapist receives further advice from his attorney or the attorney for the patient, he should not release records.

If the therapist receives a subpoena to appear for a deposition, he will probably have no choice but to appear. The therapist may be able to rearrange the time of the deposition to one that does not conflict with his schedule. As the treatment provider, the therapist will be required to appear and will be paid only a nominal fee to cover transportation costs. The therapist may seek to have the subpoena quashed through his attorney or the attorney for the patient. The therapist would be well advised to have a brief consultation with his attorney about his concerns and how to respond to a subpoena.

The therapist should immediately contact an attorney when he receives a copy of a complaint (lawsuit) which has been filed against him. He must also notify his malpractice insurance carrier within a specified time after receiving a copy of the suit, if the lawsuit is based on allegations of professional negligence (see Chapter 6, "Professional Liability"). If the suit arises out of the therapist's employment, he should immediately notify the attorney for the treatment facility. Whenever a clinician is sued, immediate notification of an attorney is critical, since the clinician will have a limited amount of time to file a formal response (answer) to the allegations in the complaint. If an answer is not filed on time, he will lose the suit by default.

The therapist may wish to contact an attorney when he is concerned about being

Table 2.2. When to Contact an Attorney

1. Upon receipt of a subpoena for records or testimony.
2. Upon receipt of a copy of a complaint.
3. When suit is likely.
4. When questions arise about the rights of the disabled.
5. When concerned about legal obligations, particularly regarding the need to breach confidentiality.
6. When seeking advice on how to deal with attorneys.
7. When a legal issues arises in private practice.

sued. This may occur when he receives threats of a lawsuit or something has happened which leads him to speculate on the possibility of litigation, such as a patient's suicide. Although consultation with an attorney cannot change the fact of an adverse result of treatment, the therapist might find it reassuring and receive suggestions on how to proceed in the future.

Legal consultation may be beneficial to determine whether the therapist is legally obligated to breach confidentiality for the public's benefit. Most notable are child-abuse-reporting statutes. Although each state has them (see Chapters 6 and 10), the requirements vary as to who must report suspected child abuse and neglect and under what circumstances. A much more ill-defined area of the law relates to the mental health professional's obligation to protect third parties from danger from their patient/client (discussed extensively in Chapter 8). In addition to obtaining a consultation from colleagues on the matter, the therapist is advised to speak to an attorney about his concerns and learn what the law requires in his state.

Business issues may arise in a professional practice which require legal consultation. These may include whether to form a partnership or a professional service corporation. Legal consultation should be sought before entering into a contractual relationship with a treatment facility or other provider. For these types of matters, the investment in legal consultation at the outset reduces the likelihood of subsequent legal problems.

The clinician may have unpleasant contacts with attorneys who are seeking confidential information from him which he is not willing to divulge without the patient's written consent. The attorney may threaten to bring the ramifications of the legal system to bear if the therapist does not cooperate with his wishes. He may threaten to bring the clinician to court, for example. Usually these are idle threats, but attorneys have learned that mental health professionals, like most people, are afraid of being involved in the legal process. Contacting an attorney can provide the therapist with the advice he needs to handle the situation confidently and competently.

Finally, the therapist should contact an attorney when he has any question about whether he needs legal advice. This contact will not only clarify for him his legal rights and obligations but may help reduce his anxiety over a particular situation. The attorney will attempt to protect the rights and interests of the therapist and ensure that he will receive all the protections guaranteed by the legal system. Many of the issues which the therapist will raise can be handled in a telephone consultation with the attorney. The therapist should expect to be billed some minimum amount for any consultation, even if it takes only a few minutes. Like mental health professionals, the attorney earns a living by selling his expertise based on the time involved.

VI. HIRING AN ATTORNEY

Now that we have discussed when the therapist will need to contact an attorney, the question arises of whom he should contact. This section will provide suggestions on how to find an attorney, and what to expect from the attorney who is hired (see Table 2.3.)

When one is seeking an attorney to advise the therapist on mental health law

Table 2.3. Hiring an Attorney

Hire an attorney with the following attributes:
1. Is highly recommended by colleagues or friends.
2. Is knowledgeable and competent in the area of legal concern.
3. Has sufficient time to handle the legal problem at issue.
4. Is interested in the legal problem.
5. Seems compatible and congenial.
6. Has affordable fees.

issues, an attorney who represents a mental health treatment facility is likely to be the most knowledgeable in this area. If the therapist is associated with a treatment facility, then he should contact the facility's attorney. If the therapist is not associated with a facility, he can find out who represents the major treatment facilities in his area. The facility attorney may be in a position to represent the therapist, or if not, he should be able to provide the names of any attorneys in the area who are knowledgeable about the issues of concern. If the therapist is employed by the treatment facility, even if only on a part-time basis, he may not want to hire the attorney for the facility if he thinks there may ever be an occasion when his interests will conflict with those of the facility.

Asking colleagues about who provides them with legal services is also likely to lead to an attorney who can meet the therapist's needs. The best advertisement an attorney can have is a satisfied client. If colleagues were pleased with the assistance they received, then this is someone with whom the clinician may be comfortable.

If the therapist has no colleagues who have experiences with attorneys or their only experiences have been unsatisfactory, he may want to ask family members or friends for the names of the attorneys they use. Although these attorneys may deal with issues that have no relationship to the therapist's practice, they may be an excellent referral source to other attorneys who are competent to handle the clinician's problems.

As a last resort, the therapist can contact the local bar association. Each bar group maintains an attorney referral service. The listing usually contains basic information about the attorney, including areas of specialization in his practice. It would be unlikely for an attorney to list mental health law as an area of practice. However, an attorney who represents health care providers or treatment facilities such as hospitals or outpatient clinics will have general knowledge about the issues most likely to be raised in practice.

The attorney–client relationship is a personal one. It is essential that the therapist interview an attorney before he hires him. During the interview he must be comfortable with the attorney, not only in terms of his competency but also in terms of his ability to communicate with him. It is critical that the therapist feel he can be open and honest with his attorney; otherwise much of the value of the attorney–client relationship will be defeated.

When interviewing attorneys, the therapist will want to learn the extent of the attorney's experience in the area of concern. Even if the attorney has never directly addressed the issues the clinician is raising, does he grasp the problem presented? Does he seem competent to research the topic sufficiently to give the therapist legal advice that he will feel comfortable with? If not, the therapist should look elsewhere.

It should be remembered that more and more attorneys are specializing, particularly in urban areas. It would probably be useless to contact an attorney with a question about the confidentiality of mental health treatment records and communications who has handled only tax problems. Therefore, the therapist must leave the interview with the belief that the attorney knows where to begin on the problems which have been presented to him.

When hiring an attorney, the therapist will also want one who has the time necessary to devote to his legal problems. If the attorney has too many clients and cannot give the clinician sufficient attention, then he needs to find someone else. However, the therapist should remember that this is one of many matters the attorney must address. In some circumstances, the therapist's problems will take precedence over those of the attorney's other clients. However, in many situations the therapist's concerns will not need immediate attention, while another client may have a legal problem that merits quick action. This should be kept in mind when the therapist contacts an attorney and establishes a reasonable time period when he should expect some response.

The attorney the therapist hires should also be someone who appears to be genuinely interested in his case, or at least in his welfare. This should be an individual who is courteous. It is also important that the attorney provide a realistic picture of the legal alternatives. The therapist should be wary of the attorney who assures the client that he will win or that there is not much to be concerned about. The most valuable service an attorney can render is his objective analysis of the case. If he promises more than he can deliver, the therapist will have unrealistic expectations, the relationship will soon sour, and the therapist will have wasted his time and money.

Finally, the therapist must find an attorney he can afford. From the outset the attorney should discuss his fees. The therapist should know not only the amount of the fee but how it was derived. The fee arrangement should be clear, and the therapist can try to negotiate a lower fee or different arrangement than the one initially proposed. The therapist will want to know what additional work will cost and the method of payment the attorney expects. Before he begins any work, the attorney should reduce the fee agreement to writing. This will prevent later misunderstandings.

VII. ATTORNEYS' FEES

Various types of fee arrangements are used by attorneys in legal cases. The type of arrangement will vary depending upon the type of case, the practice in a particular locality, and the attorney chosen. The most common type of fee arrangements include the following:

A. Flat Fee

The flat fee is a specific amount charged to handle a particular type of case. For example, the attorney will charge $400 to draft a will or $750 to represent a client in an uncontested divorce. This arrangement is common for routine legal problems that the attorney commonly handles.

B. Range Fee

In the range fee arrangement the attorney will offer a range that the case can cost. He may state, for example, that an uncontested divorce will cost between $500 and $1,000, depending upon whether there is a complex property settlement. He may state that after he has spent five hours on the case, the base of $500 will be increased by $100 per hour.

C. Hourly Fee

An hourly fee is charged when the attorney bills a specific amount for the time involved. Private attorneys' fees range from $80 to $250 or more per hour, depending upon the attorney's experience, his location, and whether he is a specialist. In urban areas, the fees are likely to be higher than in rural areas; if the attorney is a specialist, the fees are also likely to be higher. Paying higher fees to a specialist may be justified if it takes him less time to handle a matter related to his specialty. With the increasing number of attorneys in the United States, the economics of supply and demand will have a direct effect on the fees the attorney can charge.

D. Percentage Fee

The percentage fee is based upon the total value of the matter being handled. For example, an attorney may charge 5% of the value of an estate for probating it. These fee arrangements exist in some areas of the United States but not in others. They are commonly used for real estate matters and probating estates. However, the trend is to abolish such fee arrangements because it often appears that the fee is not commensurate with the amount of time the attorney spent on a case. Thus, a person involved in a costly legal matter may be paying much more than is necessary given the work involved. For example, the paperwork involved in arranging a closing on the purchase of a home is the same whether the home costs $50,000 or $500,000. With a percentage fee system, the person buying the $500,000 home will pay 10 times the legal fees paid by the person who purchased the less expensive home. On the other hand, attorneys who support such a payment scheme argue that they are exposed to greater liability under this system.

E. Contingent Fee

The contingent fee is based on the attorney's receiving some percentage of the recovery in the case. In contrast to the percentage fee, the attorney is gambling on whether there will be a recovery. This type of fee is most commonly used by plaintiffs' attorneys in personal injury, malpractice, workers' compensation, and collections cases. The fee the attorney receives may vary from 20% to 50%. The client is responsible for any costs the attorney incurs in pursuit of the litigation, such as for expert witnesses or deposition fees. Usually the client will be expected to bear these costs as they are incurred. However, when the attorney believes the plaintiff's case is strong, but the client has no funds, he may advance these expenses. When an award is entered in the client's favor either by the court or as a result of an out-of-court settlement, the attorney is entitled to his fees. For example, if the client is awarded

$110,000, the attorney's fee is 25%, and the attorney incurred $10,000 in expenses, which he advanced for the client, in bringing the suit to a conclusion, the client will receive a total of $75,000. This sum is calculated by deducting the $10,000 in advanced expenses from the award and then figuring the attorney's share and deducting this from the total.

The contingency fee structure has come under much attack, particularly by physicians, who have challenged these fees as excessive in medical malpractice actions. In reality, there are times when the plaintiff's attorney does little and earns what are excessive fees. The most obvious cases include the attorney who represents a family of a person who died in an airline crash. There is an almost guaranteed large recovery with little work. Therefore, one can question why the attorney is entitled to one third of that award.

Attorneys who work under a contingency fee arrangement argue that without this arrangement many worthwhile cases would not be filed. They further argue that the attorney should be rewarded proportionately for his efforts in obtaining a recovery for his client. In reality, experienced attorneys who handle cases on a contingency fee basis have analyzed the case carefully before accepting it to be sure that the likelihood of success is high.

In many states, legislation has been introduced, and in some instances enacted and approved by the courts, which limits the amount of the contingency fee in medical malpractice cases. With the increase in the numbers of attorneys in the United States (there are now approximately 750,000), the competition will make it possible for the astute client to arrange for the attorney to accept a lower percentage of the recovery.

VIII. THE ATTORNEY'S IMPACT ON THE MENTAL HEALTH SYSTEM

The remaining chapters of this book will illustrate some of the impact that attorneys, usually through class action litigation, have had on the mental health system. As recently as the 1960s, it was accepted that once a mentally disabled person entered a mental health or developmental disability facility he left his rights at the door and submitted himself to the complete control of the treatment staff. The public facilities providing his care were usually large, overcrowded, and understaffed. The per capita spending on patient care was relatively low. The expectation of genuine treatment or habilitation was not high, and the hope that the disabled would be able to function in the community on a long-term basis was practically nonexistent. The concept of the mentally disabled having a full set of rights which affords all the protections of the legal system was almost unknown.

Since the 1960s there has been a revolution in the rights and the care of the mentally disabled; yet, the standard by which progress is measured is quite low. This revolution has been due in large part to advances in treatment of the mentally ill with medication and to a recognition of the importance of habilitation to the developmentally disabled. The dramatic changes in the mental health system since the 1960s are due to a combination of treatment and habilitation advances and the efforts of public interest attorneys who have used the legal system to define and enforce the rights of the mentally disabled to better care in a humane environment.

The first challenges were directed against the civil commitment process. Shortly thereafter, suits were brought challenging the conditions the mentally disabled confronted within the institution. Finally, class action lawsuits challenged the notion of institutionalization itself and attempted to establish, with partial success, the need for more treatment and habilitation facilities within a community setting.

Although many mental health professionals believe that attorneys, through litigation and changes in state mental health codes, have turned the delivery of mental health services into a situation in which mental health professionals must be more concerned about the patient's legal rights than about his treatment needs, those professionals who have worked in the system for more than 20 years generally hail many of the changes which have occurred. They are aware of the increase in per patient spending, as well as the larger commitment of funds to community mental health care. They know that because of the fear of litigation, many patients receive better care in state treatment facilities than existed when no attorneys or courts were monitoring the system. Yet, few claim that most state-run facilities for the mentally disabled are ideal, and most admit the need for continuing efforts to improve the care and treatment offered in those facilities. Whether one fully agrees with all the changes brought about by litigation in the mental health field, which necessitate a book such as this one, most mental health professionals will agree that the advocacy for the mentally disabled has had a major impact on the entire delivery of mental health services.

IX. BIBLIOGRAPHY

American Bar Association. (1990). *You and the law.* Lincolnwood, IL: Publications International.

Bostick, M. R., Kirkman, G. M., & Samuel, M. B. (1983). Individual rights versus the therapeutic state: An advocacy model for respondent's counsel in civil commitment. *Capital University Law Review, 13,* 139–174.

Brakel, S. J. (1977). The role of the lawyer in the mental health field. *American Bar Foundation Research Journal, 1977,* 467–475.

Brakel, S. J. (1981). Legal advocacy for persons confined in mental hospitals. *Mental Disability Law Reporter, 5,* 274–280.

Cohen, F. (1966). The function of the attorney and the commitment of the mentally ill. *Texas Law Review, 44,* 424–469.

Galie, L. P. (1978). An essay on the civil commitment lawyer: Or how I learned to hate the adversary system. *Journal of Psychiatry and Law, 6,* 71–87.

Gallagher, B. M. (1979). *How to hire a lawyer: The consumer's guide to good counsel.* New York: Dell.

Herr, S. S. (1980). Legal advocacy for the mentally handicapped. *International Journal of Law and Psychiatry, 3,* 61–79.

Lamb, H. R. (1981). Securing patients' rights responsibly. *Hospital and Community Psychiatry, 32,* 393–397.

Landsman, S. (1983). A brief survey of the development of the advocacy system. *Ohio State Law Journal, 44,* 713–739.

Leavitt, N., & Maykuth, P. L. (1989). Conformance to attorney performance standards. *Law and Human Behavior, 13,* 217–230.

Long, L. L. (1982–1983). When the client is a child: Dilemmas in the lawyer's role. *Journal of Family Law, 21,* 607–640.

McGinn, J. C. (1977). *Lawyers: A client's manual.* Englewood Cliffs, NJ: Prentice-Hall.

Perlin, M. L. (1982). Mental patient advocacy by a patient advocate. *Psychiatric Quarterly, 54,* 169–176.

Perlin, M. L. (1992). Fatal assumption: A critical evaluation of the role of counsel in mental disability cases. *Law and Human Behavior, 16,* 39–59.

Perlin, M. L., & Sadoff, R. L. (1982). Ethical issues in the representations of individuals in the commitment process. *Law and Contemporary Problem, 45,* 161–192.

Schwartz, M. L. (1983). The zeal of the civil advocate. *American Bar Foundation Research Journal, 1983*, 543–583.
Smith, G. W. (1982). *What every client needs to know about using a lawyer* New York: Putnam.
Uphoff, R. J. (1988). The role of the criminal defense lawyer in representing the mentally impaired defendant: Zealous advocate or officer of the court? *Wisconsin Law Review, 1988*, 65–109.
Wald, P. M., & Friedman, P. R. (1978). The politics of mental health advocacy in the United States. *International Journal of Law and Psychiatry, 1*, 137–152.

3

Involuntary Hospitalization

I. Historical Perspective • **II. Admission Status** • A. Voluntary Admission • B. Informal Admission • C. Emergency Admission • D. Observational Commitment • E. Civil Commitment • **III. The State's Power to Civilly Commit** • A. *Parens Patriae* • B. Police Power • **IV. The Civil Commitment Standard** • **V. Determining When Someone Merits Commitment** • A. Mental Illness • B. Danger to Others • C. Danger to Self • D. Inability to Care for Self: Grave Disability • E. Other Commitment Criteria • **VI. Initiating the Civil Commitment Process** • A. Recommendations for Completing Commitment Papers • **VII. The Civil Commitment Hearing** • A. Rights of the Patient • B. The Role of the Prosecutor • C. Expectations of the Mental Health Professional at Trial • **VIII. Outpatient Commitment** • **IX. Duration of Commitment** • A. Clinical Indications for Discharge or Recommitment • **X. Financial Responsibility for the Costs of Institutional Care** • **XI. Commonly Asked Questions** • **Appendix** • **XII. Bibliography**

Admission to a mental health facility is often a complex and cumbersome process, particularly when the person is not entering the hospital voluntarily. This chapter will describe the various admission criteria and the rights of a mentally disabled person when civil commitment procedures are contemplated. The chapter articulates the legal theory which permits the state to involuntarily hospitalize someone. The requirements set forth by the statutes to accomplish this action are also explained. The clinical issues which arise in determining when someone meets civil commitment criteria and the expectations of the mental health professional during the process of seeking hospitalization are presented. An appendix is included to illustrate the key features of laws related to the hospitalization of the mentally ill.

I. HISTORICAL PERSPECTIVE

Laws relating to the mentally disabled are among the earliest legislation passed in the United States. In 1676, Massachusetts enacted a statute which provided that the selectmen of towns take care of dangerously distracted persons, so that "they do not damify others." In these cases, it was envisioned that the community would pay someone to keep the mentally ill person forcibly restrained. This is the first statute giving the state the authority to detain those perceived as violent, although they had not committed a crime.

For more than two centuries, the laws relating to the mentally disabled in the United States were concerned with how to remove the disabled from society, rather than with how to treat the individual with the goal of returning him to the community. The reason was in part the public's fear of the "insane" and in part that there were no known successful treatments for "insanity."

In 1751, the Pennsylvania Assembly, on a petition from Benjamin Franklin, authorized the establishment of the first general hospital to receive and cure the mentally ill and care for the sick and poor. In 1773, Virginia erected the first hospital devoted exclusively to the mentally disabled. The hospital in Willliamsburg remained the only hospital for the mentally disabled until the Eastern Lunatic Asylum was opened in Lexington, Kentucky, in 1824.

During the same period, the laws were also concerned with the ability to declare someone "*non compos mentis*" for the purpose of administering his financial affairs. As early as 1816, New York followed procedures outlined by Blackstone, the great English jurist, for declaring someone mentally incompetent. These included notice to the disabled, his appearance before a court, and the opportunity to have a jury decide his case. The notion that a disabled person should have certain procedural protections became a permanent part of the laws to declare someone incompetent as well as for involuntary hospitalization.

The hospitalization in 1860 and discharge three years later of Mrs. E. P. W. Packard had the most significant impact on the form of early civil commitment statutes. Mrs. Packard was committed to the Illinois State Hospital on the request of her husband. At that time, married women and children were not entitled to the same procedural protections or evidentiary standards as others. Upon her release, Mrs. Packard, through her frequent public lectures and books, vividly portrayed the horrors of being wrongfully placed in a mental institution. She urged that a person not be committed as insane solely on the basis of the opinions he might express and that commitment be based only on irregular conduct that indicates that the individual is so lost to reason as to render him an unaccountable moral agent. Her efforts led to the passage in Illinois of a personal liberty bill which required a jury trial before someone could be civilly committed. This law served as a model for other states which adopted civil commitment legislation. The intent of these laws was to ensure that people would not be inappropriately committed.

While Mrs. Packard crusaded for better civil commitment laws, Dorthea Lynde Dix, a Massachusetts school teacher who later became Superintendent of Nurses for the Union during the Civil War, forcefully brought to the public's attention the need for establishing and enlarging mental institutions. Her work had a profound effect on the treatment of the mentally disabled. Twenty states responded directly to Mrs. Dix's efforts with the creation of state-run mental hospitals. These efforts revolutionized the care of the mentally disabled during the 19th century. Dorthea Dix was responsible for the community's accepting the notion that it must provide institutions to care for the mentally disabled. This not only shifted the burden of caring for the mentally disabled from the family to the state but also changed the community's attitude, to expand their concern from one of self-protection from the mentally ill, to concern for the disabled members of the community.

Initially, civil commitment to an "insane asylum" was easily accomplished. It could occur in many instances solely on the request of an individual. One could approach a member of the institution's staff, and the proper papers would be signed and the person institutionalized. Mrs. Packard's efforts changed this process to include some procedural protections. These laws remained basically unchanged until about 1960. At that time legislatures not only were concerned with preventing people from being wrongfully committed but also became concerned with making it easy for the mentally disabled to receive treatment with a minimal amount of trauma. These concerns resulted in the adoption into state mental health codes of suggestions from the medical profession. These included admission on a medical certificate, the use of emergency procedures for short-term or observational commitments, and dispensing with the disabled's presence at a trial if this was considered detrimental to him.

By 1970, class action lawsuits were being initiated in various parts of the United States challenging all aspects of the civil commitment process. The most notable of these was *Lessard v. Schmidt,* which exemplified many of the issues raised in cases across the United States in the 1970s challenging civil commitment procedures. The *Lessard* decision by a federal district court in Wisconsin in 1972 served as a model for other courts which addressed the procedural guarantees appropriate for civil commitment proceedings. The reasoning and the rights recognized in *Lessard* became part of many civil commitment statutes which were revised during the 1970s in light of the litigation occurring around the country to establish the rights of the mentally disabled.

In October 1971 Alberta Lessard was picked up by two police officers and taken to a mental hospital. She was held on a "certificate of detention" filed by the officers. Two hearings were held in her absence and without her knowledge. She was ordered detained in the hospital as a result of these hearings. In her case, a class action lawsuit was brought on behalf of all adults for whom civil commitment was sought in Wisconsin. Alberta Lessard challenged that:

a. She could have been held for up to 145 days without a hearing.
b. She did not have notice of the hearings, nor was she entitled to an attorney to represent her or a jury to hear her case.
c. If she had an attorney, he was not permitted to be present during her psychiatric examinations.
d. At the hearing, hearsay evidence could be admitted and she could be forced to testify against herself.
e. She was not entitled to an independent psychiatric examination.
f. She should have known the basis for any decision to commit her and should have been committed only if the court was convinced beyond a reasonable doubt that she met the commitment criteria.

The issues raised in this case became the points of debate on how civil commitment procedures should be designed. Much of the remainder of this chapter will address these points and will explain the rights of a mentally disabled person during the civil commitment process.

II. ADMISSION STATUS

Admission to a public mental hospital, and in most states to private psychiatric treatment programs, is carefully governed by state law. This is as true for the person admitted "voluntarily" as for the one who is civilly committed. In contrast, a person may be admitted to a general hospital for medical care without state laws governing admission; the person's only status is to be a patient.

All states provide for some type of emergency or observational admission to a mental hospital, as well as procedures for civil commitment. The vast majority of state laws provide procedures for the person who wishes to enter the hospital voluntarily, and a few states permit the informal admission of patients.

A. Voluntary Admission

In 1881, the Massachusetts legislature enacted the first voluntary admission statute. Today, almost every state provides some type of voluntary or informal admission procedure for entry into a state-run mental health facility. Rarely, however, is the admission truly voluntary in the sense of the patient's entering the institution without any external pressure, and almost never is he permitted the absolute right to leave when he requests to do so. In fact, the hallmark of the voluntary admission is that generally the hospital staff has the authority to decide when the actual release will occur within legislatively mandated time frames.

Today, many state mental health codes encourage voluntary admissions. This is accomplished in a number of ways, primarily by permitting any legally competent adult to admit himself voluntarily; a growing number of states also allow adolescents to admit themselves. Most commonly this occurs for children 16 years or older, but there are states that permit 14-year-olds to sign into the hospital without parental permission. Laws in more than half the states permit an involuntary admission to be converted to a voluntary admission if the patient so desires and the facility thinks it is advisable. Finally, many courts will give the patient the option at a civil commitment hearing to sign in voluntarily if this is agreeable to the institution. As a result of these procedures, roughly half the admissions to state mental health facilities in the United States are on a voluntary basis. The proportion of voluntary admissions to private psychiatric facilities is even greater since many private facilities accept only voluntary patients.

Concern for ensuring that the patient is truly voluntarily admitted to the hospital has, in some states, resulted in provisions requiring that the person have the competency or capacity to decide to enter the treatment facility. This may mean that the patient understands that he is mentally ill, needs hospital treatment, and has certain rights. That an actively psychotic person may not in fact have the capacity to consent to a voluntary admission was litigated in a United States Supreme Court case (*Zinermon v. Burch*, 1990). In this case, a patient was allowed to voluntarily admit himself to a state hospital and then remain there for five months, even though he was apparently incapable of giving informed consent to voluntary admission because of his mental illness. He later filed a federal civil rights lawsuit against the hospital staff for depriving him of his liberty without due process of law, contending that he should have had a civil commitment hearing instead of being allowed to sign himself into the hospital. The Court held that the lawsuit could be pursued and, further, called into question the common practice of permitting the voluntary admission of decisionally incapacitated persons rather than civilly committing them.

A majority of states provide the voluntary patient with a copy of his rights specifically relating to release. At least 12 states also prohibit commitment of someone who wishes to enter the hospital voluntarily; such persons may be committed, however, if they request to be released.

The decision about whether someone will be admitted to a treatment facility voluntarily, if at all, is made by the facility. This decision is based on whether the staff determines that admission is clinically indicated, and if space is available for the patient. In private psychiatric facilities, the ability of the person to pay for his care is also a determining factor.

The shortcomings of voluntary status from the patient's perspective become clear when a patient seeks to be released from the treatment facility. Most states require that the release request be in writing. Release almost never occurs immediately upon request. The treatment facility staff has a period of time ranging from "as soon as practical" to 15 days, depending upon the state, to determine if the person can be released. Providing the staff time to evaluate the patient enables them to make a determination of whether he meets the civil commitment criteria. If he does, then the appropriate papers can be filed seeking commitment. If not, then the patient must be released. The time that elapses between the request for release and the actual discharge may give the staff time to convince the patient to rescind his release request or to arrange for appropriate outpatient care.

B. Informal Admission

Informal admission provides the patient with greater ease of entry and exit from the mental hospital than either voluntary or involuntary admission. Today, approximately 20% of the states provide for this type of admission status by statute. The salient features of an informal admission are that the person is admitted upon his oral (as opposed to written) request and can leave the hospital merely by requesting to do so. As in voluntary admission, the discretion to accept someone into the facility remains with the hospital staff. As with voluntary admissions, the statutes provide that the patient be told of his right to discharge.

Informal admission can be viewed as a more truly voluntary entry than the voluntary admission status, since the patient is discharged as soon as he requests to leave. However, in circumstances where the person has been admitted informally and he requests to leave, but he meets the civil commitment criteria, the staff would not discharge him but would begin the formal process for civil commitment. However, unlike under the voluntary admission statutes, under an informal admission the staff must make an immediate decision whether the person is committable, rather than waiting some period of time before release is mandated. Perhaps because of the lack of control of the patient by the facility staff, informal admissions occur infrequently in the states which permit them.

C. Emergency Admission

At least initially, emergency admission is a temporary measure for the expeditious processing of emergency situations. The intent of these statutes is to immediately address the behavior which is deemed to create a clear and present danger either to the individual or to others. Every state has some type of emergency detention provision. The process usually begins when someone completes a certificate or petition requesting that a mentally ill person be admitted on an emergency basis. This is usually done by a family member or friend of the disabled, or in many circumstances by a police officer. The person requesting the admission must certify that the person meets the statutory criterion, which is usually a risk of violence to himself or others, or the inability to meet his physical needs because of a mental illness. In some states, judicial approval is necessary before a law enforcement officer can forcibly remove a person from his home to a hospital for observation. In a few states, medical certification alone is sufficient to detain the person. This is based on a recent examination of the disabled person, with "recent" defined as anywhere from 24 hours in some states to 30 days in others.

An emergency admission detains the person until the emergency ends or civil commitment procedures have begun. This is the process used to admit many people to psychiatric facilities when their families are unable to convince them to enter the hospital voluntarily. The time frame permitted for this admission varies from 24 hours to as long as 20 days, with 3 to 5 days being the most common. Before the statutory time frame has elapsed, the person must either be discharged, be convinced to sign in "voluntarily," or have civil commitment proceedings commenced against him.

D. Observational Commitment

Observational commitment provides the staff of a mental hospital a specified time to observe the disabled person to determine his diagnosis and to permit limited treatment. Fewer than half the states now have such provisions, although in many states the goals of observation and limited treatment are accomplished under the emergency admission provisions. As in the emergency admission process, there is a formal application procedure. A few states limit the request to hospital personnel, but in most states the application can be filed by any adult. Court approval is required except where the person can be held for the observational period based on medical certification alone. The length of the observation period varies from 48 hours to six months. By the end of the observation period the person must either sign in voluntarily, be discharged, or have civil commitment proceedings initiated against him.

E. Civil Commitment

With few exceptions, the states provide a detailed and formal process for the civil commitment of mentally ill individuals. Since the entire process for hospitalizing and treating a person against his will has generated much legal controversy, the civil commitment process is at the heart of the debate about the rights of the mentally ill person. Much of the remainder of this chapter will focus on the specifics of this controversy and how the issues have been resolved to date.

For present purposes it is sufficient to summarize the salient features of the civil commitment process. The law of each of the states specifically sets forth the procedures required to begin initiation of civil commitment proceedings and the process by which someone is committed. In approximately two-thirds of the states, some type of medical evidence must accompany the request to begin the civil commitment proceedings. This is usually in the form of an "affidavit" or "certificate," which must be signed by a physician/psychiatrist. Many states require more than one supporting document. Usually the second document can be filled out by a psychologist or other mental health professional. Once the proper documents have been filed with the court, a civil commitment hearing is scheduled. The rights attendant on this process are described in much greater detail below in Section VII.

III. THE STATE'S POWER TO CIVILLY COMMIT

The ability of a state to civilly commit an individual is predicated on two legal theories: *parens patriae* and the police power of the state.

A. *Parens Patriae*

Parens patriae, which literally means "parent of the country," obligates the sovereign to protect those who are unable to protect themselves. They usually include the mentally ill, the physically disabled, and unsupervised minors. In the case of mentally ill individuals, their inability to care for themselves gives the state the authority to seek civil commitment as a means to provide the needed treatment. The premise for the state's having authority to make decisions for these "wards" is that they are unable to make rational decisions for themselves. Thus, the functional competency of the individual becomes the threshold question before the state can intervene in the decision-making process. Once it has been determined that the individual is unable to care for himself or is suicidal, the state has the obligation to make a decision which is in his best interests or one that most clearly reflects the decision he would have made had he been competent to do so. (See Chapter 9, "Competency and Guardianship.") The civil criteria requiring that the person is "unable to care for himself" or is "dangerous to himself" provides the *parens patriae* justification for civil commitment.

B. Police Power

The other legal theory which supports the state's power to civilly commit is its police power. Police power is a broad concept which gives the state the authority to act on behalf of the general welfare and for the public's safety. This power lets the state isolate or confine those individuals who are viewed as dangerous to the rest of society. These include not only the mentally ill but those with contagious diseases. This power also provides the justification for a broad range of statutory enactments relating to regulation of public facilities ranging from overseeing hospitals to establishing building codes. When one reviews the civil commitment criteria, the concept of *dangerousness* relates directly to the state's police power and thus provides the justification for civil commitment under this legal theory.

IV. THE CIVIL COMMITMENT STANDARD

For the state to civilly commit an individual there must be a finding that he is mentally ill. In addition, most statutes require either that he be a danger to himself or others because of his mental illness or that he be unable to provide for his basic needs. Other factors which can serve as a basis for civil commitment are set forth in the next section. The wording of these criteria may vary in minor ways. A number of states require that there be a recent overt act to indicate dangerousness. In a few states, posing a perceived danger to property may also serve as a basis for commitment if the potential danger arises out of the mental illness.

V. DETERMINING WHEN SOMEONE MERITS COMMITMENT

From a strictly legal point of view, different jurisdictions have different statutes and criteria governing civil commitment. The decision to commit a mentally ill individual to a psychiatric hospital or unit may depend upon a variety of factors beyond whether or not the patient meets commitment criteria. These factors include social, political, and familial issues; fiscal considerations; legal considerations (the fear of liability for wrongful commitment or failure to commit); and the availability of mental health professionals and mental health facilities. Geographical differences (e.g., urban versus rural setting) also frequently alter the likelihood that an individual will in fact be civilly committed to a psychiatric facility. Selective enforcement of the commitment laws by local judges, police, or state's attorneys or the variable defense of patients' rights by publicly funded mental health attorneys will also account for some differences in commitment practices in different locales. While the mental health professional must be aware of these extraclinical considerations, such factors should not unduly distract the clinician's attention from the more central clinical-legal issues in deciding whether or not to commit a patient for hospital-based psychiatric care and treatment.

Commitment statutes and criteria are often deliberately written with considerable vagueness. This provides the mental health professional with the opportunity to interpret, as well as misinterpret, the local statute in a manner consonant with the needs of the patient, staff, institution, or society at large. Thus, interpretations of legal terms in commitment laws such as *mental illness, grave disability, dangerousness, near future, serious harm,* and *ability to care for self* may differ widely. Clinicians' subjective determinations of a patient's need for treatment sometimes improperly substitute for the determination of whether involuntary hospitalization is justified according to the language of the statute. Mental health professionals may thus find themselves resentful of the law's apparent restrictiveness of the clinician's interest in providing treatment.

Nevertheless, the legal criteria for civil commitment are usually designated as the presence of (1) mental illness; (2) danger to others; (3) danger to self; and (4) inability to care for self (grave disability). Other criteria may include (1) need for treatment; (2) the treatability of the mental illness and the availability of appropriate treatment at the facility to which the patient will be committed; (3) refusal of voluntary admission; (4) lack of capacity to consent to or refuse psychiatric treatment or hospitalization; (5) future danger to property; and (6) involuntary hospitalization as the least restrictive alternative available.

A. Mental Illness

The presence of a severe mental illness is considered the threshold criterion for civil commitment. This criterion typically complements the other commitment criteria, rather than standing alone as a sufficient grounds. Yet, state statutes often fail to provide a specific definition of mental illness for the purposes of civil commitment. Particular psychiatric diagnoses are not generally listed as permissive of commitment; some statutes, however, specifically exclude patients with certain diagnostic conditions from commitment (e.g., mental retardation or other developmental disability, "senility," epilepsy, personality disorder, alcoholism, or substance abuse and dependence). Statutes often circularly define mental illness by a reference to another condition which incorporates other commitment criteria. North Carolina, for example, defines mental illness as "an illness which so lessens the capacity of the person to use self-control, judgment, and discretion in the conduct of his affairs and social relations as to make it necessary or advisable for him to be under treatment, care, supervision, guidance or control." In Michigan, "mental illness" is defined as "a substantial disorder of thought or mood which significantly impairs judgment, behavior, capacity to recognize reality, or ability to cope with the ordinary demands of life." In such cases, the mental health professional is required to make not one but a series of determinations about the nature, type, severity, and results of the mental illness in order to assess committability.

B. Danger to Others

Danger to others, as a result of a severe mental illness, has come to represent a prevalent though controversial justification for civil commitment. State commitment statutes struggle to clearly define the elements of a danger to others standard, which include (1) the nature of the future harm to others (physical or emotional injury); (2) the severity of the harm to others (bruises, fractures, life-threatening injuries); (3) the likelihood of the harm to others (possible, probable, likely, or certain); (4) the imminence of the harm to others (harmful behavior will occur in the next day, week, month, six months, etc., or the "near future"); and (5) the frequency of the harm to others (single or multiple episodes of future harm). State statutes rarely, however, denote each of these parameters of a danger to others standard or do so in a vague or general manner, for example, "the person is likely to inflict physical harm upon another."

As a result of some retrospective psychiatric research studies from the 1970s, questions have been raised about the ability of the mental health professional to accurately assess and predict future violent behavior. Nevertheless, society has called upon mental health professionals to make such determinations. To enhance the accuracy of such psychiatric predictions, some states require that an individual demonstrate some recent violent threats, attempts, or acts, beyond any general verbalizations (e.g., homicidal ideation), about future violent behavior. A few states require a recently completed violent act to demonstrate dangerousness for the purpose of civil commitment. This is sometimes referred to as the *recent overt act requirement*. Generally speaking, however, actual prior violence to others is not a premise for commitment; threats of future violence, as well as any less than violent conduct in the furtherance of such threats, when the result of a major mental illness, can justify involuntary treatment. Such behavior must usually have occurred in the recent rather than distant past. Some laws further stipulate that it must have occurred within the last 30 days.

The assessment and prediction of violence is a frequent component of assessments of committability to psychiatric hospitals. While mental health professionals have no documented ability to make reasonably certain long-term forecasts of another's possible future violent behavior, evaluations of committability require an assessment of at least the probability of a patient's violence in the near or immediate future. This section will briefly review the relevant clinical considerations in assessing an individual's short-term risk of violence.

The clinical prediction of violent behavior for purposes of civil commitment must be a multidimensional assessment of medical, psychiatric, psychological, social, demographic, and situational variables. The mental health professional must consider factors pertinent to the individual patient as well as the environment in which he lives, since violence is best assessed with respect to particular environmental factors. Finally, he must use information about the past and present condition of the patient in order to assess the patient's likely future conduct.

As much of the following data as possible should be obtained by the clinician from any sources, in addition to the patient, prior to assessing the patient's risk of future violence:

1. Demographic characteristics of the patient—age, sex, race, marital status, intelligence level, education, and employment history.
2. The patient's past history of violent behavior—prior ideation, threats, attempts, or violent acts, as well as details of the situation in which they occurred (while intoxicated, after a marital dispute, in other family or peer environments, etc.), and the outcome of the behavior (arrest, conviction, incarceration).
3. A detailed account of the presenting problem—the patient's behavior, the presence and involvement of others, and the use of weapons or intoxicants.
4. Prior relevant psychiatric history—medical or neurological disturbances (brain injury, cerebrovascular disease, seizure disorder, dementia, mental retardation, command hallucinations, manic episodes, paranoid delusions).
5. A present mental status examination—the presence of psychotic signs and symptoms, character pathology (antisocial attitudes), marked agitation, impaired sensorium, or intoxication.

Once these data are available, the mental health professional's assessment of violence depends upon the following considerations, according to Monahan (1981):

1. The prevalence of violence in the demographic group of which the patient is a member.
2. The availability of instruments of violence or weapons in the patient's environment during the time period in question.
3. The identification and availability of likely victims of the patient's violent behavior during the predicted time interval.
4. The similarity of the contexts (situations) in which the patient has used violent coping behavior in the past to the situations to which the patient is likely to be exposed in the immediate future.
5. The presence of emotional and cognitive factors which facilitate and inhibit the patient from using violent behavior as a solution to his present problems (poor behavior and impulse control, fears of arrest, retaliation, or loss of loved ones).

In most cases, the mental health professional can at best provide only a rough assessment of a patient's propensity for violent behavior in the near future. However, this is all that is required for the purpose of determining whether civil commitment is indicated on the basis of being a danger to others.

C. Danger to Self

Involuntary psychiatric hospitalization is also authorized when a person is predicted to attempt suicide as a result of mental illness. The components of a "danger to self" standard essentially parallel those described above for the "danger to others" standard. Thus, prior attempts at suicide or other intentionally physically destructive behavior such as self-mutilation may support commitment under this criterion. The applicable commitment statute may or may not state how likely or imminent is the predicted suicidal behavior. Proof of a recent suicide attempt or serious mutilation attempt may be required at the commitment hearing, as well as any suicide ideation, intention, or plan.

The clinical evaluation of suicidal behavior for the purposes of civil commitment parallels the evaluation of violent behavior reviewed above. Clinicians should inquire about the following factors about the patient and his interpersonal context:

1. Demographic variables associated with the risk of suicide (older age, male sex, single marital status, unemployment) or attempted suicide (younger age, female sex).
2. The patient's past history of self-destructive behavior, focusing particularly on the degree of lethality (prior ideation, threats, or suicide attempts) as well as the details of the context in which they occurred (e.g., while intoxicated, after a family dispute, during a psychotic episode, three months after release from a psychiatric hospital).
3. A detailed account of the presenting problem from the patient and others, regarding his behavior, his use of instruments of self-injury, or intoxication.
4. Prior relevant psychiatric history—chronic medical disease with neuropsychiatric dysfunction, severe depressive disorders, schizoaffective disorder, schizophrenia, alcohol abuse and dependence, antisocial personality disorder, and family history of self-destructive behavior.
5. A present mental status examination—hopelessness, profound dysphoria, suicide ideation/intention/plan, delusions of guilt, or significant agitation.

As noted earlier for the assessment of violent behavior, the clinician then determines the patient's risk of future suicide behavior by assessing:

1. The prevalence of suicide and attempted suicide in the patient's demographic group.
2. The availability of instruments of self-destructive behavior in the patient's environment.
3. The similarity of the context in which the patient has used self-destructive coping behavior in the past to that to which the patient is likely to be exposed in the near future.

4. The presence or absence of emotional and cognitive factors which facilitate and inhibit the patient from using self-destructive behavior as a solution to his current problems.

Again, the mental health professional can at best provide only a relatively general assessment of the patient's suicide risk for some period of time in the immediate future. This will be sufficient for purposes of initiating civil commitment, as well as for treatment planning.

D. Inability to Care for Self: Grave Disability

A person who, because of his mental illness, is unable to provide for his basic physical needs for nourishment, personal or medical care, shelter, self-protection, or safety may be involuntarily hospitalized when serious physical harm will result if the person is not hospitalized and treated. Again, the law may require that the harm occur within the near future. This commitment provision applies most often to the elderly psychiatric patient, as well as to those who are severely and chronically mentally ill and self-neglectful. An important distinguishing factor here is that there must be a potential for physical harm to the patient of a serious degree if treatment is not provided; emotional or psychological harm as a result of continued mental illness and distress is inadequate for commitment under this criterion. Thus, a mentally ill patient who is found wandering in the winter weather without coat or shoes is likely to be committable under this criterion. Finally, commitment is usually not authorized for the person if he has assistance from others so that physical harm will not ensue, even though he would not independently be able to provide for his physical needs.

E. Other Commitment Criteria

A variety of other standards are occasionally used to justify civil commitment to psychiatric hospitals. In some jurisdictions (e.g., the State of Washington), commitment is permitted in the absence of proof of physical harm to self or others under an expanded gravely disabled definition when a person "manifests severe deterioration in routine functioning evidenced by repeated and escalating loss of cognitive or volitional control over his or her actions and is not receiving such care as is essential for his or her health or safety." This represents one form of a "need for treatment" commitment criterion, usually justified under the state's *parens patriae* authority.

Another variation in commitment criteria includes the use of future property damage as grounds for commitment. Washington law, for example, provides for commitment on these grounds: "a substantial risk that physical harm will be inflicted by an individual upon the property of another, as evidenced by behavior which has caused substantial loss or damage to the property of others."

Finally, it is sometimes necessary to prove that a patient lacks the functional capacity to consent to or refuse inpatient psychiatric treatment because of his mental illness in order for commitment to occur. In such cases, the patient may not be able to understand and appreciate the presence of mental illness or the need for hospital treatment despite repeated explanations to him of his problems and the benefits of treatment. Patients who are mute or otherwise unable to make and verbalize a decision about hospitalization are also included in this category.

VI. INITIATING THE CIVIL COMMITMENT PROCESS

Included in the various state civil commitment statutes are specific requirements relating to initiation of the process and consideration of the rights of the disabled when commitment is being considered. When the disabled person has been brought to or remains in the mental health facility against his will, he is on notice that civil commitment will be sought. Most states specifically provide that he be informed of this and also provide that notice of the time of the commitment hearing and of the basis upon which commitment is sought be communicated to others, such as family members or an attorney for the disabled person. This notice is usually accomplished by copying the petition and other forms filed with the court.

Once it has been explained to the mentally ill person that commitment is being sought, he may be entitled to a warning that anything he says may be used in the commitment proceedings against him. This warning, similar to that which is required when a person is charged with a crime, is statutorily mandated in a few states. Supporters of this position argue that the constitutional privilege against self-incrimination is violated if evidence gathered during the psychiatric examination is used against the individual when he has not been warned of his right to remain silent. In those states which require the warning, a mental health professional who has not given it may be barred from testifying at the commitment hearing. The majority of states do not take this position and hold that the warning to remain silent is incompatible with the nature and purpose of civil commitment proceedings, which is to benefit the disabled person by providing him with needed treatment. In states where the warning is required, the majority of disabled people do not refuse to speak to the clinician.

A mental health professional required to give a warning should do so at the outset of the evaluation. All that need be said is that any statements the person makes may be related in court as to his clinical condition or need for treatment, and he has a right not to speak. This can be done casually, without the ceremony that accompanies a *Miranda* type of warning in criminal cases. Few patients will express any concern about this, in part because of their condition. For those who refuse to talk, speaking to them further will usually elicit some response. Even if no verbal response is forthcoming, the commitment will depend not on what is said during the examination, but on what is observed, and on the factors surrounding hospitalization.

The concern about self-incrimination also raises the issue of therapist–patient confidentiality and testimonial privilege (see Chapter 7, on "Confidentiality"). One of the almost universal exceptions to each state's confidentiality and testimonial privilege statutes is when civil commitment is sought. The notion is that by breaching a confidence the therapist is better serving the patient's need by getting him into treatment. Often, however, the therapist will not have to reveal specific patient disclosures in commitment papers or court testimony but can reveal the psychiatric history, mental status findings, and diagnosis which have led him to conclude that civil commitment was warranted.

A. Recommendations for Completing Commitment Papers

The mental health professional who certifies mentally ill persons for involuntary treatment may be confronted with a confusing array of applications and procedures. Some of the following may be of assistance in this task:

1. Be familiar with the applicable commitment law. The mental health professional who even occasionally evaluates and treats individuals subject to involuntary hospitalization must have a thorough knowledge of the relevant commitment provisions. The professional should be cognizant of the law's definitions of mental illness, dangerousness, and grave disability, as well as knowledgeable about the commitment standards and procedures. The professional should be aware of which particular mental health professionals are eligible to file papers and testify for commitment.

2. Be familiar with the applicable administrative policies. Beyond the legal requirements of the commitment law, there may be certain procedural requirements based upon the policies of some mental health agencies or responsible county offices. These may include timing of the filing of commitment papers, presentation of papers (e.g., typed or printed format), and identity of specific personnel qualified to file or review papers.

3. Perform a comprehensive psychiatric examination. Adequate completion of commitment papers is predicated upon a thorough evaluation of the patient's current mental status examination, psychiatric history, previous treatment, current risk of violence, and social supports. Information from third parties is typically useful in this evaluation.

4. Provide evidence, not simply conclusions, that the patient is mentally ill and requires hospital treatment. Record the patient's verbatim account of psychiatric and medical symptoms, as well as detailed observations of his mental status. It is not sufficient to state in conclusory terms that "The patient is psychotic and requires hospitalization." Indicate, instead, that the patient states, "My parents put oil paint in my food" and reports hearing "the voice of Satan." Use additional sheets of paper if the commitment forms do not provide enough space to permit a complete presentation of the patient's condition.

5. Provide the factual basis for any conclusions, not the conclusions alone, that the patient is dangerous to himself, others, or property. Describe in detail the patient's recent violent or self-destructive behavior, including threats or conduct in furtherance of the threats, whether the information is provided by the patient or others. Record relevant data from the patient's mental status examination which support a conclusion of imminent harm to himself or others; for example, "The patient states, 'the voice of God is telling me to kill my sister.'"

6. Describe the particular treatment needed by the patient. Indicate the nature and duration of the treatment necessary at this time and what treatment facility would be best for the patient. State, when possible, the availability of treatment at the receiving facility.

7. Complete all parts of the commitment application. Some commitment petitions require information about the patient which may not be readily available. For example, data about abnormal physical or medical conditions are sometimes relevant to the commitment process, as well as necessary to record on the petition or certificate. The commitment may subsequently be denied if all portions of the application are not adequately completed.

VII. THE CIVIL COMMITMENT HEARING

The civil commitment hearing is the culmination of the steps taken to hospitalize someone for psychiatric treatment, usually against his will. Because the individual's problem is in being alleged to be mentally disabled, the state is concerned that it not use its tremendous police or *parens patriae* power improperly. Thus, the individual has a wide range of rights prior to and during the civil commitment hearing. Not only are the rights of the alleged disabled well defined, but the role of the attorney representing the state and the expectations of the mental health professional are also well defined. This section will discuss the rights of the disabled and the expectations of the state's attorney and the mental health professional during the commitment hearing.

A. Rights of the Patient

The United States Constitution guarantees that before someone can be deprived of his life, liberty, or property, he has certain rights under the law. These due process protections guarantee that certain procedures will be followed to be sure that, before a disabled person is civilly committed and thus institutionalized against his will, he will have the opportunity to present his side of the case effectively. Because the individual is alleged to be mentally ill and the goal is to provide him treatment, he has a wide range of rights which try to ensure that he will have all the protections of the law. The rights which have been established for the mentally disabled at commitment hearings are a balance between ensuring that a person will not be unjustifiably committed and providing him with the treatment he needs. These rights include the following.

1. Notice

Notice requires that the disabled person be informed that a commitment hearing is planned to try to involuntarily institutionalize him. The time and place of the hearing must be contained in the notice as well as an indication of the basis for the action being taken. In the case of a commitment hearing the notice sets forth the allegations which the petitioner (usually the family or hospital) felt warranted civilly committing the person.

All states require that the respondent (disabled person) be given personal notice. This means that he must be handed a copy of the petition for hospitalization and told the time of the hearing. The amount of time the notice must be given before the hearing will vary from two to eight days depending upon the state, or the statute might provide for it to be given within a "reasonable time" before the hearing. The time period should be sufficient to allow the respondent to arrange for an attorney and prepare a defense.

In the vast majority of states, the notice must be provided not only to the respondent, but to his guardian, spouse, attorney, and any other relatives or friends that he designates. The point is to ensure that the disabled person will not become lost in the system and that someone will be aware of his location and the scheduled hearing.

2. *Presence at Trial*

Requiring the respondent to be present at the trial in the case of the mentally disabled person has a twofold purpose: It ensures that he will be aware of the trial and can inform his attorney of any facts which can be brought out in his favor; it also permits the court to observe the person to see if he appears to be sufficiently mentally ill to warrant commitment. The vast majority of states make the presence of the disabled at trial mandatory, at least when the respondent requests it. However, approximately 25% of the states permit his presence to be waived if the trial would be viewed as harmful from either a medical or psychiatric perspective. In many states the court will hold the hearings in an informal manner at the mental health facility. This is to make the process less traumatic to the patient and less disruptive to treatment.

3. *Representation by an Attorney*

Representation by an attorney is perhaps one of the most important rights the disabled person has at the commitment hearing and ensures that the respondent will be given all the rights to which he is entitled under the law. Through advocacy, the attorney can challenge the basis for the petition and bring out facts in his client's favor. With few exceptions, state statutes specifically provide that a person is entitled to representation when civil commitment is sought.

Since the individual has not signed into the hospital "voluntarily," he is being institutionalized against his will. By definition, he desires his attorney to contest his hospitalization. Although the attorney may believe that the person would benefit from coerced treatment, his job is to represent his client's expressed wishes. It is the responsibility of the prosecuting attorney to make the case for civil commitment. It is the responsibility of the defense attorney to bring out all the facts which will favor not committing his client. In addition, he may also attempt to present some other alternative plan for treatment, in a less restrictive setting, a private hospital, or in an outpatient program. Effective advocacy should prevent unjustified commitments.

4. *Examination of Witnesses*

When an individual is faced with a loss of liberty, the courts are concerned with ensuring that he will be afforded the full opportunity to present his side of the case and thus will not be unjustly deprived of his freedom. One of the most important ways this can be accomplished is by the individual calling his own witnesses and cross-examining the witnesses for the other side. This confrontation of the adverse witness enables the respondent to bring out any weaknesses in the state's case. The rules of evidence define the scope of the examination of all witnesses, preventing the answering of questions which are beyond the knowledge or expertise of the witness.

Hearsay is any statement made by one other than the declarant while testifying at trial and offered into evidence to prove the truth of a matter asserted at trial. Hearsay is often permitted in civil commitment hearings to serve as the basis for the opinions of the mental health professionals. The testifying professional may rely on the history of events told to someone else (e.g., the family), previous hospital records, or other information which was obtained outside the patient interview. The courts have generally permitted this type of information to serve as the basis of the mental health professional's conclusions as long as there are also personal observations which add support for the need for commitment. Recently, courts have become more willing to accept some challenges to testimony based on its being hearsay. Hearsay challenges are most likely to relate to testimony by the professional about conversations with family members or others who can personally testify at the trial. The courts, however, do not want to overburden hospital personnel and thus view much of what is in the record as a business record which will be permitted into evidence, without requiring each person who made a notation to come forward and verify the recorded information.

5. *Jury Trial*

In the majority of states the patient has a right to request a jury trial. The size of the jury may vary from 6 to 12 persons depending on state law. Attorneys representing the mentally disabled are unlikely to request such a trial. Juries are not generally sympathetic to a person who is alleged to be mentally ill and in need of hospitalization. Jurors are usually frightened of releasing such a person into the community, especially when it has been brought out that the patient has rejected the recommended psychiatric advice.

6. *Independent Examination*

A number of courts have held, and a few states by statute provide, that the respondent is entitled to an independent psychiatric examination before the civil commitment hearing. The notion is that the independent examination ensures that all avenues have been explored on behalf of the disabled. Having the examiner independent of the other mental health professionals or the treatment facility which is seeking commitment ensures an objective analysis of the respondent's need for treatment. Although the courts and some states have recognized the value of this independent opinion, there seems to be no consensus on whether the disabled person should be permitted to select the expert or can continue to obtain additional experts until he finds someone who supports his position. It also is unclear where the funds are to come from to pay for such an examination. Thus, in those states which provide this right, it is often an empty promise because of lack of adequate funds to retain an expert and lack of choice as to who it will be.

7. *Voluntary Admission*

Many states permit the respondent to sign into the hospital voluntarily before the court can find that he meets the civil commitment criteria. This position grows out of the view that it is preferable to treat someone who is hospitalized voluntarily and who is therefore more likely to participate in treatment. It also reflects the desire not to stigmatize someone with the label of being civilly committed unless this is absolutely necessary. Clinicians in some states are required to document why they have decided to commit a patient rather than respect the patient's request for a voluntary admission. Although some courts have held that someone who has consented to be voluntarily hospitalized cannot be committed, they are likely to uphold a facility's decision to refuse to accept someone's request to be a "voluntary" patient after commitment has been effected.

B. The Role of the Prosecutor

It is the responsibility of the attorney for the state to present the case as to why an individual should be civilly committed. He has the burden of proving, by at least clear and convincing evidence, that the individual meets the commitment criteria, and his goal is to accomplish commitment either for the protection of the community or for the benefit of the disabled. This will at a minimum require proving that the respondent is mentally ill and as a result of that illness is likely to pose a danger to himself or others or is unable to take care of his own needs.

The prosecutor will accomplish his goals by first reviewing the petition and medical evidence for civil commitment. He will usually meet with the petitioner, family members if they are involved in seeking commitment, and members of the staff of the treatment facility who are prepared to testify in favor of commitment. The prosecutor will call the witnesses necessary to make his case. In some states, he will even be permitted to call the respondent as an adverse witness, to bring out why he needs to be committed. After presenting his case, the prosecuting attorney will also have the opportunity to cross-examine the witnesses called on behalf of the respondent. In his concluding remarks, the prosecutor will summarize the evidence presented which justifies civilly committing the respondent.

In the vast majority of cases, civil commitment hearings are relatively brief, less than 30 minutes, and are likely to result in commitment, in part because before mental health professionals certify someone as needing commitment, they are convinced that the person meets the commitment criteria.

C. Expectations of the Mental Health Professional at Trial

Civil commitment cannot occur without supporting evidence presented at a hearing by a mental health professional. In many states there is a requirement that a psychiatrist testify at the trial. Some states require that more than one mental health professional testify and may include testimony by therapists who are not psychiatrists, such as psychologists, psychiatric social workers, or psychiatric nurses. Such testimony must be clear and concise and must describe how the observations and findings resulted in the conclusion that the respondent meets the commitment criteria.

Generally, the mental health professional and the state's attorney will meet before the hearing to discuss the clinical indications which justify the commitment. On direct examination, the prosecutor will elicit the behavior and clinical observations which point toward the need for involuntary hospitalization. As an expert witness, the mental health professional will be asked for his opinions about how the respondent's behavior formed his conclusion that the person is mentally ill and a danger to himself or others or unable to care for himself because of his illness.

In addition to staff called as expert witnesses, others, including aides, may be called to testify about specific events or behavior during the patient's hospitalization. They are fact witnesses and can state only what they saw, without drawing clinical conclusions from the patient's behavior.

At the end of the direct examination by the prosecuting attorney, the defense attorney has an opportunity to cross-examine the mental health professional as to his testimony. The goal of the defense attorney is to point out flaws in the professional's testimony in order to support his own argument that there is not sufficient clinical justification for committing his client. He may challenge the expert's credentials and the basis for his conclusions regarding the patient's present condition, need for treatment, and prognosis. The defense attorney's goal is to see that his client is not civilly committed, and he will try to make the expert's examination and conclusions appear inaccurate or biased.

Testifying at a civil commitment hearing is frightening for many mental health professionals. They may be reluctant to discuss their clinical observations in the presence of the patient and to defend their positions when under examination by attorneys. Yet this is required by law. Although the process is often burdensome to the treatment provider, it is critical to providing the disabled person the same rights any citizen would want should he be in the same situation.

The commitment hearing should be viewed as a challenge which forces one to organize one's thoughts and communicate them in a way which makes apparent the need of the disabled person to be hospitalized. Remember that the mental health professional is testifying as an expert, not an advocate. The professional's role is to enlighten the court, so that a fair decision can be made. The professional should bring his clinical skills to the hearing and let the testimony demonstrate how these skills led to the conclusion that the respondent needs to be committed. The success of the case will rest on the facts as well as in part on the skill of the involved attorneys. (See the sections in Chapter 11 on serving as an expert witness.)

VIII. OUTPATIENT COMMITMENT

A few states explicitly provide for, or at least do not prohibit, civil commitment to outpatient treatment programs. The major goal of such outpatient commitment is to reduce the likelihood of deterioration of the person's emotional functioning so that it results in hospitalization. The conditions of compulsory treatment may include taking prescribed medication, reporting to a treatment facility to monitor the person's medication compliance and mental condition, or participating in therapeutic or rehabilitation programs. Outpatient commitment may be used in conjunction with, or as an alternative to, inpatient commitment. For example, a patient may be committed to an inpatient program and then discharged by the court under an outpatient commitment. Alternatively, outpatient commitment may be initiated while the patient is in the community if, for example, a court finds that the person does not require hospitalization.

Outpatient commitment differs from conditional release in that the court, rather than treatment personnel, authorize the commitment. Outpatient commitment periods are time-limited but may sometimes be renewed. Outpatient commitment periods are often longer than statutory periods of hospital-based commitment. Typically, a patient who fails to comply with the conditions of outpatient commitment may be rehospitalized.

The standards, hearings, compliance monitoring, and revocation of outpatient commitment vary widely across the states. Some states authorize or permit outpatient commitment under less stringent commitment criteria than for inpatient commitment. In such cases, there will be no requirement of a recent act of violence or imminently expected violence to the patient or others, but only a potential of violence should the patient fail to comply with treatment. In other states, the commitment criteria for these two forms of involuntary treatment are identical.

Treatment through outpatient commitment programs presents several dilemmas for the mental health professional. In community-based commitment, when the patient fails to comply with treatment requirements, the treatment staff are confronted with the need to enforce the involuntary treatment by a variety of potential avenues, depending upon local law and practice. These include contacting the police, the mental health authorities, or the committed patient's family. They may also include coercing the patient to take medication.

Another problem in outpatient commitment is failure of communication between the committing court authority and the treatment provider. For example, a court may fail to notify the community agency that a patient has been committed to the agency for treatment. Further, the court may order outpatient commitment without the recommendation, or even against the explicit recommendation, of the clinic staff. In such cases, unwilling treatment staff are in effect ordered to treat an unwilling patient.

Outpatient commitment is not clinically appropriate for many chronically mentally ill individuals. It is more likely to be appropriate for patients who have mental disorders which have previously responded to psychotropic medication, but who have been noncompliant with medication (e.g., those with bipolar affective disorders and some schizophrenic disorders). Outpatient commitment may also be appropriate for those patients who need external structure in order to function as outpatients.

The success of an involuntary outpatient treatment program will depend upon the ability of the treatment staff to devote the resources to treating involuntary patients in the community, as well as upon the adequacy of communication among the court, the hospital staff, and the outpatient treatment provider. It will also depend upon the ability and willingness of the clinic staff to engage the enforcement authorities. Staff may not be willing to accept the responsibility for treating involuntary patients in the community, viewing hospitals as the appropriate treatment locus for such patients. Similarly, referring courts may not be able to accept the role of treatment compliance monitor for significant numbers of involuntary outpatients.

IX. DURATION OF COMMITMENT

The average length of involuntary hospitalization has decreased for more than two decades. This decrease is attributed to a variety of factors, including the development of more effective medication to treat mental illness, the availability of more facilities in the community to provide treatment, statutory demands which narrow the commitment criteria and limit the period of commitment, and decreased public and private funds for mental health care. Provisions mandating periodic review and allowing conditional release have also had an important impact on shortening lengths of involuntary admissions.

When a person has been admitted to the facility "informally" or "voluntarily," his discharge is dependent upon when he wishes to leave, when the staff determines he is ready, and in many cases the length of his insurance coverage. Although the voluntarily admitted patient cannot necessarily leave at the moment he requests release, he generally must be discharged within a short period (a week or less in most states) of requesting to be released.

For those who are civilly committed, the vast majority of states provide that commitment can only be ordered for a definite period, six months being the most common. At the end of that time period, if the staff wishes to continue the involuntary hospitalization of the patient, then a new commitment hearing must be held. The recommitments are also for finite periods, usually one and one-half to twice as long as the initial commitment period. In those states without a maximum period of commitment, there are provisions requiring periodic review of the patient's status to be sure continued hospitalization is merited. Recommitment usually requires meeting the same criteria as the initial commitment.

Involuntary patients can be discharged conditionally or absolutely. Approximately 80% of the states permit conditional discharge. The conditional release is usually premised on the patient's obtaining outpatient treatment. If this or any other conditions of the release are not met, then rehospitalization might occur. The states vary in the length of a conditional discharge, ranging from 90 days to one year. At the end of that period the person must either be rehospitalized or absolutely discharged. For rehospitalization to occur, there must be a hearing, unless an emergency exists. Even when someone is rehospitalized in an emergency situation, there must eventually be a hearing to determine that the rehospitalization is appropriate.

In the vast majority of states, the decision to discharge a patient is generally left to the superintendent of the mental health facility. In a few instances the decision must be approved by the central mental health agency. In most states the discharge decision must be reported to the committing court for record-keeping purposes. The most common discharge criterion is that the patient is no longer in need of care or treatment. The statutes also might provide that the patient no longer meets the commitment criteria or is no longer mentally ill. Some states will provide that the disabled person is no longer dangerous or likely to injure himself or others before he can be released.

In the majority of states, when the patient is dissatisfied with the facility's refusal to release him, he or someone on his behalf can request that the court determine whether he should be given an absolute discharge. Criteria for release are the same as when the discharge decision is made by the treatment facility. In cases where judicial review is sought, most states limit the number of times a person can request discharge, typically once every six months. Although a few states set no limit, others make it as infrequently as once a year. Even in states which do not specifically provide for judicial review of the decision to discharge the patient, he has the right to bring a *habeas corpus* action in state or federal court claiming that he is improperly institutionalized.

A. Clinical Indications for Discharge or Recommitment

Though in principle the decision to recommit or discharge a committed patient may be formally made by the hospital director or superintendent, in practice the decision is typically made by the attending physician or hospital treatment team. As in the initial commitment decision, a variety of considerations beyond clinical factors affects this second decision. These factors may be fiscal or social (family and neighborhood) considerations, the availability of appropriate residential facilities, and a fear of liability for commitment or release. Clinical factors will generally supersede all other considerations and include:

1. Whether the goals of the treatment plan for the patient have been realized.
2. Whether continued hospitalization at the present facility is likely to further realize those goals.
3. Whether continued hospitalization is likely to enhance or inhibit the patient's adjustment to the community whenever he is released.
4. Whether the patient continues to meet the commitment criteria of mental illness, need for treatment, danger to self, or danger to others.
5. Whether other treatment alternatives are more appropriate at this time for the patient (outpatient commitment, a residential treatment setting, sheltered care, vocational-rehabilitational services, or a transfer to another hospital facility).

X. FINANCIAL RESPONSIBILITY FOR THE COSTS OF INSTITUTIONAL CARE

Psychiatric care in a private treatment facility usually depends upon the ability to pay for that care. This is accomplished through health insurance or some type of public benefit coverage such as Medicaid or Medicare. When the care is received in a public facility, the state can hold the patient or his estate liable for the costs of that care whether he was treated voluntarily or involuntarily. Each state has laws which specify that the individual will be responsible for these costs. In all but three states (North Carolina, New Mexico, and Oregon), the family is also held legally responsible, at least to some extent. These states define which family members will be held liable; they always include a spouse, the parents of minor children, and often adult children for their parents. The trend is to set some outside limit on the length of liability, for example, 10 to 15 years, and the amount of that liability, such as $200 per month, which is determined on a sliding scale based on the relative's income. Many states also end the parents' responsibility when the child reaches 21 years of age.

Although the states have specific statutes dealing with who is responsible for the costs of institutional care, the reality is that most of the costs are borne by the taxpayers. The states will attempt to seek funds, but not at the cost of making the family bankrupt or placing them in a position of hardship. The state is most likely to attach assets which are left to the disabled person, either while he is institutionalized or once he has died. Commonly, the states will seek to be made a representative payee for persons who have been hospitalized a long time who receive social security, Veterans Administration benefits, and other types of pensions. These funds are used to offset the costs of hospitalization, with most states establishing procedures before these funds can be used, and limiting the amount of the benefit which can be applied for reimbursement of the treatment costs.

XI. COMMONLY ASKED QUESTIONS

1. *Am I liable for wrongful commitment, deprivation of civil rights, or false imprisonment if I seek to commit a patient?*

Although anyone can sue anyone else, immunity is provided to mental health professionals who in good faith seek the civil commitment of a person they believe warrants it. Immunity may not, however, preclude a suit for gross negligence in determining whether someone met the civil commitment standard or for civil rights claims. To avoid a successful suit in this area the clinician must have personally examined the respondent and attempted to take an adequate history either from him or from others. Suits based on wrongful commitment and false imprisonment are rarely filed, and even more rarely successful.

2. *Must a person be proven to have been actually violent before he can be committed to a psychiatric facility?*

In the vast majority of states, a demonstration of prior overt violence is not necessary for civil commitment to occur. The state commitment statute will set forth the standard, which may include the future likelihood of "serious harm" or a "recent overt act."

3. *Isn't it true that mental health professionals have no demonstrated capacity to predict another person's future violence? If this is true, then how can mental health professionals testify in a commitment hearing about a person's future likelihood of violence?*

There is a relatively small amount of research indicating that psychiatrists are unable to accurately predict violent behavior over the long-term future. Other work has specified the methodological flaws in the earlier research. It is also unlikely that such research can be generalized to the short-term predictions required in the civil commitment setting. Today, a clinician who has been trained in conducting risk assessments, who has evaluated the patient, reviewed his history and his current environment, and is familiar with the applicable base rates of violence should be able to assess the potential for violence in the short-term future. More importantly, the courts are looking for guidance from mental health professionals to justify providing treatment to those who need it, rather than specific numerical estimates of the likelihood and imminence of future harm.

4. *Can the mental health professional involuntarily detain a patient in the hospital who has voluntarily entered the facility?*

Yes. Most state laws provide that when a person enters the hospital voluntarily and he wishes to leave, the staff has some period of time to determine whether he should continue to be hospitalized. If at the end of this period the staff determines that the person meets the civil commitment criteria, then commitment proceedings should be initiated. Under no circumstances should a person who signed in voluntarily be discharged from the hospital upon his request to leave if the patient is clearly in need of immediate hospitalization.

5. *Can the mental health professional talk to the patient's family or friends in the process of committing the patient to the hospital even if the patient refuses?*

It is anticipated that when evaluating someone for emergency admission or for treatment, the therapist will speak with family members or friends to gain more information about the patient. This is acceptable, but the therapist must be careful what information he conveys to them about the patient. The therapist can obtain a psychiatric or social history from third parties without having to disclose confidential information (except for the fact of the hospitalization). When the patient has explicitly forbidden contacting the family or others as to his whereabouts, the therapist generally must honor that request unless good reason or a state regulation or statute would justify not complying with the patient's instruction. Courts will be sensitive to the clinician's obtaining the information he needs to be able to provide the appropriate treatment when doing so prevents serious bodily injury to the patient or others.

6. Can the mental health professional who is treating the patient refuse to testify at the commitment hearing?

No. If the treating clinician has been subpoenaed into court he must appear or he might face sanctions imposed by the court. If scheduling or other matters preclude court testimony at a certain time, the professional should attempt to contact the administrative personnel and attorneys involved in the commitment in order to make alternative arrangements if possible. Unless the clinician is paid by the patient or family for appearing in court, he is unlikely to be compensated for his time.

7. Can the mental health professional threaten to commit the patient to the hospital if the patient refuses to sign in voluntarily?

A patient should never be "threatened" with a future outcome if the professional has no grounds for commitment. It is possible, nevertheless, for the professional to inform the patient that commitment will be pursued if the patient rejects voluntary hospitalization.

8. Can the mental health professional accept the voluntary psychiatric hospitalization of a patient who is severely mentally ill and does not appear to understand his legal rights with regard to hospitalization?

As long as the patient has not been legally declared incompetent, the patient is presumed to be legally entitled to make treatment decisions for himself. Some states, however, indicate that the patient's consent for voluntary hospitalization should be a competent one to be valid; otherwise, commitment is necessary.

9. Can the mental health professional complete the commitment petitions and certificates if he is unsure whether the patient fulfills the commitment criteria, for example, when he wishes to place the responsibility for the decision to release the patient on the judge?

If after consultation with other clinicians the therapist is still unsure whether the patient meets the commitment criteria, then he should seek commitment and leave the decision to the court. Obviously, this approach should be taken only when there is truly a question in the clinician's mind about the need for commitment.

10. Should a patient be compelled to attend his commitment hearing despite his refusal?

While the patient generally has a right to attend his hearing, it is not legally required that he do so. Attendance at hearings sometimes has a psychologically harmful effect on a patient, and both the patient and the treatment staff should assess this possibility prior to the hearing.

11. Can a civil commitment ordered in one state be honored in another state?

If a person wants to involuntarily hospitalize another person, this should occur in the state where the hospital is located. Since civil commitments are authorized by state laws, which differ to some degree in commitment criteria and procedures, it is unlikely that another state will accept such a commitment at face value. Rather, the second state can then attempt to independently commit the patient according to its own law. However, transfers under the Interstate Compact on the Mentally Ill permit the return of a patient to his state of residence if he agrees and the receiving state agrees to accept him.

APPENDIX: STATE CIVIL COMMITMENT PROCEDURES

This section refers to the civil commitment standard in each state. The citation will direct the reader to its location in each state statute.

Alabama
ALA. Code 22-52-1
(1991)

"Mental illness" is defined to mean a "psychiatric disorder of thought and/or mood which significantly impairs judgment, behavior, capacity to recognize reality, or ability to cope with the ordinary demands of life. Mental illness . . . specifically excludes the primary diagnosis of epilepsy, mental retardation, substance abuse, including alcoholism, or a developmental disability."

Alaska
ALAS. Stat. 47.30.915 (12)
(1984 and Supp.1989)

"'Mental illness' means an organic, mental, or emotional impairment that has substantial adverse effects on an individual's ability to exercise conscious control of his actions or ability to perceive reality or to reason or understand; mental retardation, epilepsy, drug addiction, and alcoholism do not per se constitute mental illness, although persons suffering from these conditions may also be suffering from mental illness."

Arizona
ARIZ. Rev. Stat. Ann. 36-501 (22)
(1992)

"'Mental disorder' means a substantial disorder of the person's emotional processes, thought, cognition or memory. Mental disorder is distinguished from:

"(a) Conditions which are primarily those of drug abuse, alcoholism or mental retardation, except that persons with these conditions may also suffer from a mental disorder.

"(b) The declining mental abilities that directly accompany impending death.

"(c) Character and personality disorders characterized by lifelong and deeply ingrained antisocial behavior patterns, including sexual behaviors which are abnormal and prohibited by statute unless the behavior results from a mental disorder."

Arkansas
ARK. Code Ann. 20-47-202(J)
(1991)

"'Mental illness' refers to a substantial impairment of emotional processes, or of the ability to exercise conscious control of one's actions, or the ability to perceive reality or to reason, when the impairment is manifested by instances of extremely abnormal behavior or extremely faulty perceptions. It does not include impairment solely caused by: (1) epilepsy; (2) mental retardation; (3) continuous or noncontinuous periods of intoxication caused by substances such as alcohol or drugs; or (4) dependence upon or addiction to any substance such as alcohol or drugs."

California
CAL. Welf. and Inst. Code 5008(h)
(West 1984 and Supp.1992)

"'Gravely disabled' means . . . a condition in which a person, as a result of a mental disorder, is unable to provide for his basic personal needs for food, clothing or shelter . . . 'Gravely disabled' means a condition in which a person, as a result of impairment by chronic alcoholism, is unable to provide for his basic personal needs for food, clothing, or shelter. The term 'gravely disabled' does not include mentally retarded persons by reason of being mentally retarded alone."

Colorado
COLO. Rev. Stat. 27-10-102 (7)
(1989 and Supp.1992)

"Mentally ill person means a person with a substantial disorder of the cognitive, volitional, or emotional processes that grossly impairs judgment or capacity to recognize reality or to control behavior. Mental retardation is insufficient to either justify or exclude a finding of mental illness within the provisions of this article."

Connecticut
CONN. Gen. Stat. Ann. 319:Part II 17a-495
(1992)

"'Mentally ill person' means a person who has a mental or emotional condition which has substantial adverse effects on his or her ability to function and who requires care and treatment, and specifically excludes a person who is an alcohol-dependent person or a drug-dependent person."

Delaware
DEL. Code Ann. 16 Sec. 5001(1)
(1983 and Supp.1988)

"'Mentally ill person' means a person suffering from a mental disease or condition which requires such person to be observed and treated at a mental hospital for his own welfare and which either (i) renders such person unable to make responsible decisions with respect to his hospitalization, or (ii) poses a real and present threat, based upon manifest indications, that such person is likely to commit or suffer serious harm to himself or others or to property if not given immediate hospital care and treatment."

District of Columbia
D.C. Code Ann. 21-501
(1992)

"'Mental illness' means a psychosis or other disease which substantially impairs the mental health of a person."

Florida
FLA. Stat. Ann. 394.455 (3)
(1991)

"'Mentally ill' means an impairment of the emotional process, of the ability to exercise conscious control of one's actions, or of the ability to perceive reality or to understand, which impairment substantially interferes with a person's ability to meet the ordinary demands of living, regardless of etiology; except that, for the purposes of this act, the term does not include retardation or developmental disability, simple intoxication, or conditions manifested only by antisocial behavior or drug addiction."

Georgia
GA. Code Ann. 37-3-1 (11)
(1992)

"'Mentally ill' shall mean having a disorder of thought or mood which significantly impairs the judgment, behavior, capacity to recognize reality, or ability to cope with the ordinary demands of life."

Hawaii
HAWAII Rev. Stat. 334-1
(1992)

"'Mentally ill person' means a person having psychiatric disorder or other disease which substantially impairs the person's mental health and necessitates treatment or supervision."

Idaho
IDAHO Code 66-317(m)
(1992)

"'Mentally ill person' shall mean a person who, as a result of a substantial disorder of thought, mood, perception, orientation, or memory which grossly impairs judgment, behavior, capacity to recognize and adapt to reality, requires care and treatment at a facility.

Illinois
ILL. Compiled Stat. 405 Sec. 511-119
(1993)

"'Person subject to involuntary admission' or 'subject to involuntary admission' means:

"(1) A person who is mentally ill and who because of his illness is reasonably expected to inflict serious physical harm upon himself or another in the near future; or
"(2) A person who is mentally ill and who because of his illness is unable to provide for his basic physical needs so as to guard himself from serious harm."

Indiana
IND. Code Ann. 16-14-1-1(1)
(Burns 1990 and Supp.1992)

"A 'mentally ill person' means an individual who has a psychiatric disorder which substantially impairs his mental health, and because of such psychiatric disorder, for the welfare of such individual or for the welfare of others in the community in which such individual resides, requires care, treatment, training or detention. A psychiatric disorder means any mental illness or disease which shall include but shall not be limited to any mental deficiency, epilepsy, alcoholism, or addiction to narcotic or dangerous drugs."

Iowa
IOWA Code Ann. 229.1(7)
(1991)

"(1) 'Mental illness' means every type of mental disease or mental disorder except that it does not refer to mental retardation.
"(2) 'Serious mentally impaired' or 'serious mental impairment' describes the condition of a person who is afflicted with mental illness and because of the illness lacks sufficient judgment to make responsible decisions with respect to his or her hospitalization or treatment, and who because of that illness meets any of the following criteria:

"(a) Is likely to physically injure himself or herself or others if allowed to remain at liberty without treatment; or
"(b) Is likely to inflict serious emotional injury on members of the person's family or others who lack reasonable opportunity to avoid contact with the afflicted person if the afflicted person is allowed to remain at liberty without treatment."
"(c) Is unable to satisfy the person's needs for nourishment, clothing, essential medical care, or shelter so that it is likely that the person will suffer substantial physical injury, serious physical debilitation, or death within the reasonably foreseeable future."

Kansas
KAN. Stat. Ann. 59-2902(h)
(1991)

"'Mentally ill person' means any person who:

"(1) is suffering from a severe mental disorder to the extent that such a person is in need of treatment;
"(2) lacks capacity to make an informed decision concerning treatment; and
"(3) is likely to cause harm to self or others."

Kentucky
KY. Rev. Stat. 202 A.011(8)
(Michie 1992)

"'Mentally ill person' means a person with substantially impaired capacity to use self-control, judgment or discretion in the conduct of his affairs and social relations, associated with maladaptive behavior or recognized emotional symptoms where impaired capacity, maladaptive behavior or emotional symptoms can be related to physiological, psychological and/or social factors."

Louisiana
LA. Rev. Stat. Ann. 28:2 (14)
(West 1989 and Supp. 1991)

"'Mentally ill person' means any person with a psychiatric disorder which has substantial adverse effects on his ability to function and who requires care and treatment. It does not refer to a person suffering solely from mental retardation, epilepsy, alcoholism, or drug abuse."

Maine
ME. Rev. Stat. Ann. 34-B Sec. 3801(5)
(1991)

"'Mentally ill individual' means a person having a psychiatric or other disease which substantially impairs his mental health including persons suffering from the effects of the use of drugs, narcotics, hallucinogens or intoxicants, including alcohol, but not including mentally retarded or sociopathic persons."

Maryland
MD. Ann. Code 10-101(h)
(Michie 1990 and Supp.1992)

"(1) 'Mental disorder' means a behavioral or emotional illness that results from a psychiatric or neurological disorder.
"(2) 'Mental disorder' includes a mental illness that so substantially impairs the mental or emotional functioning of an individual as to make care or treatment necessary or advisable for the welfare of the individual or for the safety of the person or property of another.
"(3) 'Mental disorder' does not include mental retardation."

Massachusetts
MASS. Gen. Laws Ann. 104 CMR 3.01(a)
(West 1986 and Supp. 1989)

"'Mental illness' shall mean a substantial disorder of thought, mood, perception, orientation, or memory which grossly impairs judgment, behavior, capacity to recognize reality or ability to meet the ordinary demands of life, but shall not include alcoholism which is defined in M.G.L. c. 123, s. 35."

Michigan
MICH. Comp. Laws Ann. 330.1400a
(1991)

"'Mental illness' means a substantial disorder of thought or mood which significantly impairs judgment, behavior, capacity to recognize reality, or ability to cope with the ordinary demands of life."

Minnesota
MINN. Stat. Ann. 253 B.02(13)
(1991)

"'Mentally ill person' means any person who has an organic disorder of the brain or a substantial psychiatric disorder of thought, mood, perception, orientation, or memory which grossly impairs judgment, behavior, capacity to recognize reality, or to reason or understand, which

> "(a) is manifested by instances of grossly disturbed behavior of faulty perceptions; and
> "(b) poses a substantial likelihood of physical harm to self or others as demonstrated by:
>> "(i) a failure to obtain necessary food, clothing, shelter, or medical care as a result of the impairment, or
>> "(ii) a recent attempt or threat to physically harm self or others."

Mississippi
MISS. Code Ann. 41-21-61(e)
(1991)

"'Mentally ill person' means any person who has a substantial psychiatric disorder of thought, mood, perception, orientation, or memory which grossly impairs judgment, behavior, capacity to recognize reality, or to reason or understand, which (i) is manifested by instances of grossly disturbed behavior or faulty perceptions; and (ii) poses a substantial likelihood of physical harm to himself or others as demonstrated by (A) a recent attempt or threat to physically harm himself or others, or (B) a failure to provide necessary food, clothing, shelter, or medical care for himself, as a result of the impairment."

Missouri
MO. Ann. Stat. 630.005(21)
(1991)

"'Mental illness,' a state of impaired mental processes, which impairment results in a distortion of a person's capacity to recognize reality due to hallucinations, delusions, faulty perceptions or alterations of mood, and interferes with an individual's ability to reason, understand, or exercise conscious control over his actions. The term 'mental illness' does not include the following conditions unless they are accompanied by a mental illness as otherwise defined in this subdivision:

(a) Mental retardation, developmental disability or narcolepsy;
(b) Simple intoxication caused by substances such as alcohol or drugs;
(c) Dependence upon or addiction to any substances such as alcohol or drugs;
(d) Any other disorders such as senility, which are not of an actively psychotic nature."

Montana
MONT. Code Ann. 53-21-102
(1989)

"(6) 'Mental disorder' means any organic, mental, or emotional impairment which has substantial adverse effects on an individual's cognitive or volitional functions.
"(15) 'Seriously mentally ill' means suffering from a mental disorder which has resulted in a self-inflicted injury or injury to others or the imminent threat thereof or which has deprived the person afflicted of the ability to protect his life or health. For this purpose, injury means physical injury. No person may be involuntarily committed to a mental health facility or detained for evaluation and treatment because he is suffering from a mental disorder unless the condition causes him to be seriously mentally ill within the meaning of this part."

Nebraska
NEB. Rev. Stat. 83-1009
(1990)

"Mentally ill dangerous person shall mean any mentally ill person or alcoholic person or drug abusing person who presents:

"(1) A substantial risk of serious harm to another person or persons within the near future, as manifested by evidence of recent violent acts or threats of violence or by placing others in reasonable fear of such harm; or
"(2) A substantial risk of serious harm to himself within the near future, as manifested by evidence of recent attempts at, or threats of, suicide or serious bodily harm, or evidence of inability to provide for his basic human needs including food, clothing, shelter, essential medical care, or personal safety."

Nevada
NEV. Rev. Stat. 433.164
(1991)

"'Mental illness' means any mental dysfunction leading to impaired ability to maintain oneself and function effectively in one's life situation without external support."

New Hampshire
N.H. Rev. Stat. Ann. 135-C:2(x)
(1991)

"'Mental illness' means a substantial impairment of emotional processes, or of the ability to exercise conscious control of one's actions, or of the ability to perceive reality or to reason, which impairment is manifested by instances of extremely abnormal behavior or extremely faulty perceptions; it does not include impairment primarily caused by: (a) epilepsy; (b) mental retardation; (c) continuous or noncontinuous periods of intoxication caused by substances such as alcohol or drugs; (d) dependence upon or addiction to any substance such as alcohol or drugs."

New Jersey
N.J. Stat. Ann. 30:4-27.2
(West 1992)

"'Mental illness' means a current, substantial disturbance of thought, mood, perception or orientation which significantly impairs judgment, behavior or capacity to recognize reality, but does not include simple alcohol intoxication, transitory reaction to drug ingestion, organic brain syndrome or developmental disability unless it results in the severity of impairment described herein."

New Mexico
N.M. Stat. Ann. 43-1-3(o)
(1992)

"'Mental disorder' means the substantial disorder of the person's emotional processes, thought, or cognition which grossly impairs judgment, behavior or capacity to recognize reality but does not mean developmental disability."

New York
N.Y. Mental Hyg. Law 1.03(20)
(1992)

"'Mental illness' means an affliction with a mental disease or mental condition which is manifested by a disorder or disturbance in behavior, feeling, thinking, or judgment to such an extent that the person afflicted requires care, treatment and rehabilitation."

North Carolina
N.C. Gen. Stat. 122C-3(21)
(1991)

"(21) 'Mental illness' means: (i) when applied to an adult, an illness which so lessens the capacity of the individual to use self-control, judgment, and discretion in the conduct of his affairs and social relations as to make it necessary or advisable for him to be under treatment, care, supervision, guidance, or control; and (ii) when applied to a minor, a mental condition, other than mental retardation alone, that so impairs the youth's capacity to exercise age adequate self-control or judgment in the conduct of his activities and social relationships so that he is in need of treatment."

North Dakota
N.D. Cent. Code 25-03.1-02(9)
(1991)

"'Mentally ill person' means an individual with an organic, mental, or emotional disorder which substantially impairs the capacity to use self-control, judgment, and discretion in the conduct of personal affairs and social relations. 'Mentally ill person' does not include a mentally retarded or mentally deficient person of significantly subaverage general intellectual functioning which originates during the developmental period and is associated with impairment in adaptive behavior. Chemical dependency does not per se constitute mental illness, although persons suffering from these conditions may also be suffering from mental illness."

Ohio
OHIO Rev. Code Ann. 5122.01(A)
(Anderson 1989)

"'Mental illness' means a substantial disorder of thought, mood, perception, orientation, or memory that grossly impairs judgment, behavior, capacity to recognize reality, or ability to meet the ordinary demands of life."

Oklahoma
OKLA. Stat. Ann. 43A Sec.1-103(3)
(West 1990 and Supp.1992)

"'Mentally ill person' means a person afflicted with a substantial disorder of thought, mood, perception, psychological orientation or memory that significantly impairs judgment, behavior, capacity to recognize reality or ability to meet the ordinary demands of life."

Oregon
OR. Rev. Stat. 426.005(2)
(1991)

"'Mentally ill person' means a person who, because of a mental disorder, is either: (a) dangerous to himself or others; or (b) unable to provide for his basic personal needs and is not receiving such care as is necessary for his health or safety."

Pennsylvania
PA. Stat. Ann. 50 Sec.7301(a)
(1992)

"A person is severely mentally disabled when, as a result of mental illness, his capacity to exercise self-control, judgment and discretion in the conduct of his affairs and social relations or to care for his own personal needs is so lessened that he poses a clear and present danger of harm to others or to himself."

Rhode Island
R.I. Gen. Laws 40.1-5-2(13)
(1991)

"'Mental disability' means a mental disorder in which the capacity of a person to exercise self-control or judgment in the conduct of his affairs and social relations or to care for his own personal needs is significantly impaired."

South Carolina
S.C. Code Ann. 44-23-10(1)
(1991)

"'Mentally ill person' means a person afflicted with a mental disease to such an extent that, for his own welfare or the welfare of others or of the community, he requires care, treatment, or hospitalization."

South Dakota
S.D. Codified Laws Ann. 27A-1-1
(1992)

"The term 'severe mental illness'—substantial organic or psychiatric disorder of thought, mood, or perception, orientation or memory which significantly impairs judgment, or behavior; or ability to cope with the basic demands of life. Mental retardation, epilepsy, other developmental disability, or alcohol or substance abuse does not, alone, constitute mental illness."

Tennessee
TENN. Code Ann. 33-1-101(14)
(1992)

"Mentally ill individual—an individual who suffers from a psychiatric disorder, alcoholism, or drug dependency, but excluding an individual whose mental disability is mental retardation."

Texas
TEX. Rev. Civ. Stat. Ann. 571.003(14)
(Vernon 1992)

"Mental illness means an illness, disease or condition, other than epilepsy, senility, alcoholism, or mental deficiency that:

> "(A) Substantially impairs the person's thought, perception of reality, emotional process, or judgment; or
> "(B) Grossly impairs behavior as demonstrated by recent disturbed behavior."

Utah
UTAH Code Ann. 62A-12-101(5)
(Supp.1989)

"'Severe mental disorder' means schizophrenia, major depression, bipolar disorders, delusional disorders, psychotic disorders, and other mental disorders as defined by the board."

Vermont
VT. Stat. Ann. 18 Sec. 7101(14)
(1991)

"'Mental illness' means a substantial disorder of thought, mood, perception, orientation, or memory, any of which grossly impairs judgment, behavior, capacity to recognize reality, or ability to meet the ordinary demands of life, but shall not include mental retardation."

Virginia
VA. Code 37.1-1
(1992)

"'Mentally ill' means any person afflicted with mental disease to such an extent that for his own welfare or the welfare of others, he requires care and treatment; provided, that for the purposes of Chapter 2 (Sec. 37.1–63 et seq.) of this title, the term 'mentally ill' shall be deemed to include any person who is a drug addict or alcoholic."

Washington
WASH. Rev. Code Ann. 71.05.020(2)
(1991)

"'Mental disorder' means any organic, mental or emotional impairment which has substantial adverse effects on an individual's cognitive or volitional functions."

West Virginia
W.VA. Code 27-1-2
(1986 and Supp.1989)

"'Mental illness' means a manifestation in a person of significantly impaired capacity to maintain acceptable levels of functioning in the areas of intellect, emotion and physical well-being."

Wisconsin
WISC. Stat. Ann. 51.01
(1990)

"(13a) 'Mental illness' means mental disease to such extent that a person so afflicted requires care and treatment for his or her own welfare, or the welfare of others, or of the community.

"(13b) 'Mental illness,' for purposes of involuntary commitment, means a substantial disorder of thought, mood, perception, orientation, or memory which grossly impairs judgment, behavior, capacity to recognize reality, or ability to meet the ordinary demands of life, but does not include alcoholism."

Wyoming
WYO. Stat. 25-10-101(a)(ix)
(1992)

"'Mental illness' and 'mentally ill' mean a physical, emotional, mental or behavioral disorder which causes a person to be dangerous to himself or others and which requires treatment."

XII. BIBLIOGRAPHY

I. Inpatient Commitment

A. Cases—General

Rouse v. Cameron, 373 F.2d 451 (D.C. Cir. 1966).
Quesnell v. State, 517 P.2d 568 (Wash. 1968).
Bell v. Wayne County General Hospital, 456 F.2d 1062 (6th Cir. 1972).
Lessard v. Schmidt, 349 F.Supp. 1078 (E.D. Wis. 1972).
Lynch v. Baxley, 386 F.Supp. 378 (M.D. Ala. 1974).
Welsch v. Likins, 373 F.Supp. 487 (D. Minn. 1974).
Dixon v. Weinberger, 405 F.Supp. 974 (D.D.C. 1975).
Donaldson v. O'Connor, 422 U.S. 563 (1975).
New York Association for Retarded Children v. Carey, 393 F.Supp. 719 (E.D.N.Y. 1975).
Suzuki v. Quisenberry, 411 F.Supp. 1113 (D. Hawaii 1976).
Addington v. Texas, 441 U.S. 418 (1979).
Parham v. J.R., 442 U.S. 584 (1979).
Suzuki v. Yuen, 617 F.2d 175 (9th Cir. 1980).
Watkins v. Roche, 529 F.Supp. 327 (Ga. 1981).
Dick v. Watonwan County, 562 F.Supp. 1083 (Minn. 1983).
Project Release v. Prevost, 722 F.2d 960 (2nd Cir. 1983).
People v. Hays, 465 N.E.2d 98 (Ill. 1984).
State v. Smith, 692 P.2d 120 (Or.Ct.App. 1984).
In re Blair, 510 A.2d 1048 (D.C. App. 1986).
Donahue v. Rhode Island, 632 F.Supp. 1456 (R.I. 1986).
Matter of R.J., 431 N.W.2d 708 (Wis.App. 1988).
Spencer v. Lee, 864 F.2d 1376 (7th Cir. 1989).
Colorado v. District Court, County of Adams, 797 P.2d 1259 (Colo.Sup.Ct. 1990).
Goetz v. Crosson, 728 F.Supp. 995 (S.D.N.Y. 1990).
Zinermon v. Burch, 110 S.Ct. 975 (1990).
In re M.D., 596 A.2d 766 (N.J.Sup.Ct. 1991).

B. Cases-Wrongful Commitment

Reiser v. Prunty, 727 P.2d 538 (Sup.Ct.Mont. 1986).
Everett v. Florida Institute of Technology, 503 So.2d 1382 (Fla.App. 1987).
Stock v. Forbes Health System, 697 F.Supp. 1399 (W.D.Pa. 1988).
Hudgins v. Bawtinhimer, 395 S.E.2d 909 (Ga.App. 1990).
Heath v. Peachtree Parkwood Hospital, Inc., 407 S.E.2d 406 (Ga.App. 1991).
Harvey v. Harvey, 949 F.2d 1127 (11th Cir. 1992).

C. Articles and Books

American Psychiatric Association. (1982). Guidelines for the psychiatric hospitalization of minors, and four alternatives to the guidelines for the psychiatric hospitalization of minors: Clinical and legal considerations. *American Journal of Psychiatry, 139*, 971–975.

American Psychiatric Association. (1983). Guidelines for legislation on the psychiatric hospitalization of adults. *American Journal of Psychiatry, 140*, 672–679.

Bagby, R. M., & Atkinson, L. (1988). The effects of legislative reform on civil commitment rates: A critical analysis. *Behavioral Sciences and the Law, 6*, 45–62.

Brakel, S. J., Parry, J., & Weiner, B. A. (1985). *The mentally disabled and the law* (3rd ed.). Chicago: American Bar Foundation.

Chodoff, P. (1984). Involuntary hospitalization of the mentally ill as a moral issue. *American Journal of Psychiatry, 141*, 384–389.

Commission on the Mentally Disabled, American Bar Association. (1988). *Involuntary civil commitment: A manual for lawyers and judges*. Washington, DC: American Bar Association.

Conlon, P., Merskey, H., Zilli, C., & Frommhold, K. (1990). The attitudes toward committal of patients hospitalized in a psychiatric facility for the first time. *Canadian Journal of Psychiatry, 35*, 324–327.

Custer, L. B. (1970). The origins of the doctrine of *parens patriae*. *Emory Law Journal, 27*, 195–208.

Durham, M. L., & LaFond, J. Q. (1985). The empirical consequences and policy implications of broadening the statutory criteria for civil commitment. *Hospital and Community Psychiatry, 36*, 259–264.

Edelsohn, G. A., & Hiday, V. A. (1990). Civil commitment: A range of patient attitudes. *Bulletin of the American Academy of Psychiatry and the Law, 18*, 65–77.

Ensminger, J. J., & Liguori, T. D. (1978). The therapeutic significance of the civil commitment hearing: An unexplored potential. *Journal of Psychiatry and Law, 6*, 5–44.

Garcia, S. A., & Keilitz, I. (1991). Involuntary civil commitment of drug-dependent persons with special reference to pregnant women. *Mental and Physical Disability Law Reporter, 15*, 418–437.

Hiday, V. A. (1988). Civil commitment: A review of empirical research. *Behavioral Sciences and the Law, 6*, 15–44.

Knapp, S., & VandeCreek, L. (1987). A review of tort liability in involuntary civil commitment. *Hospital and Community Psychiatry, 38*, 648–651.

Livermore, J. M., Malmquist, C. P., & Meehl, P. E. (1968). On the justifications for civil commitment. *Harvard Law Review, 117*, 75–96.

McFarland, B. H., Faulker, L. R., Bloom, J. D., Hallaux, R., & Bray, J. D. (1990). Family members' opinions about civil commitment. *Hospital and Community Psychiatry, 41*, 537–540.

Miller, R. D. (1987). *Involuntary civil commitment of the mentally ill in the post-reform era*. Springfield, IL: C. C. Thomas.

Miller, R. D. (1992). Need-for-treatment criteria for involuntary civil commitment: Impact in practice. *American Journal of Psychiatry, 149*, 1380–1384.

Miller, R. D., Maier, G. J., & Kaye, M. (1985). *Miranda* comes to the hospital: The right to remain silent in civil commitment. *American Journal of Psychiatry, 142*, 1074–1077.

Miller, R. D., Maier, G. J., & Kaye, M. (1986). The right to remain silent during psychiatric examination in civil and criminal cases: A national survey and an analysis. *International Journal of Law and Psychiatry, 9*, 77–94.

Morris, G. M. (1986). The Supreme Court examines civil commitment issues: A retrospective and prospective assessment. *Tulane Law Review, 60*, 927–953.

Morse, S. J. (1982). A preference for liberty: The case against involuntary commitment of the mentally disordered. *California Law Review, 70*, 54–106.

National Center for State Courts. (1986). Guidelines for involuntary civil commitment. *Mental and Physical Disability Law Reporter, 10*, 410–514.

Parry, C. D. H., & Turkheimer, E. (1992). Length of hospitalization and outcome of commitment and recommitment hearings. *Hospital and Community Psychiatry, 43*, 65–68.

Perlin, M. L. (1989 and suppl.). *Mental disability law: Civil and criminal*. Charlottesville, VA: Michie.

Pierce, G. L., Durham, M. L., & Fisher, W. H. (1985). The impact of broadened civil commitment standards on admissions to state mental hospitals. *American Journal of Psychiatry, 142*, 104–107.

Rosenthal, M. P. (1988). The constitutionality of involuntary civil commitment of opiate addicts. *Journal of Drug Issues, 18*, 641–661.

Roth, L. H. (1979). A commitment law for patients, doctors and lawyers. *American Journal of Psychiatry, 136*, 1121–1127.

Stromberg, C. D., & Stone, A. A. (1983). A model state law on civil commitment of the mentally ill. *Harvard Journal on Legislation, 20,* 275–396.
Stone, A. A. (1975). *Mental health and law: A system in transition.* Rockville, MD: NIMH Center for Studies of Crime and Delinquency.
Treffert, D. A. (1985). The obviously ill patient in need of treatment: A fourth standard for civil commitment. *Hospital and Community Psychiatry, 36,* 259–264.
Turkheimer, E., & Parry, C. D. H. (1992). Why the gap? Practice and policy in civil commitment hearings. *American Psychologist, 47,* 646–655.
Winick, B. J. (1991). Competency to consent to voluntary hospitalization: A therapeutic jurisprudence analysis of *Zinermon v. Burch. International Journal of Law and Psychiatry, 14,* 169–214.

II. Risk Assessments of Violence

A. Articles and Books

Arkes, H. R. (1989). Principles in judgment/decision making research pertinent to legal proceedings. *Behavioral Sciences and the Law, 7,* 429–456.
Beck, J. C., White, K. A., & Gage, B. (1991). Emergency psychiatric assessment of violence. *American Journal of Psychiatry, 148,* 1562–1565.
Blomhoff, S., Seim, S., & Friis, S. (1990). Can prediction of violence among psychiatric inpatients be improved? *Hospital and Community Psychiatry, 41,* 771–775.
Dawes, R. M., Faust, D., & Meehl, P. E. (1989). Clinical versus actuarial judgment. *Science, 243,* 1668–1674.
Garb, H. N. (1989). Clinical judgment, clinical training, and professional experience. *Psychological Bulletin, 105,* 387–396.
Gutheil, T. G., Bursztajn, H., & Brodsky, B. A. (1986). The multidimensional assessment of dangerousness: Competence assessment in patient care and liability prevention. *Bulletin of the American Academy of Psychiatry and the Law, 14,* 123–129.
Hiday, V. A. (1991). Arrest and incarceration of civil commitment candidates. *Hospital and Community Psychiatry, 42,* 729–734.
Hiday, V. A. (1992). Civil commitment and arrests. *Journal of Nervous and Mental Disease, 180,* 184–191.
Janofsky, J. S., Spears, S., & Neubauer, D. N. (1988). Psychiatrists' accuracy in predicting violent behavior on an inpatient unit. *Hospital and Community Psychiatry, 39,* 1090–1094.
Klassen, D., & O'Connor, W. A. (1988). Predicting violence in schizophrenic and non-schizophrenic patients: A prospective study. *Journal of Community Psychology, 16,* 217–271.
Klassen, D., & O'Connor, W. A. (1988). A prospective study of predictors of violence in adult male mental health admissions. *Law and Human Behavior, 12,* 143–158.
McNiel, D. E., & Binder, R. L. (1987). Predictive validity of judgments of dangerousness in emergency civil commitment. *American Journal of Psychiatry, 144,* 197–200.
McNiel, D. E., & Binder, R. L. (1989). Relationship between preadmission threats and later violent behavior by acute psychiatric inpatients. *Hospital and Community Psychiatry, 40,* 605–608.
McNeil, D. E., & Binder, R. L. (1991). Clinical assessment of the risk of violence among psychiatric inpatients. *American Journal of Psychiatry, 148,* 1317–1321.
McNiel, D. E., Binder, R. L., & Greenfield, T. K. (1988). Predictors of violence in civilly committed acute psychiatric patients. *American Journal of Psychiatry, 145,* 965–970.
McNiel, D. E., Myers, R. S., Zeiner, H. K., Wolfe, H. L., & Hatcher, C. (1992). *American Journal of Psychiatry, 149,* 207–212.
Monahan, J. (1981). *The clinical prediction of violent behavior.* Rockville, MD: NIMH Center for Studies of Crime and Delinquency.
Mulvey, E. P., & Lidz, C. W. (1984). Clinical considerations in the prediction of dangerousness in mental patients. *Clinical Psychology Review, 4,* 379–401.
Mulvey, E. P., & Lidz, C. W. (1985). Back to basics: A critical analysis of dangerousness research in a new legal environment. *Law and Human Behavior, 9,* 209–219.
Otto, R. K. (1992). Prediction of dangerous behavior: A review and analysis of "second-generation" research. *Forensic Reports, 5,* 103–133.
Poythress, N. G. (1992). Expert testimony on violence and dangerousness: Roles for mental health professionals. *Forensic Reports, 5,* 135–150.
Quinsey, V. L., & Maguire, A. (1986). Maximum security psychiatric patients: Actuarial and clinical prediction of dangerousness. *Journal of Interpersonal Violence, 1,* 143–171.

Reid, W. H. (1988). Clinical evaluation of the violent patient. *Psychiatric Clinics of North America, 11*, 527–537.
Segal, S. P., Watson, M. A., Goldfinger, S. M., & Averbuck, D. S. (1988). Civil commitment in the psychiatric emergency room: 1. The assessment of dangerousness by emergency room clinicians. *Archives of General Psychiatry, 45*, 748–752.
Shah, S. A. (1978). Dangerousness: A paradigm for exploring some issues in law and psychology. *American Psychologist, 33*, 224–238.
Slobogin, C. (1984). Dangerousness and expertise. *University of Pennsylvania Law Review, 133*, 97–174.
Tardiff, K. (1992). The current state of psychiatry in the treatment of violent patients. *Archives of General Psychiatry, 49*, 493–499.
Webster, C. D., & Menzies, R. J. (1987). The clinical prediction of dangerousness. In D. Weisstub (Ed.), *Law and mental health, Vol. 3*, pp. 158–208. New York: Pergamon.

III. Outpatient Commitment

A. *Cases*

Birl v. Wallis, 633 F.Supp. 707 (Ala. 1986).
In re James, 507 A.2d 155 (D.C.App. 1986).
Matter of Guardianship of K.N.K., 407 N.W.2d 281 (Wis.App. 1987).
Rhode Island Department of Mental Health v. R.B., 549 A.2d 1028 (Sup.Ct. R.I. 1988).
Matter of Utley, 565 N.E.2d 1152 (Ind.App. 1991).
In the interest of T.J., 850 N.W.2d 850 (Sup.Ct.N.D. 1992)

B. *Articles and Books*

American Psychiatric Association. (1987). *Involuntary commitment to outpatient treatment* (Task Force Report #26). Washington, DC: American Psychiatric Association.
Fernandez, G. A., & Nygard, S. (1990). Impact of involuntary outpatient commitment on the revolving-door syndrome in North Carolina. *Hospital and Community Psychiatry, 41*, 1001–1004.
Geller, J. L. (1986). Rights, wrongs, and the dilemma of coerced community treatment. *American Journal of Psychiatry, 143*, 1259–1264.
Geller, J. L. (1990). Clinical guidelines for the use of involuntary outpatient treatment. *Hospital and Community Psychiatry, 41*, 749–755.
Hiday, V. A., & Scheid-Cook, T. L. (1991). Outpatient commitment for "revolving door" patients: Compliance and treatment. *Journal of Nervous and Mental Disease, 179*, 83–88.
Keilitz, I. (1990). Empirical studies of involuntary outpatient civil commitment: Is it working? *Mental and Physical Disability Law Reporter, 14*, 368–379.
Keilitz, I., & Hall, T. (1985). State statutes governing involuntary outpatient civil commitment. *Mental and Physical Disability Law Reporter, 9*, 378–397.
McCafferty, G., & Dooley, J. (1990). Involuntary outpatient commitment: An update. *Mental and Physical Disability Law Reporter, 14*, 277–287.
Meloy, J. R., Haroun, A., & Schiller, E. F. (1990). *Clinical guidelines for involuntary outpatient treatment.* Sarasota, FL: Professional Resource Exchange.
Miller, R. D. (1988). Outpatient civil commitment of the mentally ill: An overview and an update. *Behavioral Sciences and the Law, 6*, 99–118.
Miller, R. D. (1992). An update on involuntary civil commitment to outpatient treatment. *Hospital and Community Psychiatry, 43*, 79–81.
Mulvey, E. P., Geller, J. L., & Roth, L. H. (1987). The promise and peril of involuntary outpatient commitment. *American Psychologist, 42*, 571–584.
Schmidt, M. J., & Geller, J. L. (1989). Involuntary administration of medication in the community: The judicial opportunity. *Bulletin of the American Academy of Psychiatry and the Law, 17*, 283–292.
Schwartz, S. J., & Costanzo, C. E. (1987). Compelling treatment in the community: Distorted doctrines and violated values. *Loyola of Los Angeles Law Review, 20*, 1329–1429.

4

Rights of Hospitalized Patients

I. ***Wyatt v. Stickney*** **• II. Communication** • A. Mail • B. Visitation • C. Telephone • **III. Access to an Attorney • IV. Presumption of Competency • V. Humane Care and Treatment • VI. Least Restrictive Alternative • VII. Periodic Review • VIII. Patient Employment • IX. Right to Manage Funds** • A. Representative Payee • **X. Right to Refuse to Participate in Research • XI. Personal Possessions • XII. Religious Freedom • XIII. Voting Rights • XIV. Commonly Asked Questions • Appendix • XV. Bibliography**

Until the mid-1970s, it was accepted that, upon entering a mental health treatment facility, a person left his rights at the door and submitted himself to the complete control of the facility staff. This was as true in state mental hospitals as it was in private psychiatric treatment facilities. All aspects of the patient's daily life were controlled, from what he wore to those with whom he was permitted to communicate. The notion of the mentally ill person's having any say in his treatment was almost unknown. He was presumed to be totally incompetent and thus incapable of making rational decisions about any aspect of his daily life, including his care.

By 1975, a revolution had occurred in recognizing the rights of the hospitalized mentally ill person. These changes occurred as a result of class action lawsuits which challenged conditions at state mental institutions. State facilities were chosen because constitutional deprivations can arise only in a governmental setting. Today when someone enters a state mental health facility, he no longer leaves his rights at the door. Patient rights are now well defined in state statutes. In many states, these same rights are also guaranteed to persons receiving treatment in a private psychiatric setting. Many of these rights have helped to improve the quality of care provided to the institutionalized mentally disabled. This chapter will set forth these rights and describe the role of the mental health professional in ensuring their implementation. An appendix is provided for the reader to identify the sections of each state's law which describes the particular rights of the mentally disabled person.

I. *WYATT v. STICKNEY*

Wyatt v. Stickney sparked the revolution in establishing the rights of institutionalized mentally disabled persons—both the mentally ill and the mentally retarded. The notion that mentally disabled persons in state facilities had some rights was first raised judicially in 1970 when *Wyatt* was filed. This case, which examined all aspects of the conditions within the Alabama institutions for the mentally disabled, set the standards for what was considered the minimum required by the United States Constitution if someone were to be hospitalized for a mental disability. The case, initially brought by employees of the facilities who were being fired because of funding problems, turned into the most exhaustive examination of what the minimum care and conditions must be for those the state seeks to hospitalize involuntarily. The case involved many weeks of testimony from the country's leading experts on the needs of the mentally ill and the developmentally disabled. It resulted in a decision which set forth the minimum standards required by the United States Constitution if an institution provided involuntary hospitalization. This was accomplished through an appendix to the court's decision which detailed several aspects of the care of institutionalized persons, including establishing staff/patient ratios, and nutritional requirements, as well as defining the minimum required of the physical plant, including the numbers of showers and toilets needed for a given patient population. The reverberations from the numerous decisions surrounding the *Wyatt* case were felt in almost every state legislature and mental health agency. The rights guaranteed to the disabled in this case have become the norm in mental health codes across the United States, with many adopting the same wording that was used in the *Wyatt* decision.

II. COMMUNICATION

Perhaps the most important right a hospitalized person has is the right to communicate with those outside of the institution. This not only ensures that others will be aware of his situation but also has the beneficial effect of keeping the disabled person in contact with his community. Communication can take a variety of forms: letters to family, friends, public officials, and attorneys; personal contact with visitors; or telephone conversations. Almost all states have provisions in the patient's rights section of their mental health codes which address the right of the disabled person to communicate with those outside the institution.

A. Mail

With few exceptions, the states have adopted statutes guaranteeing the disabled person's general right to communicate by mail. Almost all the states, however, permit some restrictions to be imposed, most commonly specifying as adequate justification "good cause" or the "medical welfare of the patient." Some states permit bans on the communication when it is harassing or harmful to another party. A mentally disabled person's repeated letters threatening violence to others, for example, may prompt the facility staff to limit the person's rights in this regard. Similar cases may even constitute illegal use of the mail and represent criminal conduct. In other cases, the mentally disabled person may be deemed unable to handle mail because of his mental or physical condition.

Approximately half the states require that any limits on mail be noted in the patient's chart. This charting requirement not only specifies the limit on the person's mail and its justification, but also requires the mental health professional to carefully specify when such measures are warranted before implementing them. A valid and sufficient justification for restriction should consider the pertinent facts, including the patient's history, current condition, and prognosis. There may also be a requirement that the person be informed of any restrictions placed on his right to communicate by mail. The restriction should be no greater than is necessary to protect the particular interest in question. All restriction orders should be periodically reviewed for the necessity of continuation.

Many states also provide that certain mail cannot be censored. Several states, for example, provide that letters sent to public officials, administrators of the mental health agency, or attorneys cannot be intercepted and must be mailed. This would also be true of letters sent to the disabled person from these individuals. The few courts which have examined restrictions on outgoing mail have taken the position that the receiver of the mail can ask the post office not to deliver letters from a particular sender or they have the right not to open the letter, and that therefore the limitations should not be set by the facility staff. A mentally ill person can write irrational letters to the president, the pope, or anyone else, and the receiver can simply ignore the correspondence if desired.

An institution has a legitimate and substantial interest in preserving the therapeutic environment and the health of its patients to the fullest extent possible. For example, in circumstances where the facility staff believes that contraband such as illicit drugs or dangerous objects are arriving in the mail, the staff has the right to open the mail and search it but then must forward the letter to the disabled person. When the staff opens such packages, it is prudent to have the disabled person or the sender present to obviate charges of theft or interference with the mail.

Without access to paper, pens, and postage, the statutorily created right to communicate by mail is a hollow one. Therefore, approximately half the states have statutory provision for reasonable access to the necessary writing materials and postage. This may provide for a certain number of letters or amount of correspondence during a stated time interval. Each individual should additionally be afforded the opportunity to purchase at his expense necessary writing materials. What is reasonable has not been defined, and it is difficult to know if in those states without statutory provision for writing tools whether the right to send mail is implemented.

B. Visitation

Visitation by noninstitutionalized persons, another important means of communication, is generally guaranteed by over 90% of the states. For the mentally disabled person, face-to-face contact with visitors ensures that someone will be aware of the patient's condition and progress, something which is particularly important for the disabled person who may not be able to communicate with those outside the institution. It also permits those outside the facility to be aware of the conditions within the facility. Like the statutes relating to mail, restrictions on visitors are permitted to "protect the patient's health" or for "good cause." In approximately half the states any limitations on visitors must be charted. It is common for situations to arise in which the staff seek to limit visitation. These include cases in which the visitor is disruptive to the treatment of the mentally disabled person, to other patients or their treatment, or to the facility unit. There also may be temporary restrictions placed on a patient's visitation rights when the patient is clinically unable to tolerate visitation because of extreme agitation, hostility, delirium, or psychosis. The staff also has the right to search people entering a unit when there is probable cause to believe they may be carrying contraband items which they intend to pass to the patient. These may include drugs, potential weapons, or expensive electronic equipment. Foods and condiments which may be harmful to the health of the patient or others can also be inappropriate. Because of concerns about the types of items which are brought on the unit, visitors may have their purses checked or may be patted down. Regulations which the facility adopts to protect the patients or staff will be upheld if they are viewed as reasonable and related to patient care.

The courts, in the few cases which have addressed the issue of visitors to psychiatric units, have upheld reasonable restrictions developed by the facility but will strike down provisions which are unreasonable or excessively limit access. For example, if the facility has limited visiting hours, this may be viewed as interfering with the patient's right to communicate with others. Patients, family, and visitors should generally be informed of the visitation policy as well as any restrictions placed in a particular case. At times, it may be relevant to include the patient or family in the decision making about such restrictions.

A few states have statutory provisions for conjugal visits. Approximately one third of the states permit unrestricted visitation by clergy, and 40% of the states permit attorneys to visit without restrictions. Disputes sometimes arise about the timing and location of visits by clergy or attorneys. While a mentally disabled person may have the right to visitation by such individuals, this does not necessarily mean that a facility is no longer able to regulate such visits. Permitting visitation during daytime hours may be sufficient.

At various times the press has demanded the right to visit a psychiatric treatment facility, attend commitment hearings, or have access to the mental health records of public figures. The press argue that the First Amendment guarantee of freedom of the press guarantees their access to the facility and their attendance at hearings. The courts, however, have not permitted them to have carte blanche entry into a mental health facility. They may, however, obtain access in the ways other members of the public do, that is, by visiting specific mentally disabled persons.

Somewhat different issues are presented by on-unit visitation by other patients at the same facility, particularly when locked units are exclusively used. Visitation by other patients is typically more restricted than that by nonpatients. Such social visits from ward to ward are often restricted to one or two visitors per patient. Further, social visits must often be evaluated and approved on an individual basis by nursing and medical staff. Additional restrictions with regard to the timing, frequency and length of visits, and the search of visitors may apply as noted for nonpatient visitation. Finally, visits among patients on off-ward locations within the facility grounds will generally be permitted according to hospital policy and the clinical needs and privileges of the patients involved.

C. Telephone

Access to the telephone is particularly important for institutionalized persons who cannot write and for those whose family and friends are unable to visit because of the location of the facility or its visiting hours. The telephone thus may be important for maintaining contact with family and friends and reinforcing their support. Eighty percent of the states guarantee by statute the disabled person's right to access to the telephone. Restrictions on such telephone access, similar to those placed on access to visitors or the mail, are sometimes permitted. Limitations on telephone communication make the most sense when aimed at preventing the patient from harassing someone who has complained about previous harassment. Unlike the mail situation, in which the unwilling recipient can request that the post office not deliver a letter from a particular sender, the recipient has no way of preventing an unwanted telephone call.

Limitation of access to the telephone may be clinically justified either for making outgoing calls or for receiving incoming calls. Agitated and paranoid individuals sometimes repeatedly telephone government agencies or authorities to report a perceived conspiracy or threat of harm. Some mentally disabled individuals may be either the recipients of or offenders in telecommunications threatening serious interpersonal violence. Finally, some individuals unintentionally harass their loved ones with repeated communications so that a restriction on telephone calls, sometimes at the request of the family, becomes an important element in the individual's treatment plan.

The right to use a telephone is meaningless if there are no telephones available on the unit, or no means of making calls without funds. Thus, it is incumbent upon the facility to ensure that the statutorily created right to use the telephone becomes a reality. A facility may be required, for example, to regularly provide each mentally disabled person with a certain number of telephone calls. It is not legally necessary, however, to provide completely private facilities such as separate telephone booths or rooms for such calls; calls are typically made from hallways or other semipublic areas of the facility.

Limitations on the patient's right of access to the telephone should be explained to the patient and the patient's family. If possible, such limitations should be determined with their input.

III. ACCESS TO AN ATTORNEY

A primary reason for the many significant changes in mental health facilities since the 1960s is the advocacy of attorneys who secured individual patient rights which forced state legislatures to spend more money for the care of the mentally disabled. This advocacy occurred not only in the courtroom, but also in the state legislatures, Congress, and the news media. To sustain the achievements of the 1970s and 1980s, the mentally disabled must have access to attorneys.

In every state a disabled person has a right to be represented by a lawyer at a civil commitment hearing. This right is important to ensure that the disabled will not be improperly hospitalized (see Chapter 3). However, once the person is hospitalized, his claim to a right to an attorney greatly diminishes, as does the likelihood of receiving access to one. Yet the need for legal services does not necessarily stop once the commitment proceeding has concluded. The disabled may encounter problems while in the institution—some related to their rights while in the facility, and others of a general legal nature that affects the rest of the population.

Legal services for the mentally ill and developmentally disabled have traditionally been provided by federally funded legal aid programs. During the 1980s there was a drastic cutback in such programs, making it unlikely that an institutionalized disabled person would have access to an attorney. New York, with its Mental Health Information Service, and New Jersey stand out as notable exceptions in providing the disabled with access to attorneys. At least 20 states permit attorneys to have unrestricted access to their clients. Even in states with no such provisions, the mental health agency is hard pressed to justify denying a client/patient access to his lawyer. In fact a few cases have made it clear that the facility has the obligation to assist the disabled person in reaching his attorney via either the mail or the telephone.

Many mental health professionals assume that any dealings with attorneys must be of an adversarial nature. This is not necessarily the case. Attorneys are concerned about ensuring the rights of the client and trying to serve his best interests. In individual cases an attorney may be able to assist the staff. Often a patient will not trust the staff but will trust his attorney. If the staff explains the patient's needs to the attorney, the attorney may be in a better position to reason with the patient to accomplish the treatment goals which the staff has established. Thus, the mental health professional should try to make any contact with a patient's attorney into a constructive encounter so that it can benefit the patient as well as the facility staff.

Many mental health professionals nevertheless maintain that their experiences with patient representatives, patient attorneys, or guardianship and advocacy agency staff members are primarily antitherapeutic to the patient. Staff point to the clinical naïveté of these often young and inexperienced attorneys, and to the latter's pursuit of the patient's rights at the expense of the patient's clinical needs. Conflicts over a patient's right to refuse medical and psychiatric treatment is a common and typically heated area of disagreement between treating staff and patient attorneys. Yet, for various clinical reasons, not only are patients sometimes able to foster such conflicts by a psychological maneuver known as *splitting*, but such conflicts serve to distract both treatment staff and attorney from the clinical needs of the patient. As much as possible, both treatment staff and counsel need to minimize the antitherapeutic effect of such clinical-administrative-legal disputes.

IV. PRESUMPTION OF COMPETENCY

A judicial declaration of incompetency results in serious legal consequences in addition to the stigmatization which is so often attached. The legally incompetent individual is divested of a number of significant civil rights, including the right to vote, marry, contract, hold a driver's license, and be eligible for civil service employment and professional licensure. Freedom to make important personal decisions, such as choice of residence and refusal or acceptance of medical treatment, is often denied to the legally incompetent individual, and he may be deprived of the ability to manage financial assets. The withdrawal of these rights is based on the notion that a legally incompetent person is unable to make rational decisions as to his personal needs or financial assets (see Chapter 9, "Competency and Guardianship").

Today, involuntary hospitalization rarely results in a judicial declaration of incompetency either formally or effectively. Most states specifically provide that there is no presumption of incompetency attached to involuntary hospitalization and that incompetency must be determined in a separate hearing. A typical provision is the one set forth in *Wyatt v. Stickney:* "No person shall be deemed incompetent to manage his affairs, to contract, to hold professional or occupational or vehicle operator's licenses, to marry and obtain a divorce, to register and vote, or to make a will solely by reason of his admission or commitment to the hospital."

Notwithstanding this liberalization, some states continue to attach various restrictions to the involuntarily hospitalized patient who, at least for certain purposes, is deemed incompetent to make decisions. Usually these are restrictions on the patient's freedom to refuse medical or psychiatric treatment (see Chapter 5) and to manage his funds while hospitalized. Thus, a few state laws (for example, in Utah) provide that although the person is not considered legally incompetent, he may nevertheless be found incompetent in treatment matters, so that, for example, he does not have a right to refuse psychotropic medication.

It may seem somewhat absurd to the mental health professional to speak of preserving the freedom of the severely retarded or mentally ill to enter into contracts or to vote or hold a driver's license. This may appear to emphasize form over substance. Yet the point of not automatically declaring someone incompetent in these respects is to ensure that the person will have the right to exercise as many personal decisions as possible. This right, of course, may carry significant clinical meaning to the disabled person and assist in the treatment of the individual. In those instances where the person appears functionally incompetent to make decisions in areas of concern to his present treatment, he should be declared legally incompetent, with all the procedural protections which accompany such a declaration. This may occur, for instance, with regard to certain specialized forms of treatment such as electroconvulsive therapy, surgical procedures, unusual medications, hazardous assessment procedures, or where specific consent is required as a matter of law. (See Chapter 9 for a further explanation.)

V. HUMANE CARE AND TREATMENT

That a mentally disabled person is entitled to humane care and treatment while institutionalized seems to be so obvious as to be unworthy of comment. In fact, however, the history of the treatment of mentally disabled persons in the United States is that numerous institutions have failed to meet even minimally acceptable standards of decency. Descriptions of the depersonalization of prolonged institutional life and severe deficiencies in the conditions of confinement have generated an awareness of the possibility of harmful psychological and physical effects from long-term placement in state facilities. In response, a number of state legislatures and courts have mandated minimal standards of custody and treatment by statute or decree. *Wyatt v. Stickney* provided the model to be followed: "A patient has a right to a humane psychological and physical environment within the hospital facilities. These facilities shall be designed to afford patients with comfort and safety, promote dignity, and ensure privacy. The facilities shall be designed to make a positive contribution to the efficient attainment of the treatment goals of the hospital." This right encompasses all aspects of the institution, from the quality of the physical plant to the hands-on care provided to the disabled person.

Approximately 70% of state legislatures have enacted provisions for affording care in a safe, secure, and humane environment. Among the factors to be considered in providing an environment which ensures patient safety, comfort, dignity, and privacy are the following: hospital census and available space per patient; comfortable bed with linen and closet space; adequate number and function of toilets and shower facilities; adequately furnished dayroom and dining facilities of reasonable size; regular housekeeping and maintenance procedures; special facilities for physically handicapped individuals; adequate heating, ventilation, water, and refuse collection; and a satisfying and nutritionally adequate diet. Adequate staffing of treatment facilities for the mentally disabled is accomplished through the availability of minimum numbers of all categories of treatment personnel for each patient, as well as certification and licensing, when applicable, of treatment personnel.

Another aspect of providing humane care has been to require that individualized treatment plans be developed for each patient. This is now mandated in some states. The goal of such plans is to ensure that the staff will establish goals which will lead to the patient's discharge from the facility and will regularly review the individual's progress in meeting the treatment objectives. In the past, all patients on a unit may have been treated the same, with little recognition of their individual treatment needs. Today, the mental health professional is expected to develop a written, individualized treatment plan that is based on an assessment of the patient's clinical needs.

The patient's initial treatment plan is typically formulated within the first three days of hospitalization and is based upon an assessment of the patient's presenting problems, physical health, emotional status, and behavior. When the patient's hospital stay exceeds a week or ten days, a master treatment plan is formulated by a multidisciplinary team which considers a comprehensive assessment of the patient's needs. When appropriate, the patient and his family should participate in the development of the treatment plan. The treatment plan must consider the patient's clinical needs, specify the services required to meet those needs, and identify necessary referrals for services which are not directly provided by the facility. The master treatment plan must also contain specific goals for the patient to achieve and sustain emotional and physical health, growth, and adaptation. The written plan will also describe the treatment services and programs planned for the patient, the frequency of the planned services, and the specific personnel expected to work with the patient. Last, the treatment plan will articulate the specific criteria to be met for termination of treatment and discharge of the patient.

Whether the current statutory guarantees of humane care and treatment, with their emphasis on respect for the patient's privacy and dignity, have had any impact on the reality of institutional life is debatable. On balance, such statements serve as expressions of society's concern. They also provide benchmarks for facility administrators and judges in cases challenging substandard institutional care.

VI. LEAST RESTRICTIVE ALTERNATIVE

The doctrine of the least restrictive alternative was first applied in the mental health area to challenge the practice of institutionalizing mentally disabled individuals. It was argued that when a mentally disabled person is involuntarily institutionalized, he has a right to be treated in an environment which is the least restrictive of his liberty necessary to accomplish the treatment/habilitation goals. This concept, which has been widely accepted by both the courts and the state legislatures, often to the dismay of mental health professionals, has many applications in the area of mental health law. Initially the least-restrictive-alternative concept was inseparably linked to the right to treatment or habilitation and was used to challenge the fact of institutionalization. It has subsequently been expanded to form the basis for a challenge to the type of institution in which treatment is provided, and to the limits placed on the liberties of the institutionalized patients. It has also been relied upon as a legal justification for the asserted right to refuse certain treatments and has served as the basis for demanding alternative placements in the community for the developmentally disabled and the mentally ill.

In 1966, in *Lake v. Cameron*, a court for the first time discussed the least-restrictive-alternative concept in the context of the mentally ill. The court specifically held that before someone could be hospitalized, alternatives had to be explored. In *Covington v. Harris*, the Court of Appeals for the District of Columbia, the same court which had rendered the decision in *Lake v. Cameron*, concluded in 1969 that:

> The principle of the least restrictive alternative is equally applicable to alternate dispositions within a mental hospital. It makes little sense to guard zealously against the possibility of unwarranted deprivations prior to hospitalization, only to abandon the watch once the patient disappears behind hospital doors. The range of possible dispositions of a mentally ill person within a hospital from maximum security to outpatient status is almost as wide as that of dispositions without.

Covington thus provided the foundation not only for challenging the particular unit where the patient is placed—from a secure one to one with an open door policy—but also for questioning the privileges the patient has while hospitalized, such as grounds passes and home visits.

As in other areas of patients' rights, *Wyatt v. Stickney* set the example that would be followed by many state legislatures as well as by other courts which have heard cases dealing with the rights of the mentally disabled. Regarding the aspect of this case which related to the developmentally disabled, the court held:

> Residents shall have a right to the least restrictive conditions necessary to achieve the purposes of habilitation. To this end the institution shall make every attempt to move residents from (1) more to less structured living; (2) larger to smaller facilities; (3) larger to smaller living units; (4) group to individual residences: (5) segregated from the community to integrated into the community living; (6) dependent to independent living.

Expanding on the arguments made in *Wyatt*, advocates for the mentally disabled have sought to use the right to treatment/ habilitation in the least restrictive setting to develop community-based treatment/habilitation facilities.

With the revision of many state mental health codes during the 1970s, the concept of the least restrictive alternative has come to be embodied in the statutory prescriptions of most states. The *Wyatt* concept of humane care and treatment pursuant to an individualized treatment plan in the least restrictive setting served as the foundation for these statutory changes.

Although most citizens agree that one's liberty should not be curtailed more than necessary to accomplish treatment goals, there is likely to be disagreement as to what this means in practice. There are legitimate grounds for asking whether the least-restrictive-alternative concept requires better definition so that the restrictiveness of a given treatment setting or intervention can be more accurately measured. Many mental health professionals believe that a "linear" or continuum concept of restrictiveness does not apply to mental health treatment and that the law must come to acknowledge that more treatment is not necessarily accompanied by greater limitation of individual freedom. That is, there is no clear parallel between those forms of treatment which are more (or less) restrictive and those which are more (or less) therapeutic; restrictiveness and therapeutic efficacy or potency are distinctly different dimensions, which, at times, conflict with each other. Doubts have been raised about the validity of the assumption that being treated outside an institution is necessarily a less restrictive form of treatment. Is it more restrictive to be hospitalized in a minimum security unit of a state hospital with grounds privileges and weekend passes, or to be confined in a nursing home without grounds privileges or an opportunity to go for a walk outdoors?

For the treating professional, the concept of the least restrictive or least intrusive alternative affects daily practice in virtually every phase of the treatment process from admission to discharge. Decisions must be made about whether a person requires inpatient or outpatient treatment, which unit a person should be hospitalized on, what form of treatment should be selected in a variety of emergency and nonemergency situations (e.g., forced medication versus seclusion versus physical restraints versus behavior therapy), and which privileges should be restricted or offered on the unit.

The tension generated by the concept of the least restrictive alternative is likely to continue as litigation about mental health treatment proliferates and as state mental health departments seek to juggle shrinking budgets, political pressures, court decrees, and statutory prescriptions for the expansion of alternative placements. Although the principle of the least restrictive setting is now well accepted by both the courts and the states, it is far from self-evident which form of treatment is less restrictive. Deinstitutionalization, or a patient's ability to refuse psychotropic medications while hospitalized, for example, has not clearly resulted in more freedom or a better quality of life for the mentally disabled. Hopefully, the least-restrictive-alternative concept will provide the states with the impetus to develop meaningful alternatives which provide quality care and treatment in settings that maximize the disabled person's opportunity for liberty.

VII. PERIODIC REVIEW

Although an individual's initial confinement in a mental health facility may be justified by a variety of reasons, change in circumstances during the course of hospitalization may render further confinement invalid or even unconstitutional. Periodic review of the patient's mental condition by a multidisciplinary treatment team serves to determine whether the basis for hospitalization continues to exist, thereby ensuring that the patient's deprivation of freedom will last no longer than necessary to serve the state's interest in safety, care, and treatment.

Periodic review not only helps determine whether the patient continues to meet the standards for involuntary hospitalization but also serves to determine whether the disabled person should be treated in a less restrictive setting. It may also alert the staff to the need for a change in the patient's treatment plan or for transfer to a different facility that can better meet the treatment or habilitation needs of the patient. Requiring the staff to periodically examine why the person was institutionalized, whether he continues to need institutionalization, and what is being done for him helps to protect the disabled person from being subjected to inadequate or inappropriate treatment.

The majority of states have statutes which pertain to the periodic examination of patients; many of these statutes specify the frequency of examinations. The frequency of the review varies from every 30 days to once a year. Some states have established separate review timetables for the mentally ill and the developmentally disabled, the latter group being reviewed less frequently. This is sensible because of the relative stability of their disability and the fact that their progress in habilitation is usually much slower than that of the mentally ill patient, who often can be stabilized relatively quickly. Although most statutes do not distinguish between the periodic review of treatment plans for children and for adults, some mental health professionals assert that treatment plans for children should be reviewed more frequently to ensure that children will be hospitalized for the shortest period of time necessary to accomplish treatment goals.

Although numerous states do not provide for periodic review, fiscal considerations in administering an institution have generally led the states to be vigilant in ensuring that persons will not be unnecessarily hospitalized or treated. Although periodic review was conceived to apply to the patient receiving involuntary treatment, a number of states also require the same type of review for the voluntary patient. In private treatment facilities, hospital insurance coverage is often the most critical factor in requiring periodic review of the patient's status. Concern that the patient's care will not be covered by insurance is most likely to lead to hospitalizations that mirror the number of insured days. In addition, periodic review is mandated by the Joint Commission on Accreditation of Healthcare Organizations (JCAHO) as well as by hospital utilization review committees.

Comprehensive or master treatment plans are reviewed and updated as frequently as is clinically indicated. The nature and locus of the treatment facility will generally dictate the necessary frequency of treatment plan review and update. Treatment plan updates should be completed with the participation and consent of the patient. Some facilities require that each patient sign the written treatment plan update and receive a personal copy of it.

VIII. PATIENT EMPLOYMENT

Use of patient workers within facilities for the mentally ill and mentally retarded was an accepted practice until the 1970s. Institutionalized mentally disabled persons in large state mental facilities commonly provided a variety of services, including such activities as housekeeping, grounds maintenance, laundry, cooking, and farming. Typically the resident workers were engaged in work of minimal therapeutic value. They received little or no compensation, a practice justified on the theory that work was part of the treatment program and did not constitute employment deserving of compensation. In fact, the work often seemed to be the only available programmatic activity and often served as an excuse for not developing better treatment/habilitation approaches. Access to grounds privileges or release from the institution might be denied if the disabled person refused to perform his scheduled tasks. In some cases the institution was reluctant to release those who had become so proficient in their tasks that they were viewed as too valuable to the facility.

This situation led to challenges of *institutional peonage*, as the practice was then known. The courts, basing their decisions on a number of legal theories, concluded that uncompensated patient work is permissible in only limited circumstances. The initial court decisions barring the use of patient workers were viewed as a victory for the mentally disabled. However, the end result was that many states completely banned the use of patient workers rather than bear the cost. For many disabled people who were institutionalized for long periods, this ban eliminated work as a productive activity or therapy, with the loss of the beneficial effects of developing a sense of accomplishment and pride, increased self-esteem, relief from boredom, learning important work skills transferrable to other settings, and developing discipline.

Today approximately half the states have laws guaranteeing institutionalized mentally disabled individuals compensation for their work. Some states have specific provisions for developing patient worker programs in which the patient is paid according to the work produced, often less than the minimum wage. Compensation for work is most commonly used in workshop programs for the developmentally disabled but is also used for the mentally ill. In addition, patients can perform tasks that teach necessary skills, such as how to manage one's affairs outside the institution, without monetary compensation. The patient can also be required to perform personal housekeeping duties without compensation. For example, a patient can be required to make his bed, wash his clothes, or set his place in the dining hall. He cannot, however, be expected to make all the beds on the unit, wash all the clothes, or set the table for everyone. The patient's work responsibilities should be part of the individual treatment plan. The work should comply with relevant federal, state, and local laws and regulations about occupational conditions. It is important for mental health professionals to reexamine the use of patient workers. There are some important therapeutic and programming benefits to having patients work. This can be accomplished within the requirements of the law and without returning to the abusive system that existed in the past.

IX. RIGHT TO MANAGE FUNDS

Earlier presumptions that the mentally disabled were universally unable to manage their funds led many states to enact provisions clarifying that entry into a mental hospital does not diminish the disabled person's right to manage his funds unless he is declared legally incompetent to do so. The provisions which emphasize that the disabled person retains his right to enter into contracts are usually contained in the patient's rights section of the state mental health code. In addition, a number of states also have laws which govern the use of the person's funds while institutionalized. Typically, these statutes provide that the individual may spend "reasonable amounts" or may have "small sums" for use in buying food, toiletries, and other items sold at the institution's commissary. By regulation or statute, most states now have a formal means of accounting for funds whereby the disabled person deposits his funds in a personal account and receives periodic statements. This accounting provides both access to the funds by the patient and prevents loss or theft, a primary concern of the institution if the patient is permitted to carry large amounts of cash in the facility. Some facilities also permit a patient to open a savings account at a local financial institution in order to learn to manage his financial affairs.

Most patients who are mentally ill will not have been adjudicated incompetent and indeed are capable, at least to some extent, of managing their assets. But on relatively infrequent occasions a mentally ill person is legally declared incompetent to handle his financial affairs (see Chapter 9, "Incompetency and Guardianship"). This may occur when the person is in a severe acute psychotic episode or is severely and chronically ill and there is little likelihood of a response to treatment so that the person will be capable of managing his funds in the foreseeable future. The institutionalized mentally retarded person is even more likely than the hospitalized mentally ill person to be unable to appropriately manage his funds.

For many such patients, the family will manage any available funds until the person is discharged from the facility. In cases of persons who are severely and chronically mentally ill or profoundly retarded, and who receive benefits such as social security disability, Supplemental Security Income, or veteran's benefits, a representative payee can be appointed to manage the funds.

A. Representative Payee

A representative payee is appointed by the Social Security Administration or the Veterans Administration for the purposes of managing a beneficiary's benefits when it is determined that the beneficiary cannot act on his own behalf. Benefit payments can be made to a representative payee on behalf of a beneficiary when it appears that this method of payment is in the best interest of the beneficiary. This can occur when the beneficiary is under age 18 (except when the person is a parent and has experience in handling his own finances), legally incompetent, mentally or physically incapable of managing or directing the management of benefit payments, or medically determined to be a "drug addict or alcoholic." The representative payee concept has the advantage of avoiding the costly process of a legal declaration of incompetency and is particularly appropriate when the only assets to be managed are the benefit checks. Although this section will describe only the procedures of the Social Security Administration, similar procedures are followed by the Veterans Administration.

The appointment of a representative payee can be based on a variety of evidence. A representative payee can be appointed whether or not the disabled person has been declared legally incompetent to manage his financial affairs. A court's determination that a beneficiary is incompetent to manage his financial affairs will serve as the basis for a determination to make representative payment. Medical evidence, in the form of a written statement by a physician or other medical professional, can also be used as the basis for determining whether representative payment should occur. This can be reported on a form provided by the Social Security Administration, or by a report that, based upon a medical examination within the preceding year, the beneficiary is suffering from a mental or physical impairment, and the beneficiary's chances for recovery from the illness are such that he will remain unable to manage or direct the management of benefit payments. Statements from relatives, friends, or associates of the beneficiary will also be considered in determining whether a payee should be appointed.

Several factors are considered in the selection of potential representative payees. These include the relationship of the potential payee to the beneficiary, the degree of interest that the person shows in the beneficiary, any legal authority that the person or agency has to act on behalf of the beneficiary, whether the person has custody of the beneficiary, and whether the potential payee is in a position to look after the needs of the beneficiary. The order of preference in selecting a payee by the Social Security Administration is (1) a legal guardian, spouse, or other relative who has custody of the beneficiary, or who demonstrates a strong concern for the welfare of the beneficiary; (2) a friend who has custody of the beneficiary or demonstrates a strong concern for the beneficiary's personal welfare; (3) a public or nonprofit agency or institution which has custody of the beneficiary; (4) a licensed private institution which has custody of the beneficiary; and (5) any other person who is qualified, willing, and able to serve as a payee for the beneficiary. A person or agency who requests to be appointed the representative payee for a beneficiary must ordinarily provide information showing the relationship of the potential payee to the beneficiary, the person's concern and responsibility for the care of the beneficiary, and the availability of other potential payees.

As a result of litigation surrounding the appointment of a representative payee and the use of funds, particularly when an institutional representative has been made payee, the disabled person retains several rights with regard to representative payment. The beneficiary must receive advance notice that a determination is to be made to appoint a representative payee. The notice requests that the beneficiary notify the Social Security Administration if he objects to this form of payment or the proposed payee, and it provides the disabled person an opportunity to submit materials in his own behalf, including stating his preference for the payee. Once a determination has been made, he has a right to review the materials upon which the decision to appoint the payee is based, and to request a reconsideration.

The appointment of a representative payee often becomes a disputed matter. In the case of a person who is chronically institutionalized, the facility often prefers to be the representative payee so that the funds paid to the disabled person can be used to offset the cost of his care. Relatives of the disabled person, on the other hand, may want an opportunity to have access to the funds. Unfortunately, it is not unusual to find relatives competing to be appointed representative payee, though in the guise of acting in the best interests of the disabled person.

Once it has been determined that representative payment will occur and the payee has been selected, then the payee is directed to apply the beneficiary's payments for the beneficiary's use and benefit. Benefits are properly dispersed if they are spent for the beneficiary's current and foreseeable needs, are accumulated for specific and foreseeable purposes advantageous to the beneficiary, or are saved and invested for the beneficiary, if current needs are being met. The current needs of the beneficiary include the immediate and reasonably foreseeable essentials for living, such as shelter, food, clothing, utilities, medical care, dental care, personal hygiene, education, and rehabilitation. If the benefits are not needed for the beneficiary's current maintenance or foreseeable needs, they should be invested in insured financial instruments.

The representative payee must also maintain a continuing awareness of the beneficiary's needs and condition, notify the benefit payment source of any change in circumstances that affects the performance of his responsibilities as payee, and report any event that will alter the amount of benefit payment to the beneficiary. Written reports which account for the use of the benefit payments may also be necessary. The payee, rather than the benefit source, is responsible for any misuse of the benefits.

A treatment provider for the chronically disabled should be concerned that when a representative payee is appointed, the payee provides for the needs of the disabled person rather than misuses the funds. If misuse occurs, the agency providing the funds should be notified. It should also be borne in mind that all states require payment for the costs of the care they render, and it is appropriate for the institution to be appointed payee to use benefit funds to offset the money owed by the disabled person for his care. Generally, however, there are provisions that a certain amount of the funds paid to an institutional representative payee can be used for the disabled person for personal items of his choice. Thus, it is common for the institution to provide the disabled person a small monetary sum each month for personal spending at the facility's commissary.

X. RIGHT TO REFUSE TO PARTICIPATE IN RESEARCH

Few people question the value of human research to our society. Clearly, the only way to find help for the ills of humanity is to investigate the cause of illness and evaluate potential interventions, whether prevention or treatment. Yet, society must determine the circumstances under which the mentally disabled can serve as research subjects in this search for knowledge.

Until the early 1970s, it was accepted practice to use institutionalized populations—the mentally disabled, prisoners, and nursing home residents—as research subjects. These groups presented unique research opportunities because of the researcher's ability to carefully control and monitor the subject and his environment, and to identify subjects who willingly or unwillingly could participate in studies. These research projects, which ranged from the nonintrusive to the substantially intrusive, included a wide variety of studies aimed at obtaining information on medical and psychological problems. Few investigators questioned the propriety of including the mentally disabled in these studies.

By the early 1970s, public attention had been focused on certain research projects that were difficult to categorize as anything but abusive. It was disclosed, for example, that some retarded residents at Willowbrook State Hospital in New York had been deliberately infected with viral hepatitis and that many of them then contracted this illness. There were other revelations about inappropriate research on institutionalized individuals, and these generated concern about the use of the unconsenting mentally disabled for any research purpose. In 1974, Congress created the National Commission for the Protection of Human Subjects of Biomedical and Behavior Research to address the issues raised by human subjects research. The creation of this commission, which published the Belmont Report in 1979, along with other indications of heightened concern, later resulted in a body of restrictions regarding when an individual can be the subject of a research protocol, as well as measures to protect the person who participates in research.

In human subjects research, it is the subject alone who is at risk, while the benefits accrue to others, but only sometimes to the subject. When is it appropriate to use mentally disabled persons as research subjects? Clearly, if the research poses a low risk to the disabled person, with a high likelihood of direct benefit to him, then the research can well be justified, assuming a valid informed consent can be obtained. Controversy about the appropriateness of the mentally disabled as research subjects is particularly acute when there is no prospect of direct benefit to mentally disabled subjects and there is more than minimal risk of harm to them. The belief that each of us owes society a duty to bear minor risks for the benefit of the general welfare has been the justification for using institutionalized mentally disabled persons for research that does not directly benefit them or does not seek a cure for their illnesses. An easier case can be made for research on the causes and treatment of mental disturbance, as such research can be done only on those who in fact suffer from such disturbances.

The major underlying reservation regarding the participation of the mentally disabled in human research, whether or not it potentially offers direct benefit, is the adequacy of the informed consent process. Questions have been raised about the functional capacity or competency of the mentally disabled to consent to research procedures. These relate to the lack of consensus about the requisite threshold of decision-making capacity, and to the unreliability and lack of a standard of competency determinations by mental health researchers. Another concern, raised in a 1973 Michigan case, *Kaimowitz v. Department of Mental Health*, which considered the use of experimental psychosurgery for intractable sexual aggression, is the uncertain voluntariness of the institutionalized mentally disabled person's decision making about research participation. Questions have been raised about whether consent for research by any institutionalized individual can be genuinely voluntary and, in the case of the prison inmate, have virtually halted human research in that population. Doubt about the voluntariness of consent to research is of particular concern when the duration of institutionalization is lengthy or indeterminate.

In 1981, the United States Department of Health and Human Services published regulations regarding the conduct of research with all human subjects, though not specifically with the mentally disabled. According to these regulations, researchers conducting studies with human subjects must disclose the following to prospective subjects to obtain research consent: (1) a statement that the study involves research, including a description of the research procedures; (2) a description of any reasonably foreseeable risks; (3) a description of any benefits to the subject or others which may be expected from the research; (4) a description of the available alternative procedures; (5) a description of the extent of confidentiality available to the research subject; (6) an explanation of whether any compensation is available if injury occurs; (7) a notice about whom the subject can contact for answers to questions about the research; and (8) a statement that participation is voluntary and that refusal to participate will not deprive the subject of benefits to which he is otherwise entitled.

The regulations also assign the responsibility to approve and monitor the research consent process to the facility's institutional review board (IRB). A variety of safeguards are available to the IRB to protect vulnerable subjects (e.g., those with acute or severe physical or mental illness), including consent auditors, preconsent testing of consent forms, testing of subjects' comprehension of the research disclosures, and mandatory waiting periods after disclosures prior to the subject's written consent.

The 1981 regulations also exempt from research review certain research activities which entail minimum risk to human subjects. These include the use of educational tests or of survey and interview procedures. The regulations do not, however, provide guidance about how to assess subject competency to consent to research.

At a minimum, facilities for the mentally disabled which permit human subjects research should have written policies and procedures that protect the rights of patients involved in research projects. The written informed consent of the patient who will participate in the project usually must be obtained and a copy of the consent document included as part of the patient's record when possible. The patient has a right to withdraw from the research project at any time without prejudice to his continuing care and treatment. When necessary, and in most cases dealing with a minor or a legally incompetent adult, written informed consent should be obtained from the family or legal guardian and a copy included as part of the patient's record. The regulations provide some exceptions in the case of minors, which are detailed in Chapter 10. Ideally, the substitute decision maker should consider the prior expressed values and wishes of the incompetent adult in deciding whether to consent to research. That is, the surrogate should not consent to the subject's research participation when it is known that the subject would not have done so had he been able to decide for himself. The family member or guardian also has a right to withdraw consent to the research at any time.

XI. PERSONAL POSSESSIONS

With the trend toward making the psychiatric facility a more humane environment, many states have mandated that the mentally disabled persons be permitted to retain their possessions while institutionalized. At least half the states have enacted such provisions. Usually these statutes provide for the right of the disabled person to wear his own clothes, although they sometimes mention the right to possess toilet articles. A growing number of states provide that the disabled person shall be given storage space for private use. These statutes grow out of a recognition that it is important for the disabled person to have possession of, and control over, personal belongings while institutionalized and to feel he has some choice over what occurs in his life, even if it only involves what he will wear each day. Although there may be statutory provisions guaranteeing the patient the right to certain possessions, there are also limits to this right. The facility staff has a right to determine that certain items cannot be brought on the unit, for fear that they may either harm a patient or staff or be damaged or stolen. In the first group are items such as belts, razors, scissors, knives, lighters, matches, or other potential weapons. The second group includes expensive personal items such as televisions, radios, jewelry, or large amounts of money. The presence of either group of possessions on a facility unit may also be disruptive to the functioning of the unit and could be prohibited for this reason as well.

Upon admission the facility staff conduct a search of the patient and carefully search the personal possessions he brought with him, including the pockets of his clothing, the suitcase, and anything else which might serve to conceal medications or weapons. The facility staff also has the right to conduct searches of a patient's locker, closet, or possessions in order to serve the legitimate hospital goals of protecting patients and staff at the facility. Searches for contraband, unhealthy substances, or rotting food are proper and necessary when there is reasonable causes to believe that such items are present and could create a dangerous or unhealthy situation within the hospital. Patients should be notified of such searches or inspections, which can be conducted in the presence of the patient.

XII. RELIGIOUS FREEDOM

The freedom to practice one's religion or to refrain from religious practice is embodied in the First Amendment. Nonetheless, some states have felt the need to specifically protect this right by statute. Approximately half the states have such provisions on this topic. In addition, at least 15 states guarantee the disabled unrestricted visitation by the clergy. These statutory guarantees are particularly important for those hospitalized in private psychiatric facilities since First Amendment strictures apply only to governmental entities.

Some mentally disabled individuals refuse psychiatric treatment on the basis of their religious beliefs and practices. This refusal often presents both a challenge and a dilemma to facility staff, who are uncertain whether the refusal of treatment is a competent one or, rather, is based upon the mental disorder. A variety of factors must be considered in making this determination (see Chapters 5 and 9).

XIII. VOTING RIGHTS

Although most citizens take for granted the right to vote in local or national elections, this opportunity is often denied the institutionalized mentally disabled. The right to vote is important to the disabled person in keeping him in contact with those outside the institution and enhancing normalization. In the past the mentally disabled were usually regarded as unqualified to vote, simply by virtue of their being institutionalized, but this is no longer true. Civil commitment, which in the past typically carried with it automatic loss of the right to vote, today no longer suffices to disqualify the disabled from voting, unless the person is specifically declared incompetent to do so. Many states have enacted statutes expressly providing that an order for involuntary hospitalization does not mean the person is legally incompetent and that the patient retains all his rights, including the right to vote.

Although the right to vote is now guaranteed in many states, it means nothing if the mentally disabled person is not provided the opportunity to vote. This can be done either by taking him to his polling place on election day or by securing an absentee ballot for him. The latter approach should obviate staff concerns that a highly disorganized or disturbed individual would be disruptive to a polling place or submit an inappropriate vote. Although many hospitalized patients have no ability or desire to keep up with election issues, for others this is important and helps them feel they are participating in the world outside the facility.

XIV. COMMONLY ASKED QUESTIONS

1. *Does the facility staff have the right to search a patient's incoming mail?*

Yes. When the staff has reasonable cause to believe that the mail contains contraband, it can be searched. In some states, correspondence from attorneys and government officials cannot be opened. If mail is searched, it is advisable to do so in the patient's presence.

2. *Does the facility staff have the right to censor a patient's outgoing mail?*

Usually not. The receiver can notify the postal service not to deliver unwanted mail. Although there may clearly be detrimental consequences for patients to send threatening correspondence to government authorities, it is their right to do so, unless it constitutes a criminal offense. Staff can deal with this issue in a therapeutic manner and can also try to persuade patients not to send such mail.

3. *How should restrictions be placed upon a patient's access to the telephone or visitation?*

Facility staff should record a note in the patient's record of the extent and reason for the restrictions. In addition, those who are denied access to the patient should be informed of the restrictions and the reasons for them. It should be made clear that the patient is not being held incommunicado, and that the restrictions are in the therapeutic interests of the patient.

4. *What does the least-restrictive-alternative doctrine mandate with regard to where a patient can be hospitalized?*

Under the least-restrictive-alternative concept, a patient should be placed in the situation which least restricts his liberty, given his treatment needs. This determination requires periodic evaluation of the patient, depending upon his clinical state. A patient may need to be placed on a secure unit when he enters the hospital but may progress to off-grounds passes during the course of the hospital stay. The least-restrictive-alternative doctrine does not require an institution to create new units for the needs of specific patients. The facility staff must do the best it can with the available resources.

5. *After a committed patient's progress has been periodically reviewed by the treatment staff, must he be released if he no longer meets the civil commitment criteria?*

Some commitment laws require that a patient be discharged whenever he no longer meets commitment criteria and refuses to remain voluntarily in the hospital. Otherwise, committed patients, at the option of the treatment staff, may be retained in the hospital until the expiration of the commitment order even when they have been clinically stabilized and no longer meet commitment criteria. Particular clinical needs of the patient, the doctrine of the least restrictive alternative, and hospital utilization review procedures may argue for outpatient treatment as the patient clinically progresses.

6. *When should a representative payee be appointed?*

A representative payee should be appointed when a person receives a check from a government agency and is unable to properly manage the funds, regardless of medical or psychiatric diagnosis. When substantial assets must be managed, it is likely that the disabled person will be declared legally incompetent, and the legally appointed guardian will also serve as the representative payee.

7. How can someone request the appointment of a representative payee?

Contact the local office of the Social Security Administration or the Veterans Administration, depending on the source of the funds, for the proper applications. If an allegedly disabled person receives funds from both agencies, then applications must be completed for both.

8. When is a patient considered incompetent to consent to a research protocol?

There are no uniformly accepted criteria for a person to be either competent or incompetent to consent to medical and psychiatric research procedures. A prospective research subject should, nevertheless, understand the nature, risks, benefits, and alternatives of the research procedures in his particular case. He should also be able to decide whether to participate in the project without undue outside influence and should be able to articulate his decision and the reasons for participation with clarity and rationality.

9. Can a patient be compelled to work while hospitalized?

Yes. The patient can be required to perform tasks in the hospital which provide the skills necessary to live outside an institution. These include making his bed, cleaning his room, setting his place at the dining room table, or washing his clothes. The therapeutic need for such activities would be recorded in the patient's chart on the treatment plan. The chores cannot, however, consist of performing these tasks for the entire hospital unit. In addition, if available, a patient can participate in a workshop program but must be compensated for his work.

10. Is the patient entitled to be informed of his rights?

In the vast majority of states, and under the requirements of JCAHO, each patient is entitled to be informed of his rights while hospitalized. This is usually accomplished by having a staff member read the patient his rights upon admission, providing a written copy of his rights to the patient upon admission, and posting a copy of patient rights on each unit.

APPENDIX: PATIENTS' RIGHTS

This table refers to the rights of mentally disabled persons provided by each state. The citation will direct the reader to its location in each state statute.

State and citation	Patients' rights section
Alabama ALA. Code (1984 and Supp.1988)	None
Alaska ALAS. Stat. (1984 and Supp.1989)	47.30.825

(*continued*)

State and citation	Patients' rights section
Arizona ARIZ. Rev. Stat. Ann. (1992)	36-504 et seq.
Arkansas ARK. Code Ann. (1987 and Supp.1989)	20-47-211 20-47-220
California CAL. Welf. and Inst. Code (West 1984 and Supp.1992)	5325
Colorado COLO. Rev. Stat. (1989 and Supp.1992)	27-10-117 27-10.5-101
Connecticut CONN. Gen. Stat. Ann. (1992)	319; 17a-540 to 550
Delaware DEL. Code Ann. (1991)	16 Sec. 5161
District of Columbia D.C. Code Ann. (1992)	21-561 et seq.
Florida FLA. Stat. Ann. (1992)	394.459
Georgia GA. Code Ann. (1992)	37-3-140 et seq.
Hawaii HAWAII Rev. Stat. (1992)	334 E-2
Idaho IDAHO Code (1992)	66-346
Illinois IL Comp. Stat. (1993)	405 sec 512-100 et seq.
Indiana IND. Code Ann. (Burns 1990 and Supp. 1992)	12-27-2-1 et seq.
Iowa IOWA Code Ann. (1991)	229.23
Kansas KAN. Stat. Ann. (1991)	59-2929
Kentucky KY. Rev. Stat. (1992)	202 A.191

(continued)

State and citation	Patients' rights section
Louisiana LA. Rev. Stat. Ann. (West 1989 and Supp. 1991)	28:171
Maine ME. Rev. Stat. Ann. (1991)	34-B Sec. 3803
Maryland MD. Ann. Code (Michie 1990 and Supp.1992)	10-701
Massachusetts MASS. Gen. Laws Ann. (1992)	111 Sec. 70 E
Michigan MICH. Comp. Laws. Ann. (1991)	330.1700 et seq.
Minnesota MINN. Stat. Ann. (1992)	253 B.03
Mississippi MISS. Code Ann. (1991)	41-21-102
Missouri MO. Ann. Stat. (1991)	630.110
Montana MONT. Code Ann. (1992)	53-21-141
Nebraska NEB. Rev. Stat. (1990)	83-106
Nevada NEV. Rev. Stat. (1991)	433.482 et seq.
New Hampshire N.H. Rev. Stat. Ann. (1990 and Supp.1992)	171-A:14 135-C:57 et seq.
New Jersey N.J. Stat. Ann. (1992)	30:4-24.2
New Mexico N.M. Stat. Ann. (1978 and Supp.1987)	43-1-6
New York N.Y. Mental Hyg. Law (1992)	33.01 et seq.

(*continued*)

State and citation	Patients' rights section
North Carolina N.C. Gen. Stat. (1991)	122C-51 et seq.
North Dakota N.D. Cent. Code (1991)	25-03.1-40
Ohio OHIO Rev. Code Ann. (1991)	5122.29
Oklahoma OKLA. Stat. Ann. (West 1990 and Supp.1992)	43A Sec. 4-107
Oregon OR. Rev. Stat. (1991)	426.385
Pennsylvania PA. Stat. Ann. (1992)	50 Sec. 4423
Rhode Island R.I. Gen. Laws (1991)	40.1-5-5
South Carolina S.C. Code Ann. (1991)	44-23-1030 et seq.
South Dakota S.D. Codified Laws Ann. (1992)	27A-12-1 et seq.
Tennessee TENN. Code Ann. (1992)	33-3-104 et seq.
Texas TEX. Rev. Civ. Stat. Ann. (Vernon 1992)	572.003
Utah UTAH Code Ann. (1992)	62A-12-245
Vermont VT. Stat. Ann. (1991)	18 Sec. 7705
Virginia VA. Code (1990 and Supp.1992)	37.1-84.1 et seq.
Washington WASH. Rev. Code Ann. (1991)	71.05.360

(*continued*)

State and citation	Patients' rights section
West Virginia W.VA. Code (1992)	27-5-9
Wisconsin WISC. Stat. Ann. (1990)	51.61
Wyoming WYO. Stat. (1992)	25-10-120

XV. BIBLIOGRAPHY

I. Rights of the Mentally Disabled

A. Cases

Wyatt v. Stickney, 344 F.Supp. 373 (Ala. 1972).
Wyatt v. Aderholt, 503 F.2d 1305 (5th Cir. 1974).
Davis v. Watkins, 387 F.Supp. 1196 (Ohio 1976).
Davis v. Balson, 461 F.Supp. 842 (Ohio 1978).
Eckerhart v. Hensley, 475 F.Supp. 908 (Mo. 1979).
Sabo v. O'Bannon, 586 F.Supp. 586 (Pa. 1984).
Falter v. Veterans Administration, 632 F.Supp. 196 (N.J. 1986)[access to telephones; staff searches of mail and lockers].
Mental Health Association in California v. Deukmejian, 233 Cal.Rptr. 130 (Cal.App. 1986).
Woe v. Cuomo, 638 F.Supp. 1506 (N.Y. 1986).
Martyr v. Bachik, 770 F.Supp. 1414 (Or. 1991)[mail censorship].
Martyr v. Mazur-Hart, 789 F.Supp. 1081 (Or. 1992) [mail censorship].

B. Articles and Books

American Psychiatric Association. (1988). *Rights of the mentally disabled: Statements and standards.* Washington, DC: American Psychiatric Association.
Dowben, C. (1979). Legal rights of mentally impaired. *Houston Law Review, 16,* 833–901.
Ennis, B. J., & Emery, R. D. (1978). *The rights of mental patients.* New York: Avon.
Ferleger, D. (1988). Civil rights disability practice: Expediting institutional mistreatment litigation. *Mental and Physical Disability Law Reporter, 12,* 309–316.
Freddolino, P. P., Moxley, D. P., & Fleishman, J. A. (1989). An advocacy model for people with long-term psychiatric disabilities. *Hospital and Community Psychiatry, 40,* 1169–1174.
Friedman, P. R. (1981). *The rights of mentally retarded persons.* New York: Avon.
Geller, J. L., Fisher, W. H., Simon, L. J., & Wirth-Cauchon, J. L. (1990). Second-generation deinstitutionalization: 2. The impact of *Brewster v. Dukakis* on correlates of community and hospital utilization. *American Journal of Psychiatry, 147,* 988–993.
Geller, J. L., Fisher, W. H., Wirth-Cauchon, J. L., & Simon, L. J. (1990). Second-generation deinstitutionalization: 1. The impact of *Brewster v. Dukakis* on state hospital case mix. *American Journal of Psychiatry, 147,* 982–987.
Hannah, G. T., Christian, W. P., & Clark, H. W. (Eds.). (1981). *Preservation of client rights.* New York: Free Press.
Herr, S. S. (1983). *Rights and advocacy for retarded people.* Lexington, MA: D. C. Heath.
Herr, S. S. (1987). The future of advocacy for persons with mental disabilities. *Rutgers Law Review, 39,* 443–486.
Jones, L. R., & Parlour, R. R. (Eds.). (1981). *Wyatt v. Stickney retrospect and prospect.* New York: Grune & Stratton.

Krajewski, T. F., & Bell, C. (1992). A system for patients' rights advocacy in state psychiatric inpatient facilities in Maryland. *Hospital and Community Psychiatry, 43,* 127–131.
Leaf, P. (1977). *Wyatt v. Stickney:* Assessing the impact in Alabama. *Hospital and Community Psychiatry, 28,* 351–356.
Okin, R. L. (1984). *Brewster v. Dukakis:* Developing community services through use of a consent decree. *American Journal of Psychiatry, 141,* 786–789.
O'Reilly, J., & Sales, B. (1987). Privacy for the institutionalized mentally ill: Are court-ordered standards effective? *Law and Human Behavior, 11,* 41–53.
Perlin, M. L. (1987). Economic rights of the institutionalized mentally disabled. *International Journal of Law and Psychiatry, 10,* 187–214.
Perlin, M. L. (1989 and Suppl.). *Mental disability law: Civil and criminal.* Charlottesville, VA: Michie.
Schoenfeld, B. N. (1987). A survey of constitutional rights of mentally retarded. *Southwestern Law Journal, 32,* 605–637.
Schwartz, S. J., Fleischner, R. D., Schmidt, M. J., Gates, H. M., Costanzo, C., & Winkelman, N. (1983). Protecting the rights and enhancing the dignity of people with mental disabilities: Standards for effective legal advocacy. *Rutgers Law Journal, 14,* 541–593.
Weiner, B. A. (1985). Rights of institutionalized persons. In S. J. Brakel, J. Parry, & B. A. Weiner (Eds.), *The mentally disabled and the law* (3rd ed.). Chicago: American Bar Foundation.
Ziegenfuss, J. T., & Ziegenfuss, D. G. (1980). Rights of the mentally disabled: A bibliography. *Journal of Psychiatry and Law, 8,* 465–498.
Ziegenfuss, J. T., Charette, J., & Guenin, M. (1984). The patients rights representative program: Design of an ombudsman service for mental patients. *Psychiatric Quarterly, 56,* 3–12.
Zuckerman, M., Abrams, H. A., & Nuehring, E. M. (1986). Protection and advocacy agencies: National survey of efforts to prevent residential abuse and neglect. *Mental Retardation, 24,* 197–201.

II. Patient Funds and Representative Payee

A. Cases

McAuliffe v. Carlson, 386 F.Supp. 1245 (Conn. 1975).
McGrath v. Weinberger, 541 F.2d 249 (10th Cir. 1976).
Tidwell v. Weinberger, Nos. 73-C-3104 and 74-C-183 (N.D. Ill. June 28, 1976), cited in Mental Disability Law Reporter 1:192–193, 1976.
Vecchione v. Wohlgemuth, 558 F.2d 150 (3rd Cir. 1977).

B. Articles

Brotman, A. W., & Muller, J. J. (1990). The therapist as representative payee. *Hospital and Community Psychiatry, 41,* 167–171.
Kanter, J. (1989). Clinical case management: Definition, principles, components. *Hospital and Community Psychiatry, 40,* 361–368.
Kapp, M. B. (1978). Residents of state mental institutions and their money (or the state giveth and the state taketh away). *Journal of Psychiatry and Law, 6,* 287–356.

III. Patient Work

A. Cases

Jobson v. Henne, 355 F.2d 129 (2nd Cir. 1966).
Maryland v. Wirtz, 392 U.S. 183 (1968).
Downs v. Department of Public Welfare, 368 F.Supp. 454 (Pa. 1973).
Sounder v. Brennan, 367 F.Supp. 808 (D.C. 1973).
National League of Cities v. Usery, 426 U.S. 833 (1976).
Bayh v. Sonnenburg, 573 N.E.2d 398 (Ind.Sup.Ct. 1991).

B. Articles

Blaine, J. G., & Mason, J. H. (1986). Application of the fair labor standards act to patient work programs at mental health institutions: A proposal for change. *Boston College Law Review, 27,* 553–557.

Friedman, P. R. (1974). The mentally handicapped citizen and institutional labor. *Harvard Law Review, 87,* 567–587.

LeBar, A. B. (1976). Worker-patients: Receiving therapy of suffering peonage? *American Bar Association Journal, 62,* 219–221.

Note. (1982). From wanderers to workers: A survey of federal and state employment rights of the mentally ill. *Law and Contemporary Problems, 45,* 41–65.

Perlin, M. L. (1976). The right to voluntary compensated therapeutic work as part of the right to treatment: A new theory in the aftermath of sounder. *Seaton Hall Law Review, 7,* 298–339.

Safier, D. (1976). Patient work under fair labor standards: The issue in perspective. *Hospital and Community Psychiatry, 27,* 89–92.

IV. Voting

A. Cases

Boyd v. Board of Registrars of Voters in Belchertown, 334 N.E.2d 629 (Mass. 1975).

Manhattan State Citizens v. Bass, 524 F.Supp. 1270 (N.Y. 1981).

B. Articles

Klein, M., & Grossman, S. (1967). Voting patterns of mental patients in a community state hospital. *Community Mental Health Journal, 3,* 149–152.

Note. (1979). Mental disability and the right to vote. *Yale Law Journal, 88,* 1644–1664.

V. Least Restrictive Alternative

A. Cases

Shelton v. Tucker, 364 U.S. 479 (1960).

Lake v. Cameron, 364 F.2d 657 (D.C. Cir. 1966).

Covington v. Harris, 419 F.2d 617 (D.C. Cir. 1969).

Welsch v. Likins, 373 F.Supp. 487 (Minn. 1974).

Dixon v. Weinberger, 405 F.Supp. 974 (D.C. 1975).

Eubanks v. Clarke, 434 F.Supp. 1022 (Pa. 1977).

Morales v. Turman, 430 U.S. 322 (1977).

Wuori v. Zitnay, Civ. No. 75–80-SD (D. Maine, July 14, 1978). Cited in Mental Disability Law Reporter 2:693–696, 1978. Reprinted at Mental Disability Law Reporter 2:729–740, 1978.

Brewster v. Dukakis, 520 F.Supp. 882 (Mass. 1981); 687 F.2d 495 (1st Cir. 1982).

In interest of M.S.H., 466 N.W.2d 151 (N.D.Sup.Ct. 1991).

B. Articles and Books

Bachrach, L. L. (1980). Is the least restrictive environment always the best? Sociological and semantic implications. *Hospital and Community Psychiatry, 31,* 97–103.

Gutheil, T. G., Appelbaum, P. S., & Wexler, D. B. (1983). The inappropriateness of "least restrictive alternative" analysis for involuntary procedures with the institutionalized mentally ill. *Journal of Psychiatry and Law, 11,* 7–17.

Harris, G. T., Rice, M. E., & Preston, D. L. (1989). Staff and patient perceptions of the least restrictive alternatives for the short-term control of disturbed behavior. *Journal of Psychiatry and Law, 17,* 239–263.

Hoffman, P. B., & Foust, L. L. (1977). Least restrictive treatment of the mentally ill: A doctrine in search of its senses. *San Diego Law Review, 14,* 1100–1154.

Keilitz, I., Conn, D., & Giampetro, A. (1985). Least restrictive treatment of involuntary patients: Translating concepts into practice. *St. Louis Law Journal, 29,* 691–745.
Killebrew, J. A., Harris, C., & Kruckeberg, K. (1982). A conceptual model for determining the least restrictive treatment-training model. *Hospital and Community Psychiatry, 33,* 367–370.
Klein, J. (1983). The least restrictive alternative: More about less. *Psychiatric Quarterly, 55,* 106–114.
McGraw, B. D., & Keilitz, I. (1984). The least restrictive alternative doctrine in Los Angeles County civil commitment. *Whittier Law Review, 6,* 35–70.
Turnbull, H. R., Ellis, J. W., Boggs, E. M., Brooks, P. O., & Biklen, D. P. (1981). *The least restrictive alternative: Principles and practices.* Washington, DC: American Association on Mental Deficiency.
Woods, R. P., & Whatley, J. R. (1978). Conflict of rights: Implications for mental patients' right to adequate protection in light of the right to least restrictive treatment. *Law and Psychology Review, 4,* 191–206.
Zlotnick, D. (1981). First do no harm: Least restrictive alternative analysis and the right of mental patients to refuse treatment. *West Virginia Law Review, 83,* 375–448.

VI. Research Participation

A. *Cases*

Hyman v. Jewish Chronic Disease Hospital, 206 N.E.2d 338 (N.Y. 1965).
Kaimowitz v. Department of Mental Health for the State of Michigan. No. 73-19434-AW (Mich. Cir. Ct., Wayne County, July 10, 1973). Reprinted at *Mental Disability Law Reporter 1,* 147–154 (1976).
Knecht v. Gillman, 488 F.2d 1136 (8th Cir. 1973).
Mackey v. Procunier, 477 F.2d 877 (9th Cir. 1973).
New York Association for Retarded Children, Inc. v. Carey, 393 F.Supp. 715 (N.Y. 1975).
Scott v. Casey, 562 F.Supp. 475 (Ga. 1983).
United States v. Stanley, 107 S.Ct. 3054 (1987).
Whitlock v. Duke University, 829 F.Supp. 1340 (N.C. 1987).
Barrett v. United States, 853 F.2d 124 (2nd Cir. 1988).
Orlikow v. United States, 682 F.Supp. 77 (D.D.C. 1988).

B. *Articles and Books*

Appelbaum, P. S., & Roth, L. H. (1982). Competency to consent to research. *Archives of General Psychiatry, 39,* 951–958.
Bein, P. M. (1991). Surrogate consent and the incompetent experimental subject. *Food Drug Cosmetic Law Journal, 46,* 739–771.
Benson, P., & Roth, L. H. (1988). Trends in the social control of medical and psychiatric research. In D. Weisstub (Ed.), *Law and mental health, Vol. 4,* pp. 1–47. New York: Pergamon Press.
Benson, P., Roth, L. H., Appelbaum, P. S., Lidz, C. W., & Winslade, W. J. (1988). Information disclosure, subject understanding, and informed consent in psychiatric research. *Law and Human Behavior, 12,* 455–475.
Boruch, R. F., & Cecil, J. S. (Eds.). (1983). *Solutions to ethical and legal problems in social research.* New York: Academic Press.
Friedman, P. R. (1975). Legal regulation of applied behavior analysis in mental institution and prisons. *Arizona Law Review, 17,* 39–104.
Gallant, D. M., & Force, R. (Eds.). (1978). *Legal and ethical issues in human research and treatment.* New York, NY: Spectrum.
Greenwald, R. A., Ryan, M. K., & Mulvihill, J. E. (Eds.). (1982). *Human subjects research: A handbook for institutional review boards.* New York: Plenum Press.
Hershey, N., & Miller, R. D. (1976). *Human experimentation and the law.* Germantown, MD: Aspen Systems Corporation.
Imber, S. D., Glanz, L. M., Elkin, I., Sotsky, S. M., Boyer, J. L., & Leber, W. R. (1986). Ethical issues in psychotherapy research. *American Psychologist, 41,* 137–146.
Levine, R. J. (1986). *Ethics and regulation of clinical research* (2nd ed.). New Haven: Yale University Press.
Maloney, D. M. (1984). *Protection of human research subjects: A practical guide to federal laws and regulations.* New York: Plenum Press.
National Commission for the Protection of Human Subjects of Biomedical and Behavioral Research.

(1979, April 18). *The Belmont Report: Ethical principles for the protection of human subjects of research.* Washington, DC: U. S. Governmental Printing Office.

President's Commission for the Study of Ethical Problems in Medicine and Biomedical and Behavioral Research. (1981). *Protecting human subjects: First biennial report on the adequacy and uniformity of federal rules and policies, and their implementation, for the protection of human subjects in biomedical and behavioral research.* Washington, DC: U. S. Government Printing Office.

President's Commission for the Study of Ethical Problems in Medicine and Biomedical and Behavioral Research. (1983). *Implementing human research regulations.* Washington, DC: U. S. Government Printing Office.

Roth, L. H., & Appelbaum, P. S. (1983). Obtaining informed consent for research with psychiatric patients. *Psychiatric Clinics of North America, 6,* 551–565.

Roth, L. H., Appelbaum, P. S., Lidz, C. W., Benson, P., & Winslade, W. J. (1987). Informed consent in psychiatric research. *Rutgers Law Review, 39,* 425–441.

Sieber, J. E. (Ed.). (1984). *NIH readings on the protection of human subjects in behavioral and social science research.* Frederick, MD: University Publications of America.

Singer, R. (1977). Consent of the unfree, Part 1. *Law and Human Behavior, 1,* 1–43.

Singer, R. (1977). Consent of the unfree, Part 2. *Law and Human Behavior, 1,* 101–162.

Spicker, S. F., Alon, I., de Vries, A., & Engelhardt, H. T. (1982). *The use of human beings in research.* Dordrecht: Kluwer Academic Publishers.

U.S. Department of Health and Human Services. (1981, January 26,). Final regulations amending basic HHS policy for the protection of human research subjects. *Federal Register, 46,* 8366–8392.

Veatch, R. M. (1987). *The patient as partner: A theory of human-experimentation ethics.* Bloomington: Indiana University Press.

5

Legal Issues in Providing Treatment

I. Legal Basis for Challenging Treatment or Lack Thereof • **II. Right to Treatment** • A. Case Law • B. Present Status • C. Clinical Implications of a Right to Treatment • **III. The Right to Habilitation** • A. Case Law • B. Present Status • **IV. Informed Consent to Treatment** • A. Competency to Consent to Treatment • B. Voluntariness • C. Information • D. Implications of the Right to Refuse Treatment • **V. The Right to Refuse Treatment for a Mental Illness** • A. The Right to Refuse Psychotropic Medication • B. Legal Regulation of Electroconvulsive Therapy • C. Legal Regulation of Restraints and Seclusion • D. Legal Regulation of Behavior Modification • E. Legal Regulation of Psychosurgery • **VI. Commonly Asked Questions** • **VII. Bibliography**

Providing treatment to mentally disabled persons can be a disconcerting experience. The professional may find himself dealing with people who do not recognize their need for treatment, or who, as they begin to make progress, believe they no longer need the treatment that helped them. Because of fiscal limitations, mental health professionals who work in public facilities are often confronted with inadequate resources to accomplish their goals. Since the early 1970s, litigation has sought to establish the rights of the mentally disabled to treatment and habilitation and has advanced a right to refuse treatment. In response, many mental health professionals have come to assert that psychiatry has become discredited, and that the law has unnecessarily intruded into the clinical sphere. Many have adopted the attitude that they are "damned if they do, and damned if they don't," since no matter what they do, a lawyer will be looking over their shoulder.

This chapter will set forth the legal basis for establishing a right to treatment and habilitation, and recognizing a right to refuse treatment. The concept of informed consent will be described in detail. Since most of the litigation in these areas has surrounded the use of psychotropic medication, much of the chapter will concentrate on the current legal status of the right to refuse medication. The legal regulation of other treatment methods will also be presented.

I. LEGAL BASIS FOR CHALLENGING TREATMENT OR LACK THEREOF

The 1970s began a period when those concerned about the rights of the mentally disabled resorted to litigation as one means of attempting to establish the rights of these individuals. Class action lawsuits were brought challenging the living conditions in state operated facilities for the mentally ill and developmentally disabled. The litigation class may have been defined as all the mentally ill or developmentally disabled at a particular facility, or even as all those who were institutionalized in the facilities of a specific state. There were numerous reasons for initiating lawsuits against state institutions. First, the facilities contained large numbers of mentally disabled people, and the physical abuse or lack of care in these facilities was well documented. Second, from a tactical legal standpoint, these were the only facilities which could be effectively challenged in a courtroom. For in order to allege violations of the U.S. Constitution there must be some governmental action involved. The care of mentally disabled persons is often carried out by state or municipal mental health agencies. This state function then brings the actions taken within those facilities under the obligation to meet federal constitutional standards, as well as to comply with various federal and state laws.

This is not, however, true in the case of private mental health facilities. Although one can challenge a specific practice in a privately owned and operated facility, if the practice results in harm to the individual or violates a specific state law, there cannot be wide scale challenges to the entire facility. The notion is that since the treatment facility is private, if someone is dissatisfied with the care there, he has the right to leave.

In state facilities, the federal constitution sets forth constraints on governmental behavior. These have led to the notion that when individuals are involuntarily deprived of their liberty through civil commitment, they are entitled to certain rights, since they are being institutionalized for a disability, not criminal behavior. The protections afforded individuals in our society also apply to those who are hospitalized for a mental disability. Thus, the First Amendment's right to free speech, extended to include thoughts of any type, has been used as a basis for establishing a right to refuse medication. Other efforts at developing a right to refuse treatment have included the concept of the right to privacy, which is viewed as constitutionally protected. The Eighth Amendment's cruel-and-unusual-punishment clause has also provided a basis for recognizing a right to treatment as well as a right to refuse treatment. The development of these rights based on constitutional theory is elaborated upon later in this chapter.

II. RIGHT TO TREATMENT

In 1960, Morton Birnbaum, M.D., J.D., first proposed that the courts recognize a constitutionally protected right to treatment for institutionalized mentally ill persons based on notions of substantive due process. Viewing institutionalization without treatment in mental health facilities as tantamount to criminal incarceration, he reasoned:

> If repeated court decisions constantly remind the public that medical care in public mental institutions is inadequate, not only will the mentally ill be

> released from their mental prisons, but, it is believed that public opinion will react to force the legislatures to increase appropriations sufficiently to make it possible to provide adequate care and treatment so that the mentally ill will be treated in mental hospitals (Birnbaum, 1960, p. 503)

Birnbaum's thesis provided the foundation for later judicial developments making the right to treatment a reality.

A. Case Law

In *Rouse v. Cameron*, in 1966, a court for the first time recognized a constitutionally based right to treatment. The federal court said, "The purpose of involuntary hospitalization is treatment, not punishment." Although the court predicated its finding on a specific statute of the District of Columbia, the author of the decision, Judge David Bazelon, implied that there might also be violations of the U.S. Constitution in the procedures used for the commitment and treatment of the mentally ill. He specifically suggested that indefinite confinement without treatment of a person who has been found not criminally responsible for his actions may be cruel and unusual punishment. The court then addressed what would be required of the hospital to meet constitutional standards, concluding that "the hospital need not show that the treatment will cure or improve him, but only that there is a bona fide effort to do so." Despite its grounding on a statute whose effect applied only within the District of Columbia, the *Rouse* decision became the analytical starting point for all subsequent right-to-treatment cases.

In 1972, a federal district court in *Wyatt v. Stickney* was the first to hold that there was a constitutionally based right to treatment for civilly committed patients. The ruling resulted from a class action lawsuit challenging the conditions within Alabama's mental institutions. The court held that when patients are committed for treatment purposes, they unquestionably have "a constitutional right to receive such individual treatment as will give each of them a realistic opportunity to be cured or to improve his or her mental condition." The court noted that the purpose of involuntary hospitalization for treatment is in fact treatment and not merely custodial care or punishment, and that treatment is the only justification, from a constitutional standpoint, for civil commitment to a mental institution. In a subsequent ruling on the same case, the court, after hearing weeks of expert testimony, defined the minimum standards for constitutionally adequate treatment: (1) a humane psychological and physical environment; (2) qualified staff in numbers sufficient to administer adequate treatment; and (3) individualized treatment plans. Although *Wyatt* announced a constitutionally based right to treatment, the court did not articulate a clear legal basis for this right.

It was not until 1974, when the U.S. Court of Appeals for the Fifth Circuit decided *Donaldson v. O'Connor*, that the constitutional basis for a right to treatment was articulated. The court held that the Fourteenth Amendment to the Constitution guarantees civilly committed individuals a right to treatment. By noting that civil commitment involved the kind of massive curtailment of liberty with which the due process clause is concerned, the court then set forth a two-part theory for recognizing a constitutionally based right to treatment.

The first part of the court's theory is often referred to as the *rational relationship test*. It distinguishes between those who are committed based on the state's police power as dangerous to others and those who are committed based on a *parens patriae* rationale of being in need of treatment and unable to care for themselves. The court found that if "the rationale for confinement is the *parens patriae* rationale, that the patient is in need of treatment, the due process clause requires that minimally adequate treatment be in fact provided. This in turn requires that, at least for the nondangerous patient, constitutionally minimum standards of treatment be established and enforced." It follows, then, that if the purpose of commitment is treatment yet no treatment has been provided, the nature of the commitment bears no reasonable relationship to its purpose and the due process clause is violated.

The second part of the appellate court's theory in *Donaldson*, deemed the *quid pro quo theory*, holds that due process requires the state to extend treatment as the *quid pro quo* for its right to deprive individuals of their liberty in noncriminal proceedings. This theory requires that treatment be provided even to dangerous mentally ill individuals, whose basis for commitment is to prevent dangerous acts. In the event such individuals are untreatable, the theory as specified by the courts still requires "minimally adequate habilitation and care, beyond the subsistence level of custodial care that would be provided in a penitentiary."

In its review of the *Donaldson* case in 1975, the U.S. Supreme Court retreated from the lower court's holding. The Supreme Court unanimously agreed that "a State cannot constitutionally confine without more a nondangerous individual who is capable of surviving safely in freedom by himself or with the help of willing and responsible family members or friends" and that a "finding of mental illness alone cannot justify a State's locking a person up against his will and keeping him indefinitely in simple custodial confinement." The Supreme Court, however, noted that this case concerned not the right to or adequacy of psychiatric treatment but the propriety of involuntary confinement in an institution. Although the Supreme Court's ruling seemed to reject the Fifth Circuit's constitutional analysis of a right to treatment, the Fifth Circuit's decision has served as the basis for other lower court opinions which have recognized this right or the right to habilitation. Although the U.S. Supreme Court has never recognized a right to psychiatric treatment for mentally disabled individuals, it has also never rejected such a right.

B. Present Status

Today, the right to treatment is statutorily recognized by the majority of states for both voluntarily and involuntarily hospitalized patients. In some cases, it has been extended to the outpatient setting. Furthermore, the right appears to be widely accepted by state officials and mental health treatment providers. There remain significant problems, however, of translating the legal right to treatment into the reality of meaningful medical and psychiatric care. Budgetary constraints still limit the programs available to the mentally disabled. While most mental institutions today provide far better care and treatment than they did two decades ago, the baseline from which this progress is measured was low.

C. Clinical Implications of a Right to Treatment

A statutory or constitutional right to treatment presents several potential questions and problems for clinical and administrative personnel. Initially, there must be some definition of adequate treatment. This entails questions about the type, duration, and quality of mental health treatment, as well as consideration of the nature of the particular patient problems involved. *Treatment* in psychiatry is a term which refers to many varieties and intensities of intervention. Professional opinions often vary about the single best or preferred treatment modality for many psychiatric disorders. Does a right to treatment convey to the patient a right to select a particular treatment modality, a particular therapist, or a particular treatment setting, for a particular time period?

At least from the available case law, the right to treatment does not appear to attach to the single hypothetically best intervention, but only to adequate treatment, reasonably suitable treatment, or treatments which provide the patient a meaningful opportunity to improve. Ideally, the adequacy of treatment would be assessed according to the needs of each patient. Yet, this might be an impossible standard for the courts to enforce. The courts appear to be asking only if a patient has received an adequate amount of a carefully chosen therapeutic modality that a significant portion of mental health professionals finds appropriate for a given condition. The provision, however, of some treatment, or any treatment, is not likely to be considered adequate treatment. Any right to treatment is also likely to include a right to an assessment of the patient's therapeutic needs.

Provisions of a right to treatment may include adequate numbers of qualified staff, access to a variety of therapeutic modalities, provisions for individual treatment plans, periodic treatment reviews, record keeping, and education and rehabilitation services. Provisions may be stated generally or in considerable detail, such as standards and procedures for the administration of psychotropic medications, seclusion, restraints, and the establishment of a humane environment.

Implementation of a psychiatric patient's right to treatment presents additional problems for the treating staff. Various systems have been adopted or recommended for implementing, enforcing, and monitoring right to treatment provisions. These include judicial review, administrative review, ombudsmen, advocacy attorneys, malpractice litigation, or some combination of these systems. Each has its own set of advantages and disadvantages with regard to efficacy, as well as interference in the treatment process. The absence of articulated standards of care in many areas of psychiatric practice creates a particular problem for both treatment and enforcing personnel. Statistical requirements for a certain number of staff or other resources, for example, are unlikely to provide a meaningful assurance of a right to mental health treatment.

Clinical staff are particularly likely to resent the intrusion of judicial or administrative personnel into treatment decisions and to become distracted from their clinical responsibilities during protracted litigation. They may find themselves defensive about current treatment practices and procedures, even if inadequate, and may resist constructive change. Staff might find that legally or administratively created treatment standards are unworkable or too legalistic or interfere with clinical care. Such treatment standards rarely acknowledge or consider the treatment-resistant patient, a relatively common problem in long-term care facilities. Any of these increased legal responsibilities and risks to the staff may inadvertently drive treatment personnel out of the practice of providing mental health services in a public setting. Other professionals will welcome right to treatment provisions and litigation as an opportunity to increase the financial resources available for the care of mentally disabled persons.

III. THE RIGHT TO HABILITATION

Whereas the law speaks of the right to treatment for the mentally ill, the common phrase for the developmentally disabled is the "right to habilitation." Though the terms *habilitation* and *treatment* are sometimes used interchangeably, habilitation is distinguished by its association with the developmental model, whose aim is the remediation of the delayed learning process of the mentally retarded individual. To habilitate a person means to develop his maximum growth potential in terms of self-help, language, personal, social, educational, vocational, and recreational skills. Treatment for mental illness, based on the medical model, is by contrast aimed at a defined disease state. Although the distinction may seem one largely of language, its importance lies in its accentuation of the fact that the disorders of mentally ill and mentally retarded individuals differ with regard to etiology, symptomatology, and necessary intervention. For the mentally retarded, training in a variety of skills is a major element in making life in the community possible.

Lawsuits seeking to establish a right to habilitation initially invoked a "right to treatment" rhetoric. Indeed, the legal theories are identical, but habilitation of the retarded is usually different from the treatment requirements of the mentally ill. Although both populations require properly maintained environments and adequate staff, staff functions and program goals differ. A major thrust of today's right-to-habilitation litigation is to require programs in a community setting, rather than in large, isolated state institutions, where habilitation is considered almost impossible.

A. Case Law

Wyatt v. Stickney provided the seminal formulation of a constitutional right to habilitation for the mentally retarded person involuntarily confined in a state facility. The court defined *habilitation* as "the process by which the staff of the institution assists the resident to acquire and maintain those life skills which enable him to cope more effectively with the demands of his own person and of his environment and to raise the level of his physical, mental, and social efficiency. Habilitation includes but is not limited to programs of formal, structured education and treatment" (*Wyatt v. Stickney*, 1972, p. 395). With this standard in mind, the court asserted that "Because the only constitutional justification for civilly committing a mental retardate, therefore, is habilitation, it follows ineluctably that once committed such a person is possessed of an inviolable constitutional right to habilitation" (*Wyatt v. Stickney*, 1972, p. 390). The court then set forth the minimum conditions necessary to create an environment where habilitation can occur, which included 49 detailed provisions.

In *Welsch v. Likins*, another federal district court recognized that due process requires that civil commitment for mentally retarded individuals be accompanied by minimally adequate treatment designed to give each committed person a reasonable opportunity to be cured or to improve his or her mental condition. This case also held that Minnesota's statutory law mandated that treatment be provided in the setting least restrictive of the person's liberty.

Perhaps the most important case in establishing a right to habilitation has been *Halderman v. Pennhurst*. Over a 10-year period this case had a complicated legal history, including two reviews by the U.S. Supreme Court of various aspects of decisions of the lower courts. The result was a recognition that habilitation could not occur in a large state institution like Pennhurst. The institution was closed in 1986, and substantial funds were made available by the State of Pennsylvania for alternative types of care for the developmentally disabled, with an emphasis placed on smaller living environments and more community resources.

In 1982, in a unanimous decision, the U.S. Supreme Court, in *Youngberg v. Romeo*, recognized that an involuntarily institutionalized mentally retarded person had a right, based on the due process clause of the Fourteenth Amendment, to "minimally adequate or reasonable training to ensure safety and freedom from undue restraint." This lawsuit challenged conditions at Pennhurst State School in Pennsylvania. Nicholas Romeo, the named plaintiff, was a 33-year-old profoundly retarded man who was functioning at the level of an 18-month-old. He was injured on at least 63 occasions while in the facility and was often kept in restraints. The Court reasoned that "if it is cruel and unusual punishment to hold convicted criminals in unsafe conditions, it must be unconstitutional to confine the involuntarily committed—who may not be punished at all—in unsafe conditions." The Court recognized that to protect the liberty interest in safety and freedom from restraint, training may be necessary to avoid unconstitutional infringement of those rights.

This decision gives only scant support for a right to habilitation. It falls far short of other lower court rulings in this area. While the Court did hold that training is required in some circumstances, it mandated only the minimum amount that would enable the individual to avoid danger and unnecessary restraint and gave strong deference to the judgment of the professional caretaker. Whether *Romeo* will be viewed by the lower courts as setting constitutional maxima beyond which they will not venture, or only as articulating minima which will form the foundation for a more expansive view of habilitation rights, remains to be seen.

B. Present Status

The notion that institutionalized mentally retarded persons are entitled to habilitation and normalization has become well accepted. The present trend in most states is to develop small-group living arrangements in the community for the mentally retarded, closer to the "normal" environment. However, both the economic and the political costs of changing to community-based care are high, and the new facilities come with their own defects and inadequacies.

IV. INFORMED CONSENT TO TREATMENT

The judicial doctrine of informed consent originated as early as 1914 with the recognition that every competent individual has a right to determine what is done with his body, including the right to refuse needed medical treatment. Initially, the law was concerned with whether the patient provided consent to a particular treatment. More recently, case law and statutes in this area have related to the information that must be provided to the patient when medical treatment is sought. Informed-consent law places the burden on the treatment provider to disclose information to the patient, rather than on the patient to ask for it. In theory, prior to the acceptance of treatment, the patient must be apprised of the diagnosis, the nature of the contemplated treatment, the risks inherent in such treatment, his prognosis with and without the treatment, and any possible alternative approaches to alleviate the problem. The provision of this information does not by itself render valid an ensuing consent to treatment, for in addition to being informed, a patient must be legally competent and must give his consent voluntarily and knowingly. These elements are considered below.

A. Competency to Consent to Treatment

There are two general types of competence: (1) legal competence and (2) clinical (*de facto*) competence or decision-making ability. In addition, there is usually some specific area of competence or functioning which is addressed when a person is described as competent or incompetent (competent to consent to medical and psychiatric care, in the present context). Legal competence is at issue when a person has been declared judicially incompetent or is a minor. Every state has a procedure for declaring a person legally incompetent based upon a finding that the individual is incapable of managing his financial assets or is unable to make responsible personal decisions regarding his care and welfare. (See Chapter 9, "Competency and Guardianship," for a more extensive discussion.) Legal declarations of incompetence are often limited to certain areas of an individual's functioning. A mentally disabled person can, for example, be legally incompetent to manage his financial affairs but legally competent to consent to medical and psychiatric care. Most mentally ill persons are in fact not legally incompetent, and the statutes of most states specifically indicate that they should be presumed competent in all respects. In contrast, institutionalized mentally retarded persons are more likely to have been declared legally incompetent, because the severity of their retardation renders them unable to make competent decisions about their daily needs.

The term *clinical competence* generally refers to the functional ability of the patient to consent to or refuse medical and psychiatric intervention. There is no universally accepted standard to measure a patient's competence to consent to psychiatric treatment, and many such tests have been suggested. Most mental health professionals would agree that a mute patient who fails to respond to staff queries about his treatment would not be clinically competent to consent to or refuse treatment. A test which employs a criterion that the patient make and verbalize a treatment decision appears to be a minimal threshold of decision-making competence. A more demanding competence test inquires into the rationale for the patient's decision making (for example, was his reason for accepting or rejecting treatment rational, or was it the product of a mental disorder?). Other tests of competence to consent to treatment relate to the ability of the person to understand, or to the actual understanding of, the risks, benefits, and alternatives of the proposed treatment after these have been thoroughly explained by staff. Perhaps the most demanding test of competence to consent to treatment asks whether the patient emotionally appreciates the available treatment choices.

Treatment staff are generally free to select the test of competence to consent to treatment that they find most useful and applicable to the clinical situation in question. Occasionally, a state's mental health code or regulation will articulate a competence standard of its own, particularly when a treatment of more than usual risk is involved (e.g., electroconvulsive therapy). It may also be necessary to consider the risks and benefits of the proposed treatment when selecting a competence test. Staff are unlikely to demand that a patient be more than minimally competent to consent to the treatment when the benefit/risk ratio for the proposed treatment appears favorable to the patient. In contrast, staff are likely to demand a higher level of clinical competence to consent from a patient when the treatment presents serious risks of harm and the benefits appear uncertain.

Patients who appear to be clinically incompetent to consent to psychiatric treatment, at least by some test, but who have not been declared legally incompetent to do so, are commonly encountered in psychiatric hospitals. This situation is most likely to exist at the time of admission to a hospital, or early in the course of a hospitalization, when the person may be suffering from a psychotic disorder or severe affective disorder and has not yet begun to respond to treatment. Such relatively common situations typically stretch the limits of the doctrine of informed consent. They require the mental health professional to employ a variety of maneuvers, some not necessarily embraced by informed consent principles. These include:

1. Delaying treatment while attempting to maximize the patient's participation and competency to consent by, for example, repeatedly discussing treatment information with the patient.
2. Initiating treatment by temporarily substituting the consent of close relatives for that of the patient (a procedure which may have no technical legal validity but which may nevertheless present little liability risk to staff).
3. Substituting other treatment modalities which present a more favorable benefit/risk ratio to the patient (instead of the proposed riskier one) until his clinical condition and his capacity to assess the riskier choices improve.
4. Initiating the proposed treatment in the absence of the patient's present ability to consent to it when he has done so in the past when in a similar situation, or when the patient has provided some advanced directive authorizing such intervention should he later require it.
5. Initiating treatment in the absence of competent consent when the benefit/risk ratio appears favorable to the patient, and when it is foreseeable that the patient will soon regain his competency to consent to the treatment and will in fact consent to it at that time.
6. Applying for a court-appointed guardian or a court order to authorize necessary treatment.

While any of these strategies may at times be useful in dealing with the patient who appears unable to consent to psychiatric treatment, they each present some administrative or legal risks. They would not necessarily be applicable to the decisionally incapacitated patient who refuses treatment, which is discussed in Section V below.

B. Voluntariness

By law, an individual's consent to treatment must be made freely. This means it cannot be made under a threat of force, coercion, compulsion, fraud, duress, deceit, or some other external influence or pressure. In the context of the institutionalized mentally disabled person, the question sometimes arises of how "voluntary" any consent can be, particularly when release from the facility may depend upon the acceptance of a proposed treatment, despite a patient's reluctance to participate in it. Chronically hospitalized individuals also commonly lack interest or pleasure in their activities or treatment, so they are vulnerable to external pressure from staff, relatives, or other patients. The voluntariness issue is one that must be carefully scrutinized in the institutional setting, particularly when a proposed treatment presents significant or long-term adverse risks.

C. Information

This element of informed consent to treatment focuses on the amount and type of information which must be revealed to the patient in order for him to make an informed choice. This information generally consists of the potential risks and the expected benefits of the proposed treatment or procedure, in addition to treatment alternatives and the risks of treatment refusal. Case law or statute defines what information should be disclosed, and one of two general disclosure standards applies. The professional disclosure standard relies upon the customary practice of practitioners in a particular jurisdiction, for example, what most physicians reveal to their patients about the proposed treatment. In contrast, many jurisdictions have adopted a "reasonable patient" or "material risk" disclosure standard. In this case, the treatment provider is required to disclose to the patient the treatment information that a hypothetical "reasonable patient" or, sometimes, the particular patient in question would find significant in deciding whether to accept or reject the intervention.

There are several exceptions to these information disclosure requirements. Treatment providers must judge for themselves when and if such an exception to the disclosure rules can apply to a particular patient's case. The exceptions include:

1. An emergency, when there is insufficient time to share treatment information with the patient, or when the patient's condition renders it impossible to do so (e.g., when the patient is unconscious).
2. Waiver, when the patient voluntarily waives his right to the treatment information ("Doctor, don't tell me").
3. Therapeutic privilege, the privilege of the treatment provider not to disclose treatment information when doing so would be significantly detrimental to the patient's disorder or condition (this does not, however, permit a physician not to reveal the risks of a psychotropic medication when doing so would result in the patient's refusal of the medication).
4. Legal incompetence of the patient; in this exception, the treatment provider is required to discuss relevant treatment information with the patient's appointed guardian, rather than with the patient.

D. Implications of the Right to Refuse Treatment

When the mentally disabled individual is clinically and legally competent, has sufficient knowledge to make an informed treatment decision, and appears to be doing so voluntarily, then informed consent to treatment can be said to occur. This doctrine, which until the late 1970s was considered applicable only to medical and surgical patients who were not mentally disabled, forms the conceptual boundary within which the right to refuse psychiatric treatment has been conceived. By the end of the 1970s, the argument was made that the mentally disabled should have a similar right to make an informed decision which could result in rejecting treatment and habilitation. Proponents of this position acknowledge that the exercise of this right may result in an individual's refusing treatment that would be beneficial to him, but they find this risk outweighed by the value of giving the mentally disabled person a free choice. They point out that mentally disabled individuals cannot be presumed to be incompetent, and that some treatment or habilitation methods are harmful, exposing the person to lasting adverse consequences.

V. THE RIGHT TO REFUSE TREATMENT FOR A MENTAL ILLNESS

It is often difficult for mental health professionals to allow individuals to reject treatment which would be of great benefit and might even save their lives. It is sometimes also difficult for health care providers to appreciate that our society gives primary recognition to an individual's right to choose what is done with his body. This may mean that a person may make imprudent or foolish choices which could be fatal. Only the individual, however, has the right to decide what will be done to him. As long as the person is legally competent, society provides a right to make unwise treatment decisions, which may mean that the patient "dies with his rights on."

The recently evolving notion that an institutionalized mentally disabled person has a right to refuse treatment is one of the most divisive issues confronting the mental health field in the 1980s. It pits the medical and legal professions against each other in a way that accentuates their differing orientations, while it fails to address the larger problems of the quality of care provided in the institutions. For the health care provider, the medical best interests standard guides the decisions, with the goal to maximize the patient's life and promote the patient's health. The attorney, on the other hand, is responsible for advocating what his competent client desires, even if what he desires may not appear to be in his "best medical interests." If the client is incompetent, the attorney must try to ascertain what his client would have desired had he been competent, and the attorney then must advocate that position. This obligation is complicated by the fact that in some cases the line between competency and incompetency is an unclear one, with the client appearing competent to decide some issues and not others.

Assertion of a right of the mentally ill or mentally retarded to refuse treatment is complicated by the fact of their mental disability. In contrast to the assumption of competency governing the medical patient's decision making regarding treatment, the institutionalized mentally disabled have been thought to have no right to engage in decisions relating to their care once they are institutionalized. Until the late 1970s it was not even questioned that the institution should decide care without consulting either the disabled person or his family. Even the passage in the 1970s of the laws stating that the mentally disabled were to be considered competent to consent to treatment unless declared otherwise did not change institutional practices, since the disabled were considered clinically—albeit not legally—incompetent and accordingly could have no say in their treatment.

We are now clearly in an era when earlier assumptions about the inability of mentally disabled persons to make treatment decisions no longer apply. If the person is considered to have adequate decision-making capacity, he will be permitted to have an active role in decisions relating to his care. If the person is clearly unable to make treatment decisions for himself, then a substitute decision maker must in many cases be appointed by the court to make decisions which would be in his best medical interests or be those which the person would make if he were competent to consent. The cases challenging a patient's right to refuse medication best illustrate the arguments set forth to establish a right to refuse treatment generally and the present legal status of this right.

A. The Right to Refuse Psychotropic Medication

The introduction of psychotropic medications in the 1950s greatly altered the treatment of mentally ill individuals. Today these medications constitute an indispensable component of treatment in inpatient units. Moreover, the therapeutic effects of these medications have led to their use in facilities for the mentally retarded, as well as in juvenile detention facilities.

These medications are, however, subject to abuse in the institutional setting. Use of psychotropic medication requires careful monitoring of the patient, which may not be carried out because of staff shortages. In some cases, psychotropic medication may be more useful for behavior control or punishment than for treatment. Sometimes, psychotropic medication is used to compensate for the absence of other treatment resources, modalities, and personnel. Concern about the inappropriate use of these medications and the risk of serious side effects has led attorneys for the mentally disabled to seek judicial recognition of a right to refuse medication by the involuntarily hospitalized mentally ill person. This issue, perhaps more than any other, has brought mental health professionals and attorneys for the mentally disabled into sharp conflict.

Proponents of this right have relied primarily on constitutional law claiming that an individual's bodily integrity and personal autonomy are invaded by the coercive use of medication. This argument is supported by various constitutional rights. Patient advocates sometimes emphasize that civilly committed persons are legally competent to consent to and refuse treatment, unless specifically found not to be competent by a court, and thus have the legal right to determine what medical and psychiatric treatments they will receive. A review of the major legal cases in this area reveals that the presumption of competency to consent to treatment is the critical factor in the majority of decisions granting the mentally ill the right to refuse psychotropic medication (see Table 5.1). Finally, proponents of the right to refuse medication point to the potentially irreversible side effects (tardive dyskinesia and tardive dystonia) that may result from prolonged use of psychotropic medications.

A central concern of mental health professionals who treat involuntary patients is that if a right to refuse medication is recognized by law, they will be unable to provide the most effective treatment available to mentally disabled individuals. Second, the patient's rejection of medication may result in a long-term hospitalization of a custodial nature. Third, there may be an increased use of seclusion and physical restraints for the unmedicated patient with possible accidental injuries to him. Fourth, staff fear that treatment refusal will disrupt the therapeutic milieu of the hospital and precipitate patient violence to staff or other patients. Finally, as the case

Table 5.1. Summary Cases: Right to Refuse Medication Cases

Name	Cite	State	Holding
AE & RR v. Mitchell	724 F.2d 864 (10th Cir. 1983)	UT	Based on Utah law, a finding that a person is subject to civil commitment constitutes a determination of incompetency to make treatment decisions. A committed patient does not have the right to refuse medication.
Anderson v. Arizona	663 P.2d 570 (Ariz. 1983)	AZ	Based on Arizona law, a person who has not been adjudicated incompetent has a right to refuse nonemergency medication.
In re Boyd	403 A.2d 774 (D.C. Ct. of App. 1979)	DC	In a nonemergency situation, a legally adjudicated incompetent person can refuse medication based on religious reasons if the court determines this is what she would do if she were competent.
Davis v. Hubbard	506 F.Supp. 915 (N.D. Ohio 1980)	OH	A competent patient has a right to refuse medication except when there is probable cause to believe he poses a danger to himself or others.
Goedecke v. State	603 P.2d 123 (Colo. Sup.Ct. 1979)	CO	A legally competent patient has a right to refuse medication.
State of Washington v. Harper	110 S.Ct. 1028 (1990)	WA	A state may forcibly administer antipsychotic medication to a mentally ill prisoner without a court hearing to determine competency. The prisoner's rights are adequately protected by a hearing before a special committee of a psychiatrist, a psychologist, and an administrator, none of whom are involved in the inmate's care.
Jamison v. Farabee	No. C78-0445 WHO (N.D. Cal. April 26, 1983), reported 7 MDLR 436	CA	Consent decree which gives patient substantial rights to refuse medication but allows staff to medicate in an emergency or where patient is "substantially deteriorating."
Jarvis v. Levine	418 N.W.2d 139 (Minn. Sup.Ct. 1988)	MN	Involuntary administration of antipsychotic medications to a committed patient in a nonemergency constitutes "intrusive treatment" which requires prior judicial approval. A determination of legal incompetence, as well as the necessity and reasonableness of the treatment, must also be obtained pior to forcing medication.

(continued)

Table 5.1. (*Continued*)

Name	Cite	State	Holding
K.K.B. v. Oklahoma	609 P.2d 747 (OK Sup.Ct. 1980)	OK	Absent an emergency, a competent, involuntary patient has a right to refuse medication. Prerequisites for involuntary treatment include a judicial proceeding to declare the patient incompetent and the appointment of a guardian to make an informed decision for the patient.
In re L.R.	497 A.2d 753 (Vt. 1985)	VT	Held that a woman who refused to take medication and who had a history of suicidal and other aggressive behavior when not on medication met the Vermont civil commitment statute as a danger to herself.
In re M.P.	510 N.E.2d 645 (Ind. Sup.Ct. 1987)	IN	Based on state law, a legally competent but committed patient who refuses treatment can petition a court for review of the proposed treatment program. At this hearing, the state must prove the necessity of antipsychotic medication. There is no judicial review for medications necessary for the treatment of physical illness.
Opinion of the Justices	465 A.2d 484 (N.H. Sup.Ct. 1983)	NH	The state constitution requires a prior court determination of incompetency to consent to treatment before forcibly administering psychotropic medication to a committed patient.
People v. Medina	705 P.2d 961 (Colo. Sup.Ct. 1985)	CO	A court order must be obtained to medicate a refusing incompetent patient in a nonemergency. The court must be given clear and convincing evidence that medication is necessary to prevent significant and long-term deterioration of the patient.
Project Release v. Prevost	722 F.2d 960 (2nd Cir. 1983)	NY	Patients can be medicated despite their refusal in a nonemergency if a New York three-tiered administrative review process is followed. (Process like that adopted by New Jersey in *Rennie v. Klein*.)
R.A.J. v. Miller	590 F.Supp 1319 (N.D. Texas 1984)	TX	Court upheld a proposed rule by the Commissioner as to when medication can be given over the patient's refusal, similar to that adopted by New Jersey in *Rennie v. Klein*.

(*continued*)

Table 5.1. (*Continued*)

Name	Cite	State	Holding
Rennie v. Klein	720 F.2d 266 (3rd Cir. 1983)	NJ	The qualified right of a patient to refuse in a nonemergency can be overridden for a committed dangerously mentally ill patient "whenever in the exercise of professional judgment, such an action is deemed necessary to prevent the patient from endangering himself or others." New Jersey adopted an administrative review process which the court upheld.
Riese v. St. Mary's Hospital and Medical Center	243 Cal.Rptr. 241 (Cal.App. 1987); 774 P.2d 698 (1989).	CA	A committed patient has a statutory right to refuse antipsychotic medication in a nonemergency but can be forcibly medicated after a judicial determination of incompetency to consent to treatment. Surrogate consent must then be obtained from the responsible relative, guardian, or conservator of the patient.
Rivers v. Katz	495 N.E. 2d 337 (NY Ct.App. 1986)	NY	A legally competent, involuntarily committed patient has a right to refuse medication unless the "patient presents a danger to himself or other members of society or engages in dangerous or potentially destructive conduct within the institution." Can only medicate as long as the emergency exists. In nonemergencies, patients can be medicated despite their refusal only after a judicial determination that the patient lacks the capacity to make a treatment decision.
Rogers v. Comm of Mental Health	738 F.2d 1 (1st Cir. 1984); 458 N.E.2d 308 (Mass. Sup.Jud.Ct. 1983)	MA	Recognized a right of a competent mentally ill person to refuse medication in a nonemergency. *Emergency* defined broadly to include the "prevention of immediate, substantial and irreversible deterioration of a mental illness when even the smallest delay would be intolerable."
Guardianship of Richard Roe III	421 N.E.2d 40 (Mass. Sup.Jud.Ct. 1981)	MA	Based on state law, before medication can be given to a legally incompetent patient in a nonemergency, there must be court approval of the guardians' decision.
State ex rel. Jones v. Gerhardstein	416 N.W.2d 883 (Wisc. 1987)	WI	Involuntarily hospitalized patients may be medicated despite their

(*continued*)

Table 5.1. (*Continued*)

Name	Cite	State	Holding
			refusal only when it is necessary to prevent serious physical harm to the patient or others or if there is a court finding of probable cause to believe the individual is incompetent to refuse medication.
Stensvad v. Reivitz	601 F.Supp. 128 (WD Wisc. 1985)	WI	Upheld Wisconsin's commitment statute, which denies the patient a right to refuse medication. The court said, "Nonconsensual treatment is what involuntary commitment is all about."
U.S. v. Charters	863 F.2d 302 (4th Cir. 1988)	4th Cir.	The decision to forcibly medicate a criminal defendant found incompetent to stand trial can be made by the appropriate professionals exercising their judgment. Subsequent judicial review is available only to determine if the decision to treat was made arbitrarily.
Winters v. Miller	446 F.2d 65 (2nd Cir. 1971)	NY	In a nonemergency a competent mentally ill person has a right to refuse medication based on her religious beliefs.

law has developed, many mental health professionals justifiably worry that their time and energy will be diverted to administrative or judicial proceedings to override a patient's treatment refusal. Such resources could otherwise be used to meet the needs of those most receptive to treatment. As in the case of civil commitment contests, treatment staff and patients may assume adversarial postures in struggles over medication refusal.

In this section, we will explore the constitutional arguments in support of civilly committed patients' right to refuse psychotropic medication and will summarize the case law developments in this area. We will also address the statutory provisions which recognize such a right. We will conclude our discussion of the right to refuse medication with some comments about the clinical management of patients who refuse medication.

1. *Constitutional Basis*

Two constitutional rights have been successfully set forth as the basis for recognizing patients' right to refuse medication: (l) freedom of religion and (2) a liberty interest which guarantees a right to privacy. Although other constitutional issues were raised in the early right-to-refuse treatment cases, such as freedom of thought and freedom from cruel and unusual punishment, these concepts have not served as the basis for the decisions recognizing the right of mentally ill individuals in psychiatric hospitals to refuse medication.

a. Freedom of Religion. In New York, the First Amendment's guarantee of freedom of religion served as the basis for the first suit regarding an institutionalized mentally ill person's right to refuse medication. In *Winters v. Miller*, the court was presented with the claim of a 59-year-old practicing Christian Scientist who, upon admission to Bellevue Hospital in 1968, refused to have her blood pressure taken because of her religious beliefs and objected to being given medication for the same reason. Her objections were ignored, and the medication was administered both orally and intramuscularly. In concluding that Winters had a cause of action, the court emphasized that since she had not been declared legally incompetent, her religious views had to be honored.

Since that decision, there have been numerous other cases challenging the right of an involuntarily hospitalized mentally ill person to refuse treatment based on his religious beliefs. The courts have taken the view that freedom of religion is one of the most important guarantees in the U.S. Constitution, and that deference should be given to the practice of religion as one wishes, as long as it will not cause harm to others. In refusal-of-treatment cases based on religious beliefs, the courts will generally allow the person to follow the dictates of his religious beliefs, even if it means jeopardizing his life, such as through refusing blood transfusions. In a nonemergency situation, an adult patient's religious beliefs should be honored as long as he is competent and the religion is a recognized one and not a product of his mental disorder. The trend in the law is that even in cases where the person has been declared legally incompetent to consent to treatment, his religious objections may be followed if he has been a long-standing practitioner of that religion and his objections were known before he became incompetent. Thus, the treating professional who wishes to override a decision to refuse medication based on religious reasons would be well advised to seek a court order before doing so.

b. A Liberty Interest. The primary constitutional basis for recognizing the right of mentally disabled individuals to refuse medication is the individual's interest in liberty as protected by the due process clause of the Fourteenth Amendment. While the U.S. Supreme Court has recognized a number of liberty interests, the one of particular relevance here is the right to privacy, in the form of freedom from bodily intrusion. Two leading cases in this area, *Rennie v. Klein* and *Rogers v. Okin*, provide a good understanding of how the right to refuse psychotropic medication developed and of the different approaches finally taken by the courts. The final court decisions in these cases provide two models of the right of legally competent and civilly committed psychiatric inpatients to refuse psychiatric treatment. These cases have served as models for other state and federal courts which have addressed this issue.

(1) Rennie v. Klein. In December 1977, John Rennie, a committed mental patient at Ancora Psychiatric Hospital in New Jersey, filed suit in federal district court against the New Jersey Commissioner of Human Services alleging that the hospital's practice of forcibly medicating him with psychotropic drugs in the absence of an emergency was unconstitutional. Rennie had a long history of involuntary psychiatric hospitalizations and had been diagnosed as having a schizophrenic disorder and a manic-depressive disorder. While hospitalized, he was given numerous psychotropic medications, which had noticeable adverse side effects.

The right-to-refuse-treatment aspects of the case also had a long history. The federal district court which initially decided the case in 1978 and 1979 recognized that the right to privacy "was broad enough to protect one's mental processes from governmental interference" and "to establish an individual's autonomy over his own body." It held "that the right to refuse treatment extends to patients in nonemergent circumstances" and stated that only where the government shows some strong countervailing interest can the right to refuse treatment be qualified. The court then set forth an elaborate scheme for protecting the patient, including a formal due process hearing with representation by an attorney and an independent psychiatrist for the patient.

Upon review by the full United States Court of Appeals for the Third Circuit, the appellate court in 1981 agreed that giving medication over the patient's objection in a nonemergency situation infringed the patient's liberty interest, but it rejected the district court's requirements relating to a hearing, the use of patients' advocates, and an independent psychiatrist. The appellate court held that the procedures New Jersey had established were sufficient to meet due process protections. These are the procedures: (1) the physician attempts to inform the patient of his condition and the risks and benefits of the treatment and alternative treatments; (2) the treatment team reviews the treatment plan with the patient present, if his condition permits; and (3) if the legally competent patient continues to refuse medication despite the above, the medical director of the hospital reviews the treatment decision and, if he agrees with the necessity for medication, the medication may be administered. The medical director is also authorized to obtain an independent psychiatric consultant to evaluate the patient's need for medication and should consider his findings when reaching a conclusion about treatment.

The case was eventually argued before the U.S. Supreme Court and then was remanded back to the U.S. Court of Appeals for the Third Circuit by the Supreme Court without an opinion, based on the Supreme Court's decision in *Youngberg v. Romeo*. Upon remand, the Third Circuit in 1983 held that dangerous mentally ill patients who have been involuntarily hospitalized may be administered antipsychotic drugs "whenever, in the exercise of professional judgment, such an action is deemed necessary to prevent the patient from endangering himself or others." The court then upheld New Jersey's regulatory scheme for reviewing a patient's refusal of medication described above.

In 1990, the United States Supreme Court upheld an administrative procedure similar to New Jersey's in the context of a Washington State prisoner who had refused psychotropic medication. In *Washington v. Harper*, the Court accepted that the procedure of internal review protected the prisoner's liberty interest. The Court held that the regulation was "an accommodation between an inmate's liberty interest in avoiding the forced administration of antipsychotic drugs and the State's interests in providing appropriate medical treatment to reduce the danger that an inmate suffering from a serious mental disorder represents to himself or others."

Although the Supreme Court declined to address whether this standard would also apply to the civilly committed individual in a mental health setting, good arguments can be made that it would. The primary argument is that the individual's civil commitment is a recognition of his need for treatment, and thus the state should be able to provide treatment as long as the individual's rights are protected. In numerous other cases, the Court has held that an internal review process protects the rights of the individual. Whether or when the Court will have the opportunity to address this issue directly in the context of a civilly committed individual cannot be predicted.

(2) Rogers v. Okin. The case of *Rogers v. Okin* followed a pattern similar to the *Rennie* case: The federal district court recognized a broad right to refuse treatment for legally competent but committed patients, the U.S. Court of Appeals for the First Circuit narrowed this right, and the U.S. Supreme Court remanded the decision. *Rogers* began in 1975 as a class action suit on behalf of patients at Boston State Hospital who claimed that their constitutional rights were being violated when they received psychotropic medication over their objections in nonemergency situations. The federal district court in 1979 held that legally competent mental patients had a right to decide for themselves whether to submit to such treatment. Refusal of treatment could be overridden only in an emergency.

On appeal, the U.S. Court of Appeals for the First Circuit in 1980 recognized "an intuitively obvious proposition: a person has a constitutionally protected interest in being left free by the state to decide for himself whether to submit to the serious and potentially harmful medical treatment that is represented by the administration of antipsychotic drugs." The court accepted the right to refuse treatment based on a constitutionally protected privacy interest and ruled that a judicial determination of incapacity to make treatment decisions must be made before the state may forcibly medicate a patient in a nonemergency.

The case was subsequently argued before the U.S. Supreme Court. In 1982, the Court vacated the appellate court's judgment and remanded the case to the appellate court in light of a 1981 decision by the Massachusetts Supreme Judicial Court, *Guardianship of Richard Roe III*, which had recognized the right of a legally incompetent mentally ill person to refuse outpatient antipsychotic medication based on state law. The U.S. First Circuit Court of Appeals then certified nine questions which were answered by the Massachusetts Supreme Judicial Court. This 1983 ruling provided that legally competent but committed patients had a right to refuse medication in a nonemergency situation. In cases where the patient is deemed to be incompetent to make treatment decisions, court approval must be obtained for the use of antipsychotic medication, which would be supervised by the patient's guardian. In determining whether to authorize the use of medication despite the patient's refusal, the court must use a "substituted judgment" decision-making process. The court must consider the following factors in arriving at the medication decision: (1) the patient's expressed preferences regarding treatment; (2) his religious convictions as they pertain to his refusal of treatment; (3) the impact of the treatment decision on the patient's family; (4) the probability of adverse side effects; (5) the prognosis without treatment; and (6) the prognosis with treatment.

The Massachusetts court's decision in *Rogers* broadened the definition of emergency to provide for overriding the patient's decision when (1) he poses an imminent threat of harm to himself or others, and there is no less intrusive alternative available, or (2) when necessary "to prevent the immediate, substantial and irreversible deterioration of a serious mental illness" where even a brief delay would be intolerable.

(3) Importance of Rennie and Rogers. Until the U.S. Supreme Court directly addresses whether, and in what situations, an involuntarily hospitalized mental patient

has a right to refuse medication, the decisions reached in *Rennie* and *Rogers* provide guidance in other court interpretations of this right. While both cases recognized the right of a patient to refuse antipsychotic medication absent an emergency, based on a constitutionally protected liberty interest, each took a different approach in defining the extent of that right and in determining who has the final decision-making authority when the right to refuse medication is exercised.

In *Rennie,* the court gave deference to the determination of the treatment providers, presuming that a decision to override a patient's refusal of medication is valid unless it is a substantial departure from accepted professional judgment, practice, or standards. The court permitted an administrative review process which is deemed adequate to meet due process requirements. Other courts, including the United States Supreme Court, have followed the *Rennie* reasoning and have held that a review process similar to New Jersey's meets due process requirements.

In contrast, the court in *Rogers* took a different approach. The court held that only a court, rather than a physician or even a patient's guardian, has the ultimate authority to override a refusal of medication in nonemergency situations. A patient thought to be clinically incompetent to make treatment decisions must be formally declared incompetent to consent to treatment. The court decision, based in part on Massachusetts state law, was also unique in requiring that a guardian of an incompetent person obtain permission from the court for a treatment plan which would override the patient's medication refusal; the authorization for initiating treatment is obtained from the court, but the treating physician must report all changes in the treatment plan to the patient's guardian. Finally, the court defined *emergency* to include both imminent physical harm and psychological harm, though it sharply restricted the scope of the latter to irreversible deterioration.

2. *Statutory Basis*

Concern about the use of psychotropic medications has led at least half the states to enact laws relating to the administration of medication in facilities for the mentally disabled. A small number of states specifically recognize the right of voluntary patients to refuse medication. Some recognize that individuals may refuse treatment, including medication, based on their religious beliefs and may choose to be treated in accordance with those beliefs. A number of states provide that there shall be no excessive or unnecessary use of psychotropic medication, or that it shall not be used for the purpose of punishment. In all states where medication refusal is recognized by statute, exceptions are made for an emergency situation.

3. *Common Law*

The common law tort of battery and the doctrine of informed consent have provided non-mentally ill individuals with a right to bodily autonomy which prohibits unwanted medical or surgical procedures. These common law concepts have been put forth on behalf of the mentally disabled to argue that they are entitled to the same protection as those whose competency is not in doubt. Since the vast majority of states specifically provide that the involuntarily hospitalized person is to be presumed competent to make personal and financial decisions unless determined otherwise, the argument is made that they are entitled to the same protections as others seeking medical treatment, including the right to refuse that treatment. Proponents of such protections argue that even when an individual's refusal of treatment seems unwise and counter to his own interests, this should not justify overriding his decision; the mentally disabled person is the only one who can balance whether the potential benefits of medication outweigh its adverse effects.

The importance of these common law arguments cannot be understated. The concept that a mentally disabled person is competent to make treatment decisions until declared otherwise has been at the heart of all the decisions which have recognized that a committed mentally ill person has a right to refuse treatment. Numerous courts from Massachusetts to California have used these common law arguments to support the recognition of the right of a competent mentally ill person to refuse treatment absent an emergency.

4. *Cases Denying a Right to Refuse Medication*

Although the clear trend in the law, via both statute and case law, is to recognize that a legally competent, civilly committed person has a right to refuse psychotropic medication in a nonemergency situation, a number of states have reached a contrary conclusion. In Utah and Wisconsin, for example, the courts have held that an involuntarily hospitalized patient does not have a right to refuse medication. These decisions were based on an interpretation of state statutes.

In Utah, one of the criteria for civil commitment is that the individual "lacks the ability to engage in a rational decision-making process regarding the acceptance of mental treatment as demonstrated by evidence of inability to weigh the possible costs and benefits of treatment" (Utah Code Ann. Section 64–7-36(10)). Although not otherwise declared incompetent, the patient is deemed to be incompetent for the purposes of making treatment decisions; the decision to authorize treatment over the patient's objection is made simultaneously with the civil commitment determination. Wisconsin took a similar approach, by specifically denying a civilly committed patient a right to refuse treatment except for excessive medication, psychosurgery, or electroconvulsive therapy. Thus, the fact of commitment means that a determination has been made that treatment can be given regardless of the patient's wishes. The Wisconsin statute was challenged and upheld in a federal court (*Stensvad v. Reivitz*, 1985). The Wisconsin court noted that "civil commitment is for custody, care and treatment, and . . . that nonconsensual treatment is what involuntary commitment is all about." In 1987, however, the Wisconsin Supreme Court ruled that forcible administration of psychotropic medication can occur only when a patient has been found to be incompetent to make treatment decisions in a court hearing (*State ex rel. Jones v. Gerhardstein*).

5. *Summary of the Status of the Right to Refuse Medication*

Except in those states which specifically provide that civil commitment means the individual does not have a right to reject treatment, it is now well accepted that legally competent but involuntarily hospitalized patients, as well as voluntarily hospitalized patients, have a right to refuse psychotropic medication except in an emergency (see Table 5.1). The courts' interpretations of *emergency* vary but sometimes allow the mental health professional to define it broadly to include both impending physical and psychological harm to the patient or others.

In those instances when an individual's medication refusal can be overridden, the courts have recognized that the patient is entitled to a certain level of due process. This might include a consideration of alternative treatments, including a change in dosage or type of medication. An independent medical review of the treating physician's decision, to demonstrate that professional judgment has been properly exercised, may also be required. This review is variously conducted by a psychiatrist within the facility or by one from the community. A panel of independent clinicians and administrators may also be authorized to adjudicate treatment refusals.

States requiring a court hearing prior to the involuntary administration of psychotropic medication approach this adjudication somewhat differently. Some require that the patient be determined incapable of consenting to medication, as well as that medication be clinically indicated and the most appropriate form of treatment for the patient. Other states do not require that the patient be adjudicated incapacitated to consent to treatment prior to involuntary treatment but do require a court hearing where the appropriateness of medication is reviewed.

Courts which have addressed the authority of the guardian to consent to the use of medication for the incompetent patient have reached different conclusions. Most jurisdictions will permit substitute decision making by the guardian. In a few states, such as Massachusetts and Colorado, court approval must be obtained by the guardian to override the patient's decision to refuse medication. At least in Massachusetts, the substitute decision maker must attempt to ascertain what the patient would decide if he were competent to do so, rather than simply deciding what is in the patient's best medical interest. In these states, interpretation of the guardian's authority is based in part on specific state law.

For the mental health professional who is confronted with a treatment-refusing patient, it is critical to be aware of the current applicable law. Both law and practice in this area differ widely among jurisdictions. Reviewing the state statute or regulations will not necessarily be sufficient to understand one's obligations, authority, or limitations. The professional should become familiar with any court decisions interpreting a psychiatric patient's right to refuse medication. In states where so many patients are permitted to refuse treatment that the care of all patients is seriously compromised, the state legislature may be sensitive to modifying its civil commitment statute, similar to the practice in Utah to deny the committed patient this right.

6. *Clinical Aspects of Medication Refusal*

An inpatient's refusal of psychotropic medication often has profound implications for his treatment and that of other patients, as well as the work and morale of hospital staff. This section will discuss some of the reasons for medication refusal and some of the clinical strategies for dealing with a patient who refuses medication.

Hospitalized patients who refuse their psychotropic medication often refuse other aspects of their care and treatment. Patients may refuse to take showers, to change clothes, to eat their meals, and to attend individual and group therapy sessions. Thus, medication refusal may be one component of a much more global phenomenon, particularly when the patient is severely mentally ill.

Estimates vary widely of the prevalence of medication refusal by psychiatric inpatients. Between one quarter and one-half of patients have reportedly refused psychotropic medication at some time during their hospitalization, according to some research. Few of these patients refuse on such a continuous basis that administrative or judicial proceedings to override the refusal are required.

Little research has been performed to document the reasons for refusal of psychotropic medication, but several categories of refusal have been proposed: (1) illness-based refusals, (2) treatment-based refusals, and (3) refusals related to the doctor–patient relationship.

Many psychiatric patients refuse psychotropic medication, particularly antipsychotic medication, because of the symptomatology of their illness. This includes denial of the illness and the need for treatment, as well as specific psychiatric symptoms related to the medication: delusional thinking of a grandiose or persecutory nature, thought disturbance which interferes with the ability to accept treatment, euphoria from an affective disorder, or psychotic depression with suicide intention.

Other patients refuse medication because of factors related to the treatment itself. These include medication side effects such as movement disorders (tremor, dystonia, and tardive dyskinesia), restlessness, sedation, dysphoria, dry mouth, and weight gain, among many others caused by the antipsychotic medications. Patients may also have unrealistic fears about the route of medication administration; an intramuscular injection, for example, may be seen as a bodily assault. Further, refusal of treatment provides significant benefits to many patients of a tangible nature (continued hospitalization) and an intangible nature (maintenance of equilibrium in a psychotic state).

Finally, some patients refuse prescribed medication because of factors in their relationship with the treatment staff. These entail both transference and reality-based considerations, such as a need for emotional distance from the staff, reactions to experiences of separation and loss with regard to staff members, and staff abuse or neglect. Also included in this context are refusals stemming from the pressure of family members and other patients to avoid treatment.

Among all classes of psychotropic medication, the refusal of antipsychotic medications presents the greatest potential management problem for hospital staff. It is of interest, then, that this medication class more than any other is available to be administered by injection. In the past, physicians have been able to use this factor as an opportunity to write medication orders which authorized involuntary injections of medication when a patient refused an oral dose. Articulation of the patient's right to refuse medication in nonemergencies has, in most cases, obviated such a solution to medication refusal.

It should be clear from the above that a patient's treatment refusal initially requires a thorough exploration of the relevant issues: the illness, the treatment, and the treatment relationships. This frequently requires spending a considerable period of time with the patient, close family members, and various staff to collect and evaluate the data. Specific strategies for managing refusals will depend upon the reasons for the refusals. Some illness-related or treatment-related refusals can be relatively easily dealt with by changing medication type and dosage; other refusals clearly demand much more of a commitment in time and energy from staff. Efforts to educate the patient and the family about the nature of the illness and the need for treatment may also be helpful. Family members even more than staff are sometimes able to reassure the patient about the safety of treatment and convince him to comply with the recommended care.

Each jurisdiction's system for adjudicating medication refusals will carry its own problems and opportunities. Assessments of medical decision-making capacity and dangerousness to self or others may be required; these can be complex and require a review of prior treatment documents and sometimes consultation with colleagues. Use of independent psychiatric reviewers may decrease the patient's hostility or resistance to treatment and may provide an opportunity for increased dialogue between treatment team and staff. A requirement that patients be formally adjudicated incompetent to refuse medication, followed by appointment of a guardian, will typically entail significant delays in treatment. Staff must attempt to maintain their therapeutic alliance with the patient and persist in attempting to engage in treatment with the patient throughout this refusal period. Staff should also be alert to a patient's increased likelihood of violent or suicidal episodes because of regression during such refusals. *It should be remembered that psychotropic medication can be administered in an emergency, and in many jurisdictions, emergency is defined broadly.*

Staff need to carefully document in the record the patient data relevant to the treatment refusal and the staff's response to it. This includes the patient's stated reasons for refusal, frequency of treatment refusal, diagnostic formulation of the treatment refusal, rationale for the proposed treatment, staff attempts to achieve consent and compliance, consultations, and administrative or legal proceedings.

Managing the voluntarily admitted patient who refuses medication presents somewhat different problems. Because of long-term refusal, some patients are clearly too ill to be discharged from hospital care, though they may not meet civil commitment criteria. Pursuit of an incompetency determination may be helpful in such cases. In others, some patients simply tire of prolonged hospitalization and become compliant with medication in order to be discharged.

Finally, contending with the treatment needs of a refusing patient in an emergency situation presents other problems. As noted, emergency medication is sometimes restricted to the occurrence or threat of serious physical harm to the patient or others. More discretion is provided to the treating physician when emergency medication is authorized in psychological emergencies. In either case, the physician must determine the duration of the emergency for the purpose of authorizing medication. In the former case, a short course of emergency medication, rather than a single oral or intramuscular dose, may be permissible. However, it is important to remember that an "emergency" cannot last the entire course of the hospitalization. It should be viewed as something requiring immediate action.

7. Conclusion: Right to Refuse Medication

Although the right to refuse medication has become a highly controversial topic in the mental health law field during the past decade, it should be placed in perspective. In general, few patients consistently refuse treatment for any significant length of time. In some cases, the refusal is the patient's attempt to signal a problem with the medication or the treatment, and it presents an opportunity to review the entire treatment plan. Most courts which have adjudicated treatment refusals in particular cases have deferred to the judgment of the mental health professional, although they have recognized the constitutional right of a competent mentally ill person to refuse medication in a nonemergency situation. Given the relatively narrow definitions of a psychiatric emergency in many cases, only minimal emergency treatment can usually be accomplished, though some brief periods of treatment are possible. Even when an emergency is not present, the staff have the option of having the individual declared incompetent and seeking a court order for overriding a medication refusal. Thus, it is unlikely that state institutions will become filled with patients who are not being treated because of their refusals. It is more likely that processing and adjudicating medication refusals represent a mixed blessing: an opportunity to improve the quality of care for the patient, and interference with providing treatment, which to some extent increases the risk of physical harm to patients and staff and prolongs the patient's hospitalization.

B. Legal Regulation of Electroconvulsive Therapy

The use of electroconvulsive therapy (ECT) has provoked considerable controversy within both the legal and the medical communities for many years, in large part because of actual and alleged abuses of this procedure which occurred in the 1950s and 1960s. The public image of ECT is in part derived from film, drama, and media portrayals in which the hero is committed to a psychiatric hospital for antisocial behavior and then administered ECT as punishment when he refuses to conform to the hospital regimen. Mention of ECT to the uninformed conjures up visions of an individual with electrodes attached to his head who becomes permanently incapacitated as a result of the procedure. Many of its most energetic detractors, though, are in the medical community. Yet ECT clearly has a place as a contemporary psychiatric treatment, particularly for severe, medication-refractory depressive disorders.

Because of lingering memories of antiquated procedures and misuse, it is common to find state regulation of ECT, with an occasional attempt to ban the procedure entirely. Most such statutes provide that ECT can be administered if a written informed consent is obtained from the patient. Many provisions specifically give the patient the right to refuse its use. If the patient is incompetent, then a court order or a guardian's consent must be obtained to give the ECT over the patient's refusal. In life-threatening psychiatric emergencies in some states, ECT can be administered without a patient's or a guardian's consent, though such consent, or a court order, should then be obtained. Massachusetts and Texas limit the number of treatments that can be administered to a patient each year. Other states prescribe a set of procedures for physicians to follow prior to initiating treatment. These may include obtaining independent psychiatric reviews of the need for ECT, disclosure of specific risk and benefit information to patients, and documentation in the medical record. Some states limit the use of ECT for certain psychiatric disorders or age groups.

In recent years, some of the furor over ECT has subsided. ECT is used relatively infrequently compared to psychotropic medication, and the problems which arose in earlier years have been remedied by more advanced anesthetic techniques. Strict regulation of the use of ECT in some states has resulted in its abandonment by physicians because of inordinate procedural demands, resulting in deprivation of treatment for some patients. In other states, particularly in the public sector, lack of financial resources restricts its availability. Thus, it is unlikely that there will be much litigation in this area in the form of claims for improper treatment or negligence. In fact, the image of ECT as a dangerous treatment typically used for mildly disordered patients and punitive purposes is no longer accurate. ECT is an effective treatment which carries little medical or legal risk when administered under proper medical supervision and with proper consent. (See Chapter 6 for liability for lack of informed consent for ECT.)

C. Legal Regulation of Restraints and Seclusion

The use of physical restraints and seclusion is widely accepted in facilities for the mentally ill and the mentally retarded. Yet their value as a treatment method has been questioned by both mental health professionals and patient advocates. Significant restrictions have been imposed by both courts and state legislatures in response to real or potential abuses in their use. For those who view these practices as worthy, the restrictions in the form of procedural requirements represent troublesome interference with treatment. In contrast, for those who view restraints and seclusion as punitive, anything short of their prohibition is inadequate.

1. *The Case Law*

The use of restraints or seclusion within facilities for the mentally disabled has prompted several legal challenges in facilities for the mentally ill and for the mentally retarded. Often these challenges have been made in the context of lawsuits attacking a wide range of alleged abuses within the hospital and attempting to establish a panoply of rights for the patients of the facility. Most cases have cited specific examples of abuses in the use of restraints or seclusion. In general, the cases or consent decrees provide that restraints or seclusion can be used only when the disabled person could harm himself or others and there is no less restrictive alternative available to control this danger. Other common elements in the legal decisions are that (1) restraints and seclusion may be imposed only pursuant to a written order by a physician; (2) such orders authorizing restraints and seclusion must be limited in time; (3) the physician or nursing staff must periodically evaluate or monitor the patient's condition and document their findings in the patient's record; and (4) if orders are extended beyond the initial period, the extension must be authorized by a physician, often with mandatory review by the medical director or superintendent when restraints or seclusion have been used for several consecutive days.

The courts have held that patients have not only an interest in freedom from bodily restraint, but also an interest in their personal safety and that of other patients. The U.S. Supreme Court, in *Youngberg v. Romeo* in 1982, realized that "the question . . . is not simply whether a liberty interest has been infringed but whether the extent or nature of the restraint or lack of absolute safety is such as to violate due process." In determining whether the state's use of restraints and seclusion has unconstitutionally infringed upon a patient's liberty interest, the Court deferred to accepted professional judgment. It held that a court must be certain that "professional judgment in fact was exercised"; that is, liability for the improper use of restraints and seclusion "may be imposed only when the decision by the professional is such a substantial departure from accepted professional judgment, practice or standard as to demonstrate that the person responsible actually did not base the decision on such a judgment." Clearly, the Court attempted to avoid substituting its judgment for that of the clinician.

2. *Statutory Requirements*

Most states have enacted statutes regulating the use of restraints which generally specify the circumstances under which their use is permitted, most often when the person presents a serious risk of harm to himself or others. Some states also permit the use of restraints in nonemergencies for therapeutic purposes. Those states that do not have statutes concerning the use of restraints usually have administrative regulations on the matter. In those states with statutory law on physical restraints, administrative regulations are likely to elaborate on the procedures to be followed when restraints are employed.

Statutory regulation of the use of locked seclusion is less common than the regulation of physical restraints. Only about one-half the states have laws related to seclusion. Statutory provisions include the necessity for a physician's or psychologist's order to initiate locked seclusion and monitoring of the patient in seclusion. The staff must also document the reasons for using seclusion.

Voluntarily admitted patients may also require restraints and seclusion in emergency situations. It may then be necessary to certify the patient for involuntary admission, depending upon local regulation and statute, since a voluntary patient is presumed to have a right to refuse treatment and to request discharge from the hospital. In other jurisdictions, use of short-term emergency seclusion or restraint for voluntary patients is permissible without certification and subsequent commitment.

3. *Clinical Guidelines for Meeting Legal Requirements*

The use of physical controls over mentally disabled individuals in hospitals or emergency rooms is clinically indicated in several situations: (1) to prevent serious imminent harm to the patient or others when other preventive techniques are inappropriate or ineffective; (2) to prevent serious physical damage to the hospital environment or significant disruption of the treatment program; (3) as a component of a behavior therapy treatment program; and (4) at the request of a patient.

Emergency locked seclusion and restraints to prevent serious physical harm to patients and staff are sometimes used in several types of situations. Emergency controls may be used following an actual, attempted, or threatened violent incident, or when violent behavior is imminent. Controls may also be used in the absence of a recent history of violence when future violent behavior is imminent, though clinical inaccuracies in predicting future conduct make this use more problematic. A patient's sudden and severe clinical regression may suggest such an outcome. Use of physical controls after an episode of violent behavior but without an expectation of imminent future violence would be inappropriate as it would be punitive.

The requirement that locked seclusion and restraints be the least restrictive of the patient's rights presents several problems for mental health professionals who manage violent and disruptive patients. As noted in Chapter 4, there is no clear parallel between the "restrictiveness" of interventions and their therapeutic efficacy. There are likely to be divergent views among mental health professionals, for example, about the hierarchy of intrusiveness of locked seclusion, restraints, and involuntary/injected antipsychotic medication. In many cases, there are also likely to be differing clinical opinions about the choice of treatment for a disruptive or violent patient. Clinicians in such cases are encouraged to clearly conceptualize and document the reasons for their treatment choices whatever they may be.

Use of locked seclusion and restraints in a behavior treatment program in nonemergency situations is more complex from both a clinical and a legal perspective. A behavior technique which uses seclusion and restraint to reduce target behaviors consisting of disruptive and violent behavior is more easily justified from a legal standpoint than a behavior program which is used for other purposes. Treatment plans should specify when seclusion and restraints will be used in a behavior treatment program. In any event, there may be questions about a competent patient's right to refuse the physical controls in a nonemergency. Such dilemmas may be partially addressed by informed-consent procedures or statutory authorization for seclusion and restraint in behavior modification programs.

Clinicians who use restraints or seclusion are well advised to be familiar with the specific requirements of the law and regulations in their jurisdiction. Many state regulations dictate the procedures that are required for ordering physical controls and monitoring their use. In their absence, clinicians should use promulgated standards in the mental health professions. A 1985 American Psychiatric Association Task Force Report, for example, reviewed the indications, contraindications, and techniques of the psychiatric use of seclusion and restraints. According to these standards, a patient placed in seclusion or restraints for the first time should be personally evaluated by a physician within three hours of the initiation of the seclusion or restraint episode. The physician should reevaluate the patient at least every 12 hours, while nursing staff observations of the patient should be made every 15 minutes. Use of such guidelines, in conjunction with repeated careful clinical assessment of the patient's physical and emotional functioning, is likely to be a significant protection against a patient's subsequent claim of negligence or violation of civil rights, as well as against an injured party's claim of negligent failure to protect. Thorough documentation in the patient's medical record, by all evaluators and consultants, of the indications for physical controls, lack of contraindications, and absence of treatment alternatives is mandatory.

D. Legal Regulation of Behavior Modification

As noted above, behavior modification procedures employ a series of techniques to alter specific behavior. These techniques assume various forms and are used in a variety of settings, including psychiatric institutions, facilities for the developmentally disabled, prisons, and classrooms. In some settings, techniques such as aversive conditioning may raise questions of appropriateness and efficacy.

Several lawsuits have challenged the use, within prisons and mental institutions, of behavior modification techniques, most commonly the aversive procedures, in which an unpleasant event is imposed each time the individual exhibits inappropriate behavior. Particular targets of the litigation have been the administration of electrical shock and drugs that cause nausea and vomiting. One issue has been whether the objective of the procedure is indeed behavior modification or is punishment that is disproportionate to the violation of the rules.

At present, there is relatively little regulation of the use of specific behavioral treatment techniques. A few states regulate aversive techniques, while more states regulate restraints and seclusion as part of a behavior modification program. With the exception of a few challenges to the use of token economies, there has been almost no litigation in this area. The therapist who employs behavior modification techniques should make them part of the patient's treatment plan and treatment program. The technique employed should not be physically harmful to the patient, and its effectiveness in terms of the treatment goals should be apparent. The patient's or guardian's informed consent to a behavioral treatment should also be obtained.

E. Legal Regulation of Psychosurgery

Psychosurgery is the application of surgical techniques to the treatment of psychiatric problems. These techniques may include brain surgery, implantation of electrodes, destruction or stimulation of brain tissue, or the direct application of substances to the brain. These techniques are not ordinarily considered the same as the surgical treatment of demonstrated neurologically based mental disorders such as seizure disorder, brain tumors, and parkinsonism. At present, psychosurgery is viewed as a hazardous procedure for the treatment of mental illness. Its efficacy is undocumented, though it is perhaps more accepted as a treatment for intractable pain. Psychosurgical procedures of the 1940s and 1950s, such as frontal lobotomy or prefrontal leucotomy, have been superseded by stereotactic limbic leucotomy, subcaudate tractotomy, and amygdalotomy. Psychosurgical techniques have been used for the treatment of affective disorders, anxiety disorders, schizophrenic disorders, sexual deviations, and behavior disorders.

In the early 1970s, a proposal to use psychosurgery on a hospitalized person in Michigan brought the public's attention to this issue. In this case, *Kaimowitz v. Department of Mental Health (Michigan)*, the court ruled that "psychosurgery should never be undertaken upon involuntarily committed populations, when there is a high risk–low benefits ratio" as was demonstrated in that case. The court then forbade the procedure.

Kaimowitz resulted in a great deal of legal commentary about psychosurgery and resulted in the majority of states' enacting laws restricting its use. Most of the laws provide that psychosurgery may not be performed without the patient's written, informed consent, thereby foreclosing the debate on whether a mentally disabled individual can refuse treatment. Other states require that if the patient is incompetent to consent to treatment, then psychosurgery can be performed only with the consent of the court. Patients who refuse psychosurgical procedures are highly unlikely to be coerced to undergo such treatment.

At this time, psychosurgery is not a customary form of treatment for functional psychiatric disorders in North America. With rapid advances in medicine, however, it is possible that, in the future, some form of psychosurgery will become an accepted procedure for treating some mental disturbances. Once the benefits of the surgery are clear and the risks to the patient are minimal, or the surgery appears to provide the only opportunity for treatment, then it will become easier to perform psychosurgery without as much concern about legal regulation or restriction.

VI. COMMONLY ASKED QUESTIONS

1. How long can psychotropic medication be administered during a psychiatric emergency?

Probably no state law delineates the duration of a psychiatric emergency for the purpose of overriding a patient's refusal of psychotropic medication. In effect, psychotropic medication can be administered for as long as the emergency exists. The determination of how long the emergency lasts is a clinical one. The practice of administering only a single dose of antipsychotic medication following an episode of violent behavior in a severely mentally ill individual may represent inadequate treatment of that emergency. On the other hand, use of a long-acting, depot form of antipsychotic medication may be more questionable, since such use represents treatment for a prolonged period of time, perhaps two to six weeks, possibly extending beyond the emergency period. Staff should document in the record the reason for defining the situation as an emergency. If the emergency continues for more than 24 hours, there should continue to be sufficient documentation supporting the clinical finding of an "emergency."

2. Can a hospitalized patient refuse customary medical procedures like blood tests and physical examinations?

Routine diagnostic medical procedures such as physical examination and phlebotomy are usually necessary upon admission to a psychiatric hospital, and they may need to be repeated subsequently during the hospitalization if the patient's medical condition significantly changes. Depending upon local regulation or statute, it is likely that a mentally ill person hospitalized on an emergency basis or civilly committed has no right to refuse such accepted and relatively innocuous measures. A legally competent and voluntarily admitted patient usually has the right to refuse such procedures, except in an emergency situation. Voluntarily or involuntarily hospitalized, legally competent patients can refuse more invasive medical diagnostic procedures (e.g., lung biopsy, bone marrow biopsy), and a court determination of decision-making incapacity must usually be obtained.

3. Must the hospital staff retain a voluntary patient in the hospital when he continually refuses psychotropic medication?

There is probably no law which requires hospital staff to either retain or discharge a voluntarily admitted patient from the hospital when the patient persistently refuses antipsychotic medication. The staff's course of conduct should, however, be dictated by standard psychiatric practice. Staff should first carefully assess the patient's mental status and behavior to determine whether civil commitment is appropriate. At the commitment hearing in some jurisdictions, staff can request a court order for compulsory medication. If commitment is not appropriate, staff should assess the patient's ability to function outside of the hospital and consider involuntarily discharging the patient. Clinicians should be familiar with the available resources in the community in determining whether the patient can safely manage to live outside the hospital. In some cases, rather than discharge the patient, it may be clinically necessary to proceed to override the patient's refusal through the appropriate administrative and judicial procedures when the patient appears incompetent to refuse the medication.

4. *Should hospital or clinic staff inform a patient about the risk of tardive dyskinesia when antipsychotic medication is prescribed?*

The legal doctrine of informed consent requires that a patient be informed of the risks, benefits, and alternatives to psychiatric treatment, including the use of psychotropic medication. State law will not specify which risks of treatment must be disclosed to a psychiatric patient when he is treated with antipsychotic medication. Because of the relative frequency and seriousness of tardive dyskinesia following the long-term use of antipsychotic medication, however, it may be considered either negligence or a failure to obtain valid informed consent if one fails to disclose this risk to the patient. Because patients appear to have difficulty in acknowledging this risk, as well as the presence of tardive dyskinesia, it is usually necessary to repeatedly discuss this possibility with the patient. Such disclosures should also be made to the guardian of a legally incompetent patient who is treated with antipsychotic medication, including minors and the mentally retarded. Because a patient may be unable to understand this risk of treatment when he is initially admitted to a hospital, it is usually acceptable to defer disclosing this risk for a brief period of time until the patient has stabilized, particularly when the patient has received little or no prior exposure to antipsychotic medication. Such informed-consent discussions should be repeated on a periodic basis, depending on the clinical situation, perhaps every three to six months.

5. *Must patients sign written informed consent forms for psychotropic medication?*

As a result of consent decrees or state law, patients hospitalized in a psychiatric facility are sometimes required to sign written informed consent forms to the voluntary use of psychotropic medication, including lithium carbonate, tricyclic antidepressants, and antipsychotic medication. When not required by law, however, such documents are not recommended for the treatment of patients with psychotropic medication. Consent forms are typically used to document the informed consent to medical diagnostic and therapeutic procedures of an intrusive nature. Unfortunately, such forms are mistakenly used to substitute for the process of informed consent to treatment, rather than to serve as evidence of it. Without genuine communication between staff and the patient, they may fail to protect hospital or clinic staff against allegations of failure to obtain informed consent. Documentation of informed consent discussions should be recorded in the patient's medical record when they occur.

6. *Can hospital psychiatrists write medication "as needed" orders?*

The use of medication as needed (prn) orders by hospital medical and nursing staff raises problems. It may be unclear, for example, whether the medication is to be administered when the staff determine that it is indicated, or upon the patient's request. Use of prn medications administered intramuscularly often represents involuntary treatment which may be impermissible in a nonemergency. A patient's right to refuse antipsychotic medication applies equally to medication administered on the basis of a standing order and to medication administered "as needed."

7. Does the right to psychiatric treatment mean that an involuntarily hospitalized patient can select his own therapist from the hospital or the outside community?

If the patient is hospitalized in a publicly funded treatment facility, he will not be able to select the members of his treatment team. The right to treatment or habilitation has been construed to require some form of acceptable psychiatric evaluation and treatment, not one that may be ideal, nor one determined by the patient. The courts are concerned that a reasonable form of treatment be provided, rather than that the patient be satisfied with the treatment provider. However, if the patient has been hospitalized in a private facility, he may be able to select certain staff members who will be responsible for his care.

8. Can ECT be administered without a court order?

If the patient can provide an informed consent to treatment, then there is no need to obtain substituted consent. When the patient cannot provide informed consent to treatment with ECT, state laws require the consent of a surrogate decision maker. This may be a patient's family member, a legal guardian, or a specific court order. Even when the patient can give an informed consent, it is advisable to have a written consent from the closest relative.

9. Can a staff member file civil or criminal charges against a patient who has injured him?

Any injured person has the legal right to file charges against the party who caused the injury. It may be difficult, however, to prosecute the case because of the unwillingness of a prosecuting attorney to go forward with a criminal case. Similarly, a plaintiff's attorney may refuse to accept the case because the patient might not have the financial resources to pay a civil judgment. Civil or criminal prosecution of a patient may have a beneficial effect on the patient, other patients, the staff's willingness to work with difficult patients, and the hospital milieu, though it may interfere with the therapeutic alliance. Other clinical and administrative interventions to deter violent behavior in the hospital are also useful.

10. Can staff discharge their obligations to obtain informed consent to treatment from a patient by only answering the patient's questions?

No. The informed consent doctrine requires that the therapist adequately inform the patient about the proposed treatment. The therapist bears the burden to inform, rather than the patient. The patient may not think to ask the proper questions, or may be afraid to do so. The therapist should answer any questions, but not rely on the patient to ask them in the first place.

VII. BIBLIOGRAPHY

I. Right to Treatment

A. Cases

Rouse v. Cameron, 373 F.2d 451 (D.C. Cir. 1966).
Wyatt v. Stickney, 325 F.Supp. 781 (1971); 344 F.Supp. 373 (Ala. 1972); 344 F.Supp. 387 (Ala. 1972).
Donaldson v. O'Connor, 493 F.2d 507 (5th Cir. 1974).

Wyatt v. Aderholt, 503 F.2d 1305 (5th Cir. 1974).
O'Connor v. Donaldson, 422 U.S. 563 (1975).
State v. Brosseau, 470 A.2d 869 (N.H. 1983).
Arnold v. Arizona Dept. of Health Services, 775 P.2d 521 (Ariz. 1989).
K.C. v. State, 771 P.2d 774 (Wyo. 1989).
Mahoney v. Lensink, 569 A.2d 518 (Sup.Ct. Conn. 1990).

B. *Articles and Books*

Baldwin, D. (1975). *O'Connor v. Donaldson:* Involuntary civil commitment and the right to treatment. *Columbia Human Rights Law Review, 7,* 573–589.
Birnbaum, M. (1960). The right to treatment. *American Bar Association Journal, 46,* 499–505.
Freddolino, P. P., Moxley, D. P., & Fleishman, J. A. (1989). An advocacy model for people with long-term psychiatric disabilities. *Hospital and Community Psychiatry, 40,* 1169–1174.
Garvey, J. H. (1981). Freedom and choice in constitutional law. *Harvard Law Review, 94,* 1756–1794.
Geller, J. L., Fisher, W. H., Simon, L. J., & Wirth-Cauchon, J. L. (1990). Second-generation deinstitutionalization: 2. The impact of *Brewster v. Dukakis* on correlates of community and hospital utilization. *American Journal of Psychiatry, 147,* 988–993.
Geller, J. L., Fisher, W. H., Wirth-Cauchon, J. L., & Simon, L. J. (1990). Second-generation deinstitutionalization: 1. The impact of *Brewster v. Dukakis* on state hospital case mix. *American Journal of Psychiatry, 147,* 982–987.
Hoffman, P. B., & Dunn, R. C. (1976). Guaranteeing the right to treatment. *Psychiatric Annals, 6,* 258–282.
Jones, L. R., & Parlour, R. R. (Eds). (1981). *Wyatt v. Stickney retrospect and prospect.* New York: Grune & Stratton.
Katz, J. (1969). The right to treatment-an enchanting legal fiction? *University of Chicago Law Review, 36,* 755–783.
Kaufman, E. (1979). The right to treatment suit as an agent of change. *American Journal of Psychiatry, 136,* 1428–1432.
Leaf, P. (1977). *Wyatt v. Stickney:* Assessing the impact in Alabama. *Hospital and Community Psychiatry, 28,* 351–369.
Lipscomb, N. I. (1975–1976). "Without more": A constitutional right to treatment. *Loyola Law Review, 22,* 373–383.
Mills, M. J. (1982). The right to treatment: Little law but much impact. In L. Grinspoon (Ed.), *Psychiatry 1982 annual review.* Washington, DC: American Psychiatric Association.
Nordwind, B. L. (1982). Developing an enforceable "right to treatment" theory for the chronically mentally disabled in the community. *Schizophrenia Bulletin, 8,* 642–651.
North, B. S. (1974). A patient involuntarily civilly committed to a state mental hospital has a constitutional right to treatment. *Villanova Law Review, 20,* 214–225.
Okin, R. L. (1984). *Brewster v. Dukakis:* Developing community services through use of a consent decree. *American Journal of Psychiatry, 141,* 786–789.
Rapson, R. (1980). The right of the mentally ill to receive treatment in the community. *Columbia Journal of Law and Social Problems, 16,* 193–268.
Spece, R. G. (1978). Preserving the right to treatment: A critical assessment and constructive development of constitutional rights to treatment theories. *Arizona Law Review 20,* 1–47.
Stone, A. A. (1975). Overview: The right to treatment-comments on the law and its impact. *American Journal of Psychiatry, 132,* 1125–1135.
Weiner, B. A. (1985). Treatment rights. In S. J. Brakel, J. Parry, & B. A. Weiner (Eds.), *The mentally disabled and the law* (3rd ed.). Chicago: American Bar Foundation.
Wolpe, P. R., Schwartz, S. L., & Sanford, B. (1991). Psychiatric inpatients' knowledge of their rights. *Hospital and Community Psychiatry, 42,* 1168–1169.

II. Right to Habilitation

A. *Cases*

Wyatt v. Stickney, 344 F.Supp. 387 (M.D. Ala. 1972).
Davis v. Watkins, 384 F.Supp. 1196 (N.D. Ohio 1974).
Welsch v. Likins, 373 F.Supp. 487 (D. Minn. 1974).

New York Association for Retarded Citizens v. Carey, 393 F.Supp. 715 (1975).
Youngberg v. Romeo, 457 U.S. 307 (1982).
Halderman v. Pennhurst State School and Hospital, 446 F.Supp. 1295 (E.D. Pa. 1977); 612 F.2d 84 (3rd Cir. 1979); 101 S.Ct. 1531 (1981); 673 F.2d 647 (3rd Cir. 1982); 104 S.Ct. 900 (1984); 610 F.Supp. 1221 (D.C.Pa. 1985); 901 F.2d 311 (3rd Cir. 1990); 784 F. Supp. 215 (E.D.Pa. 1992).
Jackson v. Fort Stanton Hospital & Training School, 757 F.Supp. 1243 (N.M. 1990).

B Articles and Books

Breck, D. S. (1982). The "right" to habilitation: *Pennhurst State School & Hospital v. Halderman* and *Youngberg v. Romeo. Connecticut Law Review, 14*, 557–583.
Dietz, P. P. (1984). The constitutional right to treatment in light of *Youngberg v. Romeo. Georgetown Law Journal, 72*, 1785–1816.
Esposito, V. M. (1980). The constitutional right to treatment services for the noncommitted mentally disabled. *University of San Francisco Law Review, 14*, 675–705.
Ferleger, D. (1983). Anti-institutionalization and the Supreme Court. *Rutgers Law Journal, 14*, 595–636.
Gallo, L. V. (1982). *Youngberg v. Romeo:* The right to treatment dilemma and the mentally retarded. *Albany Law Review, 47*, 179–213.
Herr, S. S. (1983). *Rights and advocacy for retarded people.* Lexington, MA: D. C. Heath, Lexington Books.
Herr, S. S., Arons, S., & Wallace, R. E. (1983). *Legal rights and mental health care.* Lexington, MA: Lexington Books.
Kindred, M., Cohen, J., Penrod, D., & Shaffer, T. (Eds.). (1976). *The mentally retarded citizen and the law.* New York: Free Press.
Mason, B. G., Menolascino, F. J., & Galvin, L. (1976). Mental health: The right to treatment for mentally retarded citizens. *Creighton Law Review, 10*, 124–166.
Symposium. (1979). Mentally retarded people and the law. *Stanford Law Review, 31*(4), 541–829.

III. Informed Consent

A. Cases

Salgo v. Leland Stanford Jr. University, 317 P.2d 170 (Cal.App. 1957). [aortography]
Woods v. Brumlop, 377 P.2d 520 (N.M. 1962). [ECT]
Mitchell v. Robinson, 334 S.W.2d 11 (Mo. 1960), affirmed after retrial, 360 S.W.2d 673 (Mo. 1962). [insulin coma]
In the matter of W.S., Jr., 377 A.2d 969 (N.J. 1977). [ECT]
Truman v. Thomas, 62 P.2d 902 (Cal. 1980). [diagnostic testing]
Gundy v. Pauley, 619 S.W.2d 730 (Ky. 1981). [ECT]
Clites v. Iowa, 322 N.W.2d 917 (Iowa 1982). [medication]
Lojuk v. Quandt, 706 F.2d 1456 (7th Cir. 1983). [ECT]
Lillian F. v. Superior Court, 206 Cal.Rptr. 603 (1984). [ECT]
In re Fadley, 205 Cal.Rptr. 572 (1984). [ECT]
In the matter of Kinzer, 375 N.W.2d 526 (Minn. 1985). [ECT]
Barclay v. Campbell, 704 S.W.2d 8 (Tex. 1986). [medication]
Frasier v. Department of Health, 500 So.2d 858 (La. 1986). [medication]
San Diego v. Waltz, 227 Cal.Rptr. 436 (1986). [ECT]
In re Schuoler, 723 P.2d 1103 (Wash. 1986). [ECT]
Shinn v. St. James Mercy Hospital, 675 F.Supp. 94 (W.D. N.Y. 1987). [medication]
Whittle v. U.S., 669 F.Supp. 501 (D.D.C. 1987). [medication]
Dooley v. Skodnek, 529 N.Y.S.2d (A.D. 1988). [medication]
Adams v. Allen, 783 P.2d 635 (Wash.App. 1989). [medication]
Nolen v. Peterson, 544 So.2d 863 (Sup.Ct. Ala. 1989). [medication]
Barnhart v. United States, 884 F.2d 295 (7th Cir. 1989). [medication]
Steck v. Henderson Mental Health Center, Inc., 539 So.2d 1173 (Fla.App. 1989). [medication]
In the Matter of Zuckerman, 477 N.W.2d 523 (Minn.App. 1991). [CT scan and blood test]
Annotation: Modern status of views as to general measure of physician's duty to inform patient of risks of proposed treatment, 88 A.L.R.3rd 1008.

B. Articles and Books

Appelbaum, P. S. (1984). Informed consent. In D. N. Weisstub (Ed.), *Law and Mental Health, Vol 1*, pp. 45–83. New York: Pergamon Press.
Appelbaum, P. S., & Grisso, T. (1988). Assessing patients' capacities to consent to treatment. *New England Journal of Medicine, 319*, 1635–1638.
Appelbaum, P. S., & Roth, L. H. (1981). Clinical issues in the assessment of competency. *American Journal of Psychiatry, 138*, 1462–1467.
Appelbaum, P. S., Lidz, C. W., & Meisel, A. (1987). *Informed consent*. New York: Oxford University Press.
Benson, P. R. (1984). Informed consent: Drug information disclosed to patients prescribed antipsychotic medication. *Journal of Nervous and Mental Disease, 172*, 642–653.
Clary, C., Dever, A., & Schweizer, E. (1992). Psychiatric inpatients' knowledge of medication at hospital discharge. *Hospital and Community Psychiatry, 43*, 140–144.
Cohen, D. L., Kessel, R. W. I., McCullough, L. B., Apostolides, A. Y., & Heiderich, K. J. (1990). Informed consent and the "medical student psychiatrist." *Academic Medicine, 65*, 127–128.
Culver, C. M., & Gert, B. (1982). *Philosophy in medicine: Conceptual and ethical issues in medicine and psychiatry*. New York: Oxford University Press.
Drane, J. F. (1985). The many faces of competency. *Hastings Center Report, 15*, 17–21.
Faden, R. F., & Beauchamp, T. L. (1986). *A history and theory of informed consent*. New York: Oxford University Press.
Grisso, T., & Appelbaum, P. S. (1991). Mentally ill and non-mentally ill patients' abilities to understand informed consent disclosures for medication. *Law and Human Behavior, 15*, 377–388.
Gurian, B. S., Baker. E. H., Jacobson, S., Lagerbom, B., & Watts, P. (1990). Informed consent for neuroleptics with elderly patients in two settings. *Journal of the American Geriatrics Society, 38*, 37–44.
Gutheil, T. G., & Bursztajn, H. (1986). Clinicians' guidelines for assessing and presenting subtle forms of patient incompetence in legal settings. *American Journal of Psychiatry, 143*, 1020–1023.
Gutheil, T. G., Bursztajn, H., & Brodsky, A. (1984). Malpractice prevention through the sharing of uncertainty. *New England Journal of Medicine, 311*, 49–51.
Handelsman, M. M., & Galvin, M. D. (1988). Facilitating informed consent for outpatient psychotherapy: A suggested written format. *Professional Psychology: Research and Practice, 19*, 223–225.
Handelsman, M. M., Kemper, M. B., Kesson-Craig, P., McLain, J., & Johnsrud, C. (1986). Use, content, and readability of written informed consent forms for treatment. *Professional Psychology: Research and Practice, 17*, 514–518.
Katz, J. (1977). Informed consent—A fairy tale? *University of Pittsburgh Law Review, 39*, 137–174.
Katz, J. (1984). *The silent world of doctor and patient*. New York: Free Press.
Kennedy, N. J., & Sanborn, J. S. (1992). Disclosure of tardive dyskinesia: Effect of written policy on risk disclosure. *Psychopharmacology Bulletin, 28*, 93–100.
Lidz, C. W., Appelbaum, P. S., & Meisel, A. (1988). Two models of implementing informed consent. *Archives of Internal Medicine, 148*, 1385–1389.
Lidz, C. W., Meisel, A., Zerubavel, E., Carter, M., Sestak, R. M., & Roth, L. H. (1984). *Informed consent: A study of decisionmaking in psychiatry*. New York: Guilford Press.
Meisel, A. (1979). The "exceptions" to the informed consent doctrine: Striking a balance between competing values in medical decisionmaking. *Wisconsin Law Review*, 413–488.
Meisel, A., Roth, L. R., & Lidz, C. W. (1977). Toward a model of the legal doctrine of informed consent. *American Journal of Psychiatry, 134*, 285–289.
Pavlo, A. M., Bursztajn, H., & Gutheil, T. G. (1987). Christian Science and competence to make treatment choices: Clinical challenges in assessing values. *International Journal of Law and Psychiatry, 10*, 395–401.
Pavlo, A. M., Bursztajn, H., Gutheil, T. G., & Levi, L. M. (1987). Weighing religious beliefs in determining competence. *Hospital and Community Psychiatry, 38*, 350–352.
Quaid, K. A., Faden, R. R., Vining, E. P., & Freeman, J. M. (1990). Informed consent for a prescription drug: Impact of disclosed information on patient understanding and medical outcomes. *Patient Education and Counseling, 15*, 249–259.
Quill, T. E. (1989). Recognizing and adjusting to barriers in doctor-patient communication. *Annals of Internal Medicine, 111*, 51–57.
Roth, L. H., Meisel, A., & Lidz, C. W. (1977). Tests of competency to consent to treatment. *American Journal of Psychiatry, 134*, 279–284.
Rozovsky, F. A. (1990). *Consent to treatment: A practical guide* (2nd ed.). Boston: Little, Brown.

Schwartz, H. I., & Blank, K. (1986). Shifting competency during hospitalization: A model for informed consent decisions. *Hospital and Community Psychiatry, 37*, 1256–1260.
Shugrue, R. E., & Linstromberg, K. (1991). The practitioner's guide to informed consent. *Creighton Law Review, 24*, 881–928.
Shultz, M. M. (1985). From informed consent to patient choice: A new protected interest. *Yale Law Journal, 95*, 219–299.
Stone, A. (1979). Informed consent: Special problems for psychiatry. *Hospital and Community Psychiatry, 30*, 321–327.
Twerski, A. D., & Cohen, N. B. (1988). Informed decision making and the law of torts: The myth of justiciable causation. *University of Illinois Law Review*, 607–665.
Wettstein, R. M. (1988). Informed consent and tardive dyskinesia. *Journal of Clinical Psychopharmacology, 8* (Suppl.), 65S-70S.
Wilcoxon, S. A. (1986). One-spouse marital therapy: Is informed consent necessary? *American Journal of Family Therapy, 14*, 265–270.

IV. Right to Refuse Treatment for a Mental Illness

A. *Cases*

Winters v. Miller, 446 F.2d 65 (2nd. Cir. 1971).
In re Boyd, 403 A.2d 774 (D.C. Ct.App. 1979).
Goedecke v. Colorado, 603 P.2d 123 (Colo. Sup.Ct. 1979).
Davis v. Hubbard, 506 F.Supp. 915 (N.D. Ohio 1980).
In re Mental Health of K.K.B., 609 P.2d 747 (Okla. Sup.Ct. 1980).
Wolfe v. Maricopa County General Hospital, 619 P.2d 1041 (Ariz. 1980).
Guardianship of Richard Roe, III., 421 N.E.2d 40 (Mass. Sup.Jud.Ct. 1981).
People v. Freeman, 636 P.2d 1334 (Colo.App. 1981).
A.E. & R.R. v. Mitchell, 724 F.2d 864 (10th Cir. 1983).
Anderson v. Arizona, 663 P.2d 570 (Ariz. 1983).
Jamison v. Farabee, No. C780445 WHO (N.D. Cal. 1983).
Opinion of the Justices, 465 A.2d 484 (N.H. Sup.Ct. 1983).
Rennie v. Klein, 462 F.Supp. 1131 (D.C. N.J. 1978); 476 F.Supp. 1294 (D.C. N.J. 1979); 653 F.2d 836 (3rd Cir. 1981); 720 F.2d 266 (3rd Cir. 1983).
Johnson v. Silvers, 742 F.2d 823 (4th. Cir. 1984).
Kolocotronis v. Ritterbusch, 667 S.W.2d 430 (Mo.App. 1984).
R.A.J. v. Miller, 590 F.Supp. 1319 (N.D.Tex. 1984).
Rogers v. Okin, 478 F.Supp. 1342 (Mass. 1979); 634 F.2d 650 (1st Cir. 1980); 102 S.Ct. 2442 (1982); 458 N.E.2d 308 (Mass Sup. Jud. Ct. 1983); 738 F.2d 1 (1st Cir. 1984).
Weiss v. Missouri Department of Mental Health, 587 F.Supp. 1157 (E.D. Mo. 1984).
Colorado v. Medina, 705 P.2d 961 (Colo. Sup.Ct. 1985).
In re L.R., 497 A.2d 753 (Vt. 1985).
Stensvad v. Reivitz, 601 F.Supp. 128 (Wis. 1985).
In re M.P., 500 N.E.2d 216 (Ind. Sup.Ct. 1986).
Rivers v. Katz, 495 N.E.2d 337 (N.Y. Ct.App. 1986).
Dautremont v. Broadlawns Hospital, 827 F.2d 291 (8th Cir. 1987).
In the Matter of Kolodrubetz, 411 N.W.2d 528 (Minn.App. 1987).
Riese v. St. Mary's Hospital, 243 Cal.Rptr. 241 (App. 1987).
State ex rel. Jones v. Gerhardstein, 416 N.W.2d 883 (Wis. Sup.Ct. 1987).
Hopkins v. Colorado, 772 P.2d 624 (Colo.App. 1988).
Jarvis v. Levine, 418 N.W.2d 139 (Minn. Sup.Ct. 1988).
In the Matter of Jeffrey Orr, 531 N.E.2d 64 (Ill.App. 1988).
U.S. v. Charters, 863 F.2d 302 (4th Cir. 1988).
Walters v. Western State Hospital, 864 F.2d 695 (10th Cir. 1988).
Colorado v. Gilliland, 769 P.2d 477 (Colo. Sup.Ct. 1989).
Matter of Lambert, 437 N.W.2d 106 (Minn.App. 1989).
Matter of Peterson, 446 N.W.2d 669 (Minn.App. 1989).
Matter of Steen, 437 N.W.2d 101 (Minn.App. 1989).
Nolen v. Peterson, 544 So.2d 863 (Sup.Ct. Ala. 1989).
Bee v. Greaves, 910 F.2d 686 (10th Cir. 1990).[prisoner refusal]
Matter of Axelrod, 560 N.Y.S.2d 573 (A.D.1990).

Washington v. Harper, 110 S.Ct. 1028 (1990).[prisoner refusal]
Williams v. Wilzack, 573 A.2d 809 (Md.Ct.App. 1990).
Bradshaw v. Idaho, 816 P.2d 986 (Idaho Sup.Ct. 1991).
Guardianship of Weedon, 565 N.E.2d 432 (Mass. Sup.Jud.Ct. 1991).
Matter of Mary Ann D, 578 N.Y.S.2d 622 (A.D. 1992)[lithium carbonate administered by nasogastric tube].
Guardianship of Roe, 583 N.E.2d 1282 (Mass. Sup.Jud.Ct. 1992).

B. Articles and Books

American Bar Association Commission on the Mentally Disabled. (1986). *The right to refuse antipsychotic medication*. Washington, DC: American Bar Association.
Appelbaum, P. S. (1988). The right to refuse treatment with antipsychotic medications: Retrospect and prospect. *American Journal of Psychiatry, 145*, 413–419.
Appelbaum, P. S., & Hoge, S. K. (1986). The right to refuse treatment: What the research reveals. *Behavioral Sciences and the Law, 4*, 279–292.
Ayd, F. J. (1985). Problems with orders for medication as needed. *American Journal of Psychiatry, 142*, 939–942.
Beck, J. C. (1987). Right to refuse antipsychotic medication: Psychiatric assessment and legal decision making. *Mental and Physical Disability Law Reporter, 11*, 368–372.
Brooks, A. D. (1980). The constitutional right to refuse antipsychotic medications. *Bulletin of the American Academy of Psychiatry and the Law, 8*, 179–221.
Brooks, A. D. (1987). The right to refuse antipsychotic medications: Law and policy. *Rutgers Law Review, 39*, 339–376.
Ciccone, J. R., Tokoli, J. F., Clements, C. D., & Gift, T. E. (1990). Right to refuse treatment: Impact of *Rivers v. Katz*. *Bulletin of the American Academy of Psychiatry and the Law, 18*, 203–215.
Cichon, D. E. (1989). The Eighth Circuit and professional judgment: Retrenchment of the constitutional right to refuse antipsychotic medication. *Creighton Law Review, 22*, 889–953.
Clayton, E. W. (1987). From *Rogers* to *Rivers*: The rights of the mentally ill to refuse medication. *American Journal of Law and Medicine, 13*, 7–52.
Cournos, F. (1989). Involuntary medication and the case of Joyce Brown. *Hospital and Community Psychiatry, 40*, 736–740.
Cournos, F., McKinnon, K., & Adams, C. (1988). A comparison of clinical and judicial procedures for reviewing requests for involuntary medication in New York. *Hospital and Community Psychiatry, 39*, 851–855.
DeLand, F. H., & Borenstein, N. M. (1990). Medicine Court: 2. *Rivers* in practice. *American Journal of Psychiatry, 147*, 38–43.
Doudera, A. E. & Swazey, J. P. (Eds.). (1982). *Refusing treatment in mental health institutions-values in conflict*. Ann Arbor, MI: AUPHA Press.
Faden, R., & Faden, A. (1977). False belief and the refusal of medical treatment. *Journal of Medical Ethics, 3*, 133–136.
Farnsworth, M. G. (1991). The impact of judicial review of patients' refusal to accept antipsychotic medications at the Minnesota Security Hospital. *Bulletin of the American Academy of Psychiatry and the Law, 19*, 33–42.
Ford, M. D. (1980). The psychiatrist's double bind: The right to refuse medication. *American Journal of Psychiatry, 137*, 332–339.
Gelman, S. (1984). Mental hospital drugs, professionalism, and the Constitution. *Georgetown Law Journal, 72*, 1725–1784.
Gurian, B. S., Baker, E. H., Jacobson, S., Lagerbom, B., & Watts, P. (1990). Informed consent for neuroleptics with elderly patients in two settings. *Journal of the American Geriatrics Society, 38*, 37–44.
Gutheil, T. G. (1985). *Rogers v. Commissioner:* Denouement of an important right to refuse treatment case. *American Journal of Psychiatry, 142*, 213–216.
Gutheil, T. G., & Appelbaum, P. S. (1983). "Mind control," "synthetic sanity," "artificial competence," and genuine confusion: Legally relevant effects of antipsychotic medication. *Hofstra Law Review, 12*, 77–120.
Gutheil, T. G., & Appelbaum, P. S. (1985). The substituted judgment approach: Its difficulties and paradoxes in mental health settings. *Law, Medicine and Health Care, 13*, 61–64.
Harmon, L. (1990). Falling off the vine: Legal fictions and the doctrine of substituted judgment. *Yale Law Journal, 100*, 1–71.

Hoge, S. K., Appelbaum, P. S., Lawlor, T., Beck, J. C., Litman, R., Green, A., Gutheil, T. G., & Kaplan, E. (1990). A prospective, multicenter study of patients' refusal of antipsychotic medication. *Archives of General Psychiatry, 47*, 949–956.
Litman, J. (1982). A common law remedy for forcible medication of the institutionalized mentally ill. *Columbia Law Review, 82*, 1720–1751.
McKinnon, K., Cournos, F., & Stanley, B. (1989). *Rivers* in practice: Clinicians' assessments of patients' decision-making capacity. *Hospital and Community Psychiatry, 40*, 1159–1162.
Mills, M. J. (1980). The rights of involuntary patients to refuse pharmacotherapy: What is reasonable? *Bulletin of the American Academy Psychiatry and the Law, 8*, 313–324.
Perlin, M. (1989 and Suppl.). *Mental disability law: Civil and criminal*. Charlottesville, VA: Michie.
Rhoden, N. K. (1980). The right to refuse psychotropic drugs. *Harvard Civil Rights—Civil Liberties Law Review, 15*, 363–413.
Roth, L. H. (1986). The right to refuse treatment: Law and medicine at the interface. *Emory Law Journal, 35*, 139–161.
Schmidt, M. J., & Geller, J. L. (1989). Involuntary administration of medication in the community: The judicial opportunity. *Bulletin of the American Academy of Psychiatry and the Law, 17*, 283–292.
Schouten, R., & Gutheil, T. G. (1990). Aftermath of the *Rogers* decision: Assessing the costs. *American Journal of Psychiatry, 147*, 1348–1352.
Schwartz, H. I., Vingiano, W., & Perez, C. B. (1988). Autonomy and the right to refuse treatment: Patients' attitudes after involuntary medication. *Hospital and Community Psychiatry, 39*, 1049–1054.
Veliz, J., & James, W. S. (1987). Medicine court: *Rogers* in practice. *American Journal of Psychiatry, 144*, 62–67.
Winick, B. J. (1989). The right to refuse mental health treatment: A First Amendment perspective. *University of Miami Law Review, 44*, 1–103.
Winick, B. J. (1991). Competency to consent to treatment: The distinction between assent and objection. *Houston Law Review, 28*, 15–61.
Zito, J. M., Craig, T. J., & Wanderling, J. (1991). New York under the *Rivers* decision: An epidemiologic study of drug treatment refusal. *American Journal of Psychiatry, 148*, 904–909.
Zito, J. M., Haimowitz, S., Wanderling, J., & Mehta, R. M. (1989). One year under *Rivers*: Drug refusal in a New York State psychiatric facility. *International Journal of Law and Psychiatry, 12*, 295–306.

V. Legal Regulation of Electroconvulsive Therapy

A. *Cases*

Wyatt v. Hardin, Civil Action 3195-N (Ala. 1975).
Aden v. Younger, 129 Cal.Rptr. 535 (1976).
McDonald v. Moore, 323 So.2d 635 (Fla. 1976).
Price v. Sheppard, 239 N.W.2d 905 (Minn. 1976).
In re Fadley, 205 Cal.Rptr. 572 (1984).
Lillian F. v. Superior Court, 206 Cal.Rptr. 603 (1984).
Gowan v. United States, 601 F.Supp. 1297 (Or. 1985).
Northern California Psychiatric Society v. Berkeley, 223 Cal.Rptr. 608 (1986).
In re Schuoler, 723 P.2d 1103 (Wash. 1986).

B. *Articles and Books*

American Psychiatric Association, Task Force. (1990). *The practice of electroconvulsive therapy*. Washington, DC: American Psychiatric Association.
Baxter, L. R., Roy-Byrne, P., Liston, E. H., & Fairbanks, L. (1986). Informing patients about electroconvulsive therapy: Effects of a videotape presentation. *Convulsive Therapy, 2*, 25–29.
Culver, C. M., Ferrell, R. B., & Green, R. B. (1980). ECT and special problems of informed consent. *American Journal of Psychiatry, 137*, 586–591.
Guze, B. H., Baxter, L. R., Liston, E. H., & Roy-Byrne, P. (1988). Attorneys' perceptions of electroconvulsive therapy: Impact of instruction with an ECT videotape demonstration. *Comprehensive Psychiatry, 29*, 520–522.

Kaufmann, C. L., & Roth, L. H. (1981). Psychiatric evaluation of patient decision making: Informed consent to ECT. *Social Psychiatry, 16,* 11–19.
Kramer, B. A. (1990). ECT use in the public sector: California. *Psychiatric Quarterly, 61,* 97–103.
Martin, B. A., & Jacobsen, P. M. (1986). Electroconvulsive therapy and brain damage: The Ontario Supreme Court hearing of the evidence. *Canadian Journal of Psychiatry, 31,* 381–386.
Mills, M. J., Pearsall, D. T., Yesavage, J. A., & Salzman, C. (1984). Electroconvulsive therapy in Massachusetts. *American Journal of Psychiatry, 141,* 534–538.
Morrissey, J. P., Burton, N. M., & Steadman, H. J. (1979). Developing an empirical base for psycholegal policy analyses of ECT: A New York State survey. *International Journal of Law and Psychiatry, 2,* 99–111.
Note. (1976). Regulation of electroconvulsive therapy. *Michigan Law Review, 75,* 363–412.
Roy-Byrne, P., & Gerner, R. H. (1981). Legal restrictions on the use of ECT in California: Clinical impact on the incompetent patient. *Journal of Clinical Psychiatry, 41,* 300–303.
Slawson, P. (1985). Psychiatric malpractice: The electroconvulsive therapy experience. *Convulsive Therapy, 1,* 195–203.
Slawson, P. (1989). Psychiatric malpractice and ECT: A review of national loss experience. *Convulsive Therapy, 5,* 126–130.
Taub, S. (1987). Electroconvulsive therapy, malpractice, and informed consent. *Journal of Psychiatry and Law, 15,* 7–54.
Tenenbaum, J. (1983). ECT regulation reconsidered. *Mental Disability Law Reporter, 7,* 148–211.
Weitzel, W. D. (1977). Changing law and clinical dilemmas. *American Journal of Psychiatry, 134,* 293–295.
Winslade, W. J., Liston, E. H., Ross, J. W., & Weber, K. D. (1984). Medical, judicial, and statutory regulation of ECT in the United States. *American Journal of Psychiatry, 141,* 1349–1355.

VI. Legal Regulation of Restraints and Seclusion

A. *Cases*

Dusine v. Golden Shores Convalescent Center, Inc., 249 So.2d 40 (Fla.App. 1971).
Youngberg v. Romeo, 102 S.Ct. 2452 (1982).
Walters v. Western State Hospital, 864 F.2d 695 (10th Cir. 1988).
Clark v. Ohio Department of Mental Health, 573 N.E.2d 794 (Ohio Ct.Cl. 1989). [restraints used punitively]
Kuster v. State of New York, 560 N.Y.S.2d 301 (1989).
Hopper v. Callahan, 562 N.E.2d 822 (Mass. Sup.Jud.Ct. 1990). [death in seclusion]

B. *Articles and Books*

American Psychiatric Association. (1985). *Seclusion and restraint, the psychiatric uses, Task Force Report* (Report No. 22). Washington, DC: American Psychiatric Association.
Antoinette, T., Iyengar, S., & Puig-Antich, J. (1990). Is locked seclusion necessary for children under the age of 14? *American Journal of Psychiatry, 147,* 1283–1289.
Davidson, N. A., Hemingway, M. J., & Wysocki, T. (1984). Reducing the use of restrictive procedures in a residential facility. *Hospital and Community Psychiatry, 35,* 164–167.
Fassler, D., & Cotton, N. (1992). A national survey on the use of seclusion in the psychiatric treatment of children. *Hospital and Community Psychiatry, 43,* 370–374.
Favell, J. E., McGimsey, J. F., Jones, M. C., & Cannon, P. R. (1981). Physical restraint as positive reinforcement. *American Journal of Mental Deficiency, 85,* 425–432.
Johnson, S. H. (1990). The fear of liability and the use of restraints in nursing homes. *Law, Medicine, and Health Care, 18,* 263–273.
Kapp, M. B. (1992). Nursing home restraints and legal liability. *Journal of Legal Medicine, 13,* 1–32.
Moss, R. J., & La Puma, J. L. (1991). The ethics of mechanical restraints. *Hastings Center Report, 21,* 22–25.
Saks, E. R. (1986). The use of mechanical restraints in psychiatric hospitals. *Yale Law Journal, 95,* 1836–1856.
Soliday, S. M. (1985). A comparison of patient and staff attitudes toward seclusion. *Journal of Nervous and Mental Disease, 173,* 282–286.

Tardiff, K. (Ed.). (1984). *The psychiatric uses of seclusion and restraint.* Washington, DC: American Psychiatric Press, Inc.
Tinetti, M. E., Liu, W. L., & Ginter, S. F. (1992). Mechanical restraint use and fall-related injuries among residents of skilled nursing facilities. *Annals of Internal Medicine, 116,* 369–374.

VII. Legal Regulation of Behavior Modification

A. Cases

Knecht v. Gillman, 488 F.2d 1136 (8th Cir. 1973).
K.P. v. Albanese, 497 A.2d 1276 (N.J. 1985).
Green v. Baron, 925 F.2d 262 (8th Cir. 1991).

B. Articles and Books

American Medical Association. (1987). Aversion therapy. *Journal of the American Medical Association, 258,* 2562–2566.
Foxx, R. M., McMorrow, M. J., Bittle, R. G., & Bechtel, D. R. (1986). The successful treatment of a dually-diagnosed deaf man's aggression with a program that included contingent electric shock. *Behavior Therapy, 17,* 170–186.
Ludwig, A. M., Marx, A. J., Hill, P. A., & Browning, R. M. (1969). The control of violent behavior through faradic shock. *Journal of Nervous and Mental Disease, 148,* 624–637.
Martin, R. (1975). *Legal challenges to behavior modification.* Champaign, IL: Research Press.
Singer, R. (1977). Consent of the unfree, Part 1. *Law and Human Behavior, 1,* 1–43.
Singer, R. (1977). Consent of the unfree, Part 2. *Law and Human Behavior, 1,* 101–162.
Stolz, S. B. (1978). *Ethical issues in behavior modification.* San Francisco, CA: Jossey Bass.
Wexler, D. B. (1973). Token and taboo: Behavior modification, token economies, and the law. *California Law Review, 61,* 81–109.
Wexler, D. B. (1975). Behavior modification and other behavior change procedures: The emerging law and the proposed Florida guidelines. *Criminal Law Bulletin, 11,* 600–636.

VIII. Legal Regulation of Psychosurgery

A. Cases

Kaimowitz v. Michigan Department of Mental Health, Civil No. 73–19, 434-AW (Cir. Ct. Wayne Co., Mich. 1973).
Aden v. Younger, 129 Cal.Rptr. 535 (1976).
Kapp v. Ballantine, 402 N.E.2d 463 (Mass. 1980).

B. Articles and Books

Kleinig, J. (1985). *Ethical issues in psychosurgery.* London: Allen & Unwin.
Kopesky, J. P. (1979). Psychosurgery and the involuntarily confined. *Villanova Law Review, 24,* 949–991.
Robitscher, J. B. (1974). Psychosurgery and other somatic means of altering behavior. *Bulletin of the American Academy of Psychiatry and the Law, 2,* 7–33.
Shuman, S. I. (1977). *Psychosurgery and the medical control of violence: Autonomy and deviance.* Detroit: Wayne State University Press.
Valenstein, E. S. (Ed.). (1980). *The psychosurgery debate: Scientific, legal, and ethical perspectives.* San Francisco: Freeman.
Valenstein, E. S. (1986). *Great and desperate cures: The rise and decline of psychosurgery and other radical treatments for mental illness.* New York: Basic Books.

6

Professional Liability

I. Malpractice • A. Negligence • B. Attorney's Analysis of a Malpractice Case • C. Proving Professional Negligence • **II. Potential Areas of Malpractice Liability** • A. Suicide and Attempted Suicide • B. Failure to Diagnose • C. Negligent Release • D. Sexual Activity with a Patient • E. Improper Psychotherapy • F. Abandonment • G. Negligent Administration of Medication • H. Electroconvulsive Therapy • I. Negligent Psychological Evaluation • J. Social Worker Negligence • **III. Problems in Proving Liability against Mental Health Professionals** • **IV. Other Causes of Liability** • A. Lack of Informed Consent • B. Breach of Confidentiality • C. Duty to Protect Third Parties • D. Failure to Report Child Abuse • E. Civil Rights Suits • **V. Hospital or Agency Liability** • **VI. Suits against Supervisory Personnel** • **VII. Suits against State Employees** • **VIII. Malpractice Insurance** • **IX. Record Keeping** • A. Record Keeping Functions • B. Contents of Records • **X. Malpractice Prevention** • A. Communication • B. Empathy • C. Limitations • D. Informed Consent • E. Fees • F. Comprehensive Evaluation • G. Consultation • H. Continuity of Care • I. Knowing the Relevant Law and Institutional Policies • **XI. Responding to a Malpractice Lawsuit** • **XII. Coping with a Malpractice Lawsuit** • **XIII. Conclusion** • **XIV. Commonly Asked Questions** • **XV. Bibliography**

Concern about professional liability is an issue facing every professional. National attention has been drawn to the "malpractice crisis" and its potential effect on patient care. This increased attention on liability has made it a real issue for most professionals. The thought of being sued for negligence in our professional work frightens most of us. Yet the reality is that mental health professionals are infrequently sued, although the number and types of liability actions are increasing.

Fear of liability has affected patient care both positively and negatively. On the positive side, clinicians are involving patients in the decision-making process to a greater extent. On the negative side, the clinician may be unnecessarily cautious or defensive in the actions he takes. This may increase the cost of providing mental health services. Additionally, he will be concerned about the likelihood that his actions will result in a lawsuit and increased malpractice insurance premiums. These concerns have been translated into greater interest by mental health professionals in the legal process and how to avoid liability.

This chapter examines professional liability from the perspectives of the clinician and the attorney. It begins with an introduction to malpractice and explains how an attorney analyzes a case. The common areas in which suits against mental health professionals are brought are discussed, along with an explanation of the difficulty of proving negligence by mental health professionals. Other areas of potential liability are set forth. Specific suggestions are given on how to avoid being sued, and what to do if you are sued. Suits based on a "duty to warn" or "negligent release" merit a separate chapter because of the growth in litigation in this area and the amount of concern by mental health professionals over these types of actions. This topic is covered in Chapter 8. Chapter 7 provides a detailed discussion of issues related to confidentiality.

I. MALPRACTICE

A. Negligence

To understand malpractice one must understand negligence. Negligence is conduct which falls below the standard established by society for the protection of others against unreasonable risk of harm. Each adult is expected to conduct himself in a way that other ordinary and reasonable persons would act. When behavior falls below this standard and someone is harmed, negligence has occurred. The injured person would then have the right to bring a lawsuit against the person who harmed him, claiming his negligent behavior was the proximate cause of the injury the plaintiff (the person bringing the suit) suffered. This type of suit derives from tort law, the law of civil wrongs.

Claims of negligence are unintentional torts. This means that the person who committed the harm did not intend to do harm, but it occurred as a result of his negligent behavior. There are many types of negligence actions. When litigation is initiated as a result of an injury to a person, it is called a *personal injury case*. Most common are cases as a result of automobile accidents. Most relevant to our discussions are suits brought as a result of injuries inflicted by a health care provider. These tort actions are malpractice cases.

Malpractice is negligence in the execution of professional duties. Any type of professional can be accused of malpractice. Medical malpractice is a suit against a physician, although the term is often applied to the broad range of health care providers. Attorneys, architects, engineers, and accountants can also be sued for malpractice. As in the case of health care providers, there has been an increase in litigation against these professionals and in their insurance rates.

Throughout this discussion of malpractice, it is important for the mental health professional to remember two things: First, the clinician does not guarantee a specific result (i.e., successful treatment) and is expected only to provide services in a manner which is consistent with his training and the standard of practice within the field. The mere fact that an injury occurred or a bad result was obtained does not mean that there was negligence. Second, each specialist is to be judged by the standards for his specialty. This means that a psychologist will be measured against the expectations of other psychologists, a social worker against other social workers, and so on.

To succeed in any negligence action, the plaintiff (the injured party) must prove four elements: (1) duty, (2) breach of duty, (3) damages, and (4) causation between the breach of the duty and the damages. When a personal injury suit is brought, the plaintiff must prove by a preponderance of the evidence that these elements existed.

The plaintiff's argument must be more convincing than the defendant's for the plaintiff to prevail. These elements are explained below.

1. *Duty*

The first element in proving malpractice is establishing the existence of a duty by the provider to the injured party. The duty has two components: the duty to perform and the concomitant duty to do so in an acceptable manner. Duty is proven by showing that there was a professional relationship between the mental health professional and the injured party. There are two legal theories which support the existence of the provider–patient relationship. The first is based on the concept that the parties entered into a contract. In return for a fee, paid either directly or indirectly by a third party, the provider agrees to provide services. The second theory holds that by providing care, a professional relationship is created and a duty of care arises.

Proving that a duty existed to the injured party is the easiest element in a malpractice action. If the injured party sought care from the professional and it was given, then a relationship arose and the duty existed. Several professionals who are providing care may simultaneously have a duty to the patient. For example, a person may have sought psychiatric help, and the psychiatrist may have utilized a team of a social worker, a psychiatric nurse, and a psychologist to perform part of the services. In this case, the professional relationship between each member of the team is implied because of their delivery of services. Thus, in an action against the psychiatrist for negligent care, it is likely that the other members of the team will be joined in the lawsuit.

2. *Breach of Duty*

Establishing a breach of duty requires proving that the professional's behavior fell below the standard of care expected of a similarly trained professional. This breach may be a result of the professional's failure to do something that should have been done (omission) or his doing something that should not have been done (commission). Breach of duty is usually the most difficult element to prove in a malpractice action. In the absence of obvious negligence (for example, where the surgeon amputates the wrong arm), an expert witness will be required to establish the standard of care and its breach. (This is discussed at length in Section C below.)

3. *Damages*

For the plaintiff to win a malpractice action, he must show how he was damaged. Damages require some measurable injury, whether physical, emotional, or both. The plaintiff must prove the cost to him as a result of the injury. Documentation will be provided to recover the cost of past and expected future medical expenses. How the injury damaged the plaintiff's life and his income potential will be presented. There will also be a request for a monetary reward for the "pain and suffering" this injury has caused the plaintiff.

4. *Causation*

Finally, the plaintiff must establish that the injury he suffered was proximately caused by the negligent behavior of the defendant. The defendant will not be liable if the injury was not proximately caused by his negligence, but by the plaintiff's own conduct or that of some third party. In medical malpractice actions, establishing causation is complicated by the fact that the patient has usually sought care because of some preexisting problem. Generally, expert testimony will be required to establish causation and to separate the preexisting injury from the posttreatment damage. There are two commonly used tests to establish causation. The "but for" test requires proving that it is more probable than not that "but for" the actions of the defendant, the plaintiff's injury would not have occurred. The other test is a "substantial factor" test. In this test, the defendant's conduct has to have been a substantial factor in producing the injury.

In suits against mental health professionals, establishing causation is often difficult. The preexisting condition which required seeking treatment can have a major impact on the later injury which is blamed on the health care provider. One of the reasons for the relatively few suits against mental health professionals is the difficulty of proving that the professional caused the harm.

B. Attorney's Analysis of a Malpractice Case

When a prospective plaintiff brings a potential malpractice case to an attorney, the attorney has a professional duty to the client to properly evaluate the case to determine its likely success. In deciding whether to accept a malpractice case, the attorney for the plaintiff completes a five step analysis, which includes determining whether the case can be filed within the statute of limitations, and then reviewing the four elements required to prove a negligence action.

1. *Statute of Limitations*

Malpractice actions, like all lawsuits, must be filed within a certain time period, established by law, known as the *statute of limitations*. For malpractice, the time period varies from two to five years depending on the state and the legal cause of the action. When the case involves a minor, the time period is usually tolled until the minor reaches 18 years of age, and then it begins to run, though the various states vary widely in this area. For example, in states with a two-year statute of limitations, the plaintiff must file a lawsuit within two years of when he became aware or should have become aware of the malpractice. If the suit is not filed in a timely manner, the case will be dismissed, and the plaintiff will have no further recourse. An attorney will not accept a case which occurred too long ago to fall within the statute of limitations. In fact, an important basis for malpractice suits against attorneys is accepting cases and not filing them within the statute of limitations.

2. *Duty*

Was there a therapist–patient relationship? If the answer is no or it is unclear, then the case is weak. The law of negligence is based on proving that the defendant had an obligation to the injured party.

3. *Breach of Duty*

Did the defendant clearly fail to meet the standard of care expected of one in his specialty? To determine this, the attorney will refer the records of the case to one or more mental health professionals who can advise him on whether they think the care provided was substandard or questionable. If the experts consulted by the attorney conclude that the therapist performed as expected, even though a bad result occurred, the attorney will be unlikely to accept the case because he will conclude that the provider did not deviate from acceptable practice.

4. *Damages*

In many ways, the value of the case is the crucial factor for the attorney in determining whether the case is worth pursuing. Since many personal injury attorneys work on a contingency fee basis (where they receive a percentage of the fee award), they are interested only in cases which have a high probability of recovery. They may invest a great deal of time and resources in developing a case in the hopes that it will have been worthwhile. Often it is five years from the time the case is filed until it is finally settled or goes to trial. The contingent fee arrangement causes greater selectivity for the attorney in cases than would an hourly fee arrangement, in which the attorney is paid regardless of the outcome of the case.

Determining how much damage has been done depends on many factors. There is a maxim in the law which says, "You take your victim as you find him." Clearly, some victims are much more expensive to harm than others. In addition, the nature of the harm, its permanence, and the level of negligence by the defendant are all factors in determining the extent of damages. For example, in a hospital suicide case in which the victim was a plastic surgeon who jumped out of the window while on suicide precautions, who was 37 years old, and who had three children, the extent of the damages would be substantial. If, however, the victim was a 70-year-old, never employed, chronic schizophrenic individual who had been in and out of the state mental health system, the case would have a much lower potential award. If, in the case of the surgeon, he survived but remained in a persistent vegetative state, damages would take into account these expenses and would be even more substantial.

When determining damages, the goal of tort law is to try to "make the victim whole." This may require a great deal of monetary compensation. In cases of serious medical problems that will require expensive long-term medical care, the costs will be substantial. Add to this the lost income and the loss to the family of the benefits of having a husband and father, and juries will be willing to compensate in any way they can for such a tragedy. When these factors are combined with the obvious negligence of having an openable window on a psychiatric unit, and having a patient on suicide precautions in a situation where he is unsupervised and able to get out of that window, there will be great jury appeal.

Even if a case is less clearly negligent, an attorney may decide to accept the case with the expectation that the insurance company will settle the case quickly. This settlement will be based on the view that negligence clearly occurred, and the defendant would be held liable if the case went to trial.

5. *Causation*

Was the injury proximately caused by the acts of the defendant? If it is clear to the plaintiff's attorney that the defendant's behavior resulted in direct harm to the plaintiff, this is a strong case. If, however, the plaintiff is alleging harm, and it is difficult to see that it was caused by the acts of the defendant, then the case is much weaker. Causation is particularly a problem in cases involving mental health professionals, because the harm alleged may have a psychological element. Since the person sought treatment for some type of mental problem, it is easy for the defendant to argue that the problem was preexisting, and that any harm that the plaintiff is claiming is not due to the defendant's actions.

In the mental health area, suits are often brought as a result of suicide or attempted suicide. In a case in which the person was an outpatient and expressed suicidal thoughts but seemed to have no specific plans of suicide and commits suicide, it may be difficult to establish that the therapist was negligent. In contrast, if the person was hospitalized and on suicide precautions, but the staff allowed him a room with a window which could be opened, and the patient jumped and died, this would result in clear liability against the hospital and the treating staff. From a plaintiff's attorney's perspective this is an attractive case. The duty of care and the breach of that duty to the patient are clear. Permitting a patient with suicidal behavior in a room with an openable window without supervision would be substandard practice and clearly negligent behavior. With regard to causation, the failure of the staff to install locked windows and supervise the patient would be a substantial factor in the death of the patient.

These five factors determine whether an attorney will accept the plaintiff's case. The attorney's evaluation of these factors determines how vigorously the case will be pursued, what documentation will be needed to make his points clear, and what amount of damages will be sought. For the attorney who is approached to take a personal injury case, the accuracy of the initial analysis will determine whether he is likely to be financially successful on the case.

At the same time that a plaintiff's attorney is going through these steps, an attorney for the defendant will also be going through the same process. His goal will be to determine whether the case should be settled quickly and for how much or whether it is a close case and should not be settled. The more obvious the negligence, and the more serious the injury to the patient, the more eager the defense attorney will be to settle the matter as quickly as possible to avoid a trial and reduce legal fees. In the examples of hospital suicides by jumping out a window, a settlement offer would likely be made quickly.

The clinician must appreciate that the attorney for either the plaintiff or the defendant has a duty to his client to act in a professional manner throughout the litigation. Just as the patient seeks the services of the mental health professional with regard to his emotional problems, the client seeks the services of the plaintiff's attorney because he believes that he has been subjected to negligent care and that the attorney is his means to its redress in the courts. The attorney's role is not to find "great" cases for himself but to represent the legal interests of the client in the most effective way possible. The clinician's role, likewise, is to provide standard care without being distracted by the "value" of the patient's economic interests or losses.

C. Proving Professional Negligence

There are two ways to prove professional negligence. The first is by direct evidence. This is accomplished by describing the injury-producing act and having an expert witness explain why the behavior was negligent. The second way, which is applicable only in limited circumstances, is by using circumstantial evidence. This approach is known as the doctrine of *res ipsa loquitur*.

1. *Res Ipsa Loquitur*

Res ipsa loquitur literally translated means, "The thing speaks for itself." This is a doctrine of circumstantial proof. It means that negligence may be inferred from the fact of an unexplained injury of a type that does not normally occur in the absence of negligence. An illustration is a surgeon's removing the wrong arm or leaving his scalpel in the patient's abdomen, causing medical complications and eventual death. In these cases, the negligence is so obvious that the fact of the injury makes further evidence unnecessary as to its causation.

For the doctrine of *res ipsa loquitur* to be satisfied, three elements must be proven:

1. The event must be of a kind which ordinarily does not occur in the absence of someone's negligence.
2. It must be caused by something within the exclusive control of the defendant.
3. It must not have been due to any voluntary action or contribution on the part of the plaintiff.

Once the facts are presented, the defendant has the burden of establishing that the injury was not due to his negligence. Suits based on *res ispa loquitur* are infrequent. When such a case arises, the defendant will be anxious to settle the matter as quickly as possible, since the liability is obvious. There are, however, few of these types of cases involving mental health professionals. Some psychotropic medication cases could give rise to a *res ipsa loquitur* action. For example, if the patient is given a lethal dosage of the wrong medication, the negligence is clear. In this type of case there may be a dispute as to who is the guilty defendant. It may be the physician who wrote a prescription for the wrong medication or in a manner the pharmacist could not read. It may be the pharmacist who filled the prescription incorrectly, or it may be the nurse who administered the lethal dosage. In any event, there is clearly a defendant who is liable, and the attorney will join all the parties who may have been responsible for the wrong medication having been given to the deceased.

In *res ipsa* cases, the case speaks for itself. An expert witness is not needed because the negligence is so apparent that the average person can easily understand how the standard of care was violated.

2. *Establishing the Standard of Care*

Establishing a violation of the standard of care is perhaps the most crucial element in a malpractice case. This generally must be done with the testimony of expert witnesses. Expert witnesses are necessary in any case in which the matter is not within the common knowledge of the layman. The defendant's conduct will be evaluated in terms of his specialty. The standard of care will be determined by professional custom (community standards) or by what would be expected of a similarly trained practitioner in a similar clinical situation.

a. Selecting an Expert Witness. For the attorney the choice of his expert witness is critical to the likelihood that the case will be successful. There are certain factors that will be essential if the attorney is to successfully convey how the standard of care was followed if he represents the clinician, or how it was negligently breached if he represents the plaintiff. (See the section in Chapter 11, Section III on serving as an expert witness.)

The first factor in choosing an expert will be finding a reputable practitioner from the same specialty as the defendant. Psychiatrists will be held to the standard expected of psychiatrists, psychologists to the standard expected of psychologists, and so on. For example, in a case against a psychiatrist, the expert witness will typically be a psychiatrist. He will be needed to establish the standard of care in the particular type of case, how the standard of care was breached in this case, and how the deviation from the standard of care was the proximate cause of the injuries to the plaintiff.

One of the problems for the plaintiff in establishing the applicable standard of care in mental health cases is the availability of a variety of treatment approaches. A clinician is not negligent in selecting among two or more recognized methods of treatment. This raises the issue of whether the expert witness must be from the same school of therapy as the defendant. With a multitude of schools of treatment, it may be possible to argue that one should be judged only by someone from the same school of thought. Although few courts have addressed this issue, it is likely that there are certain basic principles common to the various therapeutic approaches which will serve to establish the applicable standard of care in a specific case. A major consideration will be whether the treatment approach employed is one used by at least a substantial minority of mental health professionals. Under the so-called "respected [or respectable] minority rule," a therapist may use a treatment technique employed by a minority of practitioners and still satisfy the standard of care.

The expert witness will also need to be someone who is familiar with the treatment which should be employed for the plaintiff's illness. Ideally, the expert from each side should have experience in treating the specific illness. The expert will testify as to what type of care would be expected given the circumstances of the plaintiff's case. Since the defendant is not liable for making a wrong decision, if the care rendered was within the acceptable range of treatment alternatives, then the defendant was not negligent even though a bad result occurred.

In the past, the defendant/clinician was governed by the accepted clinical standard in his community. With the growing standardization of practice across wide geographical areas, the wide availability of literature to update the clinician on recent developments in his field, and the ability to attend continuing education seminars, the requirement that an expert witness be from the same locality as the defendant no longer applies in most jurisdictions. Where the standard of care is stated with reference to a particular locality, the expert witness must be able to state that he is familiar with the standard of practice within that community, even though he may not have practiced there.

The expert witness is expected to educate the court as to what type of care would be expected under a given set of circumstances. This expectation does not turn on what the expert would have done under the circumstances, but whether what was done was within the range of what is deemed to be clinically acceptable by similarly trained clinicians.

b. Use of Professional Guidelines. Another way in which the attorney can establish a deviation from the standard of care is via the guidelines of professional organizations, the literature distributed by drug manufacturers, and the professional literature on the topic. These items will be brought to the attention of the court through the expert witness.

Many organizations of health care professionals have developed guidelines for the practice of their respective professions. These are variously referred to as practice parameters, practice standards, practice policies, or practice options. They may have been developed for varying purposes including defining optimal care, providing for quality assurance, determining reimbursement, or controlling the costs of care. These may be general or specific, and easy or difficult to apply to particular clinical situations. These standards may be of use in a particular case of malpractice litigation by either the plaintiff or the defendant. For example, the American Psychiatric Association has formulated recommendations for clinical practice in electroconvulsive therapy (ECT). If the defendant significantly deviated from these recommendations in the patient's treatment, this deviation could be used at trial as evidence of the defendant's negligent behavior. However, most practice parameters are designed to be flexible rather than absolute standards of care.

In cases involving medication, the pharmaceutical manufacturer's package insert, or the statements in the *Physician's Desk Reference* (PDR), will be admissible in most courts to establish the standard of care, along with expert testimony. Deviation from the recommendations does not necessarily prove the defendant was negligent, particularly if there exists a body of professional literature to support the use of the drug in the manner used under the circumstances presented by the case.

Treatises and other recognized works in the field can be used as a powerful statement as to the negligence of the defendant. This approach will be successful only when the conduct of the defendant is clearly in conflict with the principles set forth in the textbooks. Since there is so much published in the health care fields, it is often easy to find literature which refute the position put forth by one side. For this reason, the professional literature may be of questionable value when there are several respectable treatment approaches to the case.

3. *Damages*

Assuming the plaintiff's attorney has proven that all the elements of a negligence case existed (duty, breach of duty, and injury which was proximately caused by the defendant's actions), the case is not completed until the attorney proves how his client was specifically damaged. In personal injury cases, the plaintiff is entitled to all costs which will be required to "make him whole" again. These will include all costs of care, past, present, and future. They will also include recovery for lost wages, both past and future. The plaintiff will not be entitled to recover the costs of his attorney's fees, nor will he be eligible for lost interest on the money expended thus far.

The attorney will introduce evidence to prove the expenses incurred by the plaintiff. Expert witnesses will testify as to expected future expenses given the plaintiff's prognosis. Attempts will be made to document lost future income, through the use of actuarial consultants. The actuary will testify as to what someone with the plaintiff's background and experience would earn over the course of a normal work life. Efforts will be made to show how the pain and suffering caused by the defendant's negligent actions have impacted on the daily life of the plaintiff and have affected him and his family. A value will be placed on this amount. Once this testimony has been presented, the plaintiff's attorney will request a specific amount of money as damages. The defendant's attorney will dispute the amount requested, often with his own actuarial witnesses.

The defense attorney will try to establish that the plaintiff in some way contributed to his own harm. He might argue, for example, that he did not follow the clinician's directions or did not notify the clinician of problems caused by medication. If the plaintiff may have contributed to his own injury, the defense will argue that any award should be reduced by the amount of fault attributable to the plaintiff.

After hearing all the evidence the jury will make an award of damages. Only in rare instances, when the conduct of the defendant has been outrageous, will punitive damages be awarded. An award of punitive damages is a statement by the court or jury that the defendant engaged in gross and willful misconduct. It is their way of punishing the defendant for his behavior. Most malpractice insurance policies do not provide coverage for punitive damages, so that the defendant would be personally responsible for them.

II. POTENTIAL AREAS OF MALPRACTICE LIABILITY

Suits against mental health professionals are still quite infrequent. A recent survey revealed that claims against psychiatrists represented only 0.3% of all malpractice claims filed against physicians. Approximately 2% to 4% of psychiatrists have claims filed against them annually. The majority of these relate to improper treatment, especially medication. It is even less common for psychologists, social workers, or nurses to be sued. This low incidence of malpractice suits results in relatively less expensive malpractice insurance premiums for mental health professionals, though these rates have risen by substantial percentages in recent years. With the greatly increasing number of professionals who offer mental health services, and the variety of actions which can lead to a suit, there is an increased concern about malpractice litigation. This section begins with a discussion of suits which can be brought against mental health professionals. Always bear in mind that a poor outcome is not sufficient to establish negligence. Even when negligence occurs, there must be a compensable injury.

A. Suicide and Attempted Suicide

One of the most common reasons for malpractice suits against mental health professionals is the patient's suicide or attempted suicide. Neither patients nor families expect that the patient will die or seriously injure himself during the course of treatment for a mental disorder. Families maintain this expectation even in the face of the patient's repeated self-destructive behavior. When a suicide occurs, the family may bring a wrongful death action. Unlike in other personal injury suits, where the injury is blamed on the actions of the defendant, liability in a suicide case is based on the therapist's failure to take any action to prevent the suicide. The fact of a suicide or attempted suicide does not by itself indicate negligence. Clinicians are not liable for errors of clinical judgment; they are liable only for departures from the relevant standard of care, given the clinical situation. In fact, short of gross misconduct, it may be difficult to find the therapist liable for the self-injury. The low reliability and validity of clinical judgments and predictions of a patient's suicide risk are well known to clinicians, well documented in the literature, and routinely the subject of testimony in such cases at trial. The courts now recognize that the prediction of suicidal behavior is inherently uncertain.

The therapist's liability for suicide or attempted suicide may arise in one of three contexts. A patient may injure or kill himself (1) during hospitalization; (2) while on a temporary pass or official discharge, or during an escape from the hospital; or (3) during or after outpatient treatment.

Death or serious injury occurring during hospitalization is the most likely occasion for filing a suit based on suicide or attempted suicide. In these cases, the suit will be brought against the treating physician, members of the treatment team, and the hospital itself. A suicide or attempted suicide on an inpatient unit does not *per se* mean that negligence occurred. Liability can result when the staff negligently failed to evaluate the patient's suicide risk, or to do so as frequently as necessary. This negligence can include failure of the staff to obtain an adequate and accurate history of previous self-destructive behavior from the patient or third parties.

Liability can also occur when the staff has failed to take adequate precautions to manage an identified suicide risk. Common examples including failing to place a patient on suicide precautions, failure to use the appropriate level of supervision, and failure to communicate information to other staff regarding the patient's suicide potential. In the absence of obvious negligence, such as allowing a patient with suicidal intent to have access to lethal instruments (e.g., sharp objects, nonbreakaway shower rods, open windows, door keys, or unlocked doors on a secure unit), it may be difficult to prove liability against a hospital or its staff because of the fact of a patient suicide.

When a suicide occurs while the patient is temporarily away from the hospital, similar arguments will be presented as to why the hospital staff should be held liable. Treating staff may have negligently failed to assess the patient's suicide risk upon release or may have negligently concluded that the benefits of release outweighed its risks. Included in this category are cases where the patient requests a discharge from the hospital and the staff negligently concludes the patient is not subject to involuntary hospitalization.

Cases involving suicide by individuals who are in outpatient treatment, or who have recently been discharged from outpatient treatment, also involve questions about the adequacy of the suicide assessment process, as well as the management of suicide risk. Here clinicians are commonly confronted with individuals with past suicide attempts, current suicide ideation, depressed mood, hopelessness, pessimism, or impaired therapeutic alliance due to a personality disorder. In contrast to the suicide cases involving hospitalized patients, the outpatient clinician typically has limited control over the suicidal individual. Changes in the type or intensity of psychotherapy or the addition of psychotropic medication can be implemented when the patient's suicide risk appears to have increased. However, in the absence of involuntary hospitalization, such measures may provide little chance of actually preventing self-injury. The courts have been reluctant to impose liability for the suicides of outpatients.

Perhaps the best defense a clinician has in most suicide cases is his testimony of the potential harm which would occur to the patient if the therapist had applied increased suicide precautions when they were unnecessary. Such harms include prolonged hospitalization, excessive treatment with medication, decreased self-esteem, stigma, rage, and increased dependence on others.

The courts have recognized that the clinician must balance the benefits and risks of suicide precautions and restrictions for each patient in striving to help the patient function independently. The courts often defer to the clinician's judgment about the appropriateness of release decisions. Additionally, there is likely to be less liability the further removed in time the self-injury is from the treatment.

Clinicians can successfully defend themselves against charges of negligent suicide when the suicide appears to be an independent act of a competent patient, or when the patient has concealed his suicide ideation, intention, or plan from the therapist. In both situations, the patient acted voluntarily and competently, and his own behavior is the proximate cause of his injury. Clinicians who have involved the patient in the decision making about his suicide status (e.g., necessary levels of supervision, passes, privileges, and discharge), in conformity with the doctrine of informed consent, can also successfully defend themselves in suicide litigation.

There also may be intervening factors which the therapist could not predict or control. A man, for example, visits his hospitalized wife and tells her he is filing for divorce and will be moving from the marital residence when she is discharged. When a suicide occurs shortly after a visit or telephone call, it is important to try to document what occurred during the visit or call which may have precipitated the suicide.

When a patient suicide does occur, it is important for the treating staff to convey concern for the survivors. The therapist should not make any statements which would indicate lack of diligence on his part. It is also important for the therapist to convey to the family that they are not to blame for the patient's death. Often suits are initiated after a suicide because the family are unable to tolerate their guilt for the act and need to externalize blame for the unexpected death.

B. Failure to Diagnose

Failure to diagnose the patient's illness is another basis for malpractice liability against mental health professionals. Generally this should be thought of as a misdiagnosis or missed diagnosis of an illness. A typical example is the therapist's failure to exclude medical causes for the person's behavior, such as a thyroid disorder or a brain tumor. Failure to diagnose the patient as having a major depressive disorder which can be treated, given the patient's subsequent suicide, is another example of possible liability.

Although there is an expectation that psychiatrists will identify nonpsychological causes for disturbed behavior because of their medical training, nonmedical mental health professionals are expected to seek a medical or psychiatric consultation when there is a question about the etiology of the behavior.

To find a mental health professional negligent for failure to diagnose would require that the plaintiff prove that the professional should have made the diagnosis or at least considered it. Further, the plaintiff must demonstrate that the medical problem was the cause of his behavior, and that had it been properly diagnosed at the time he sought help from the mental health professional, he would not have been injured, or at least not to the extent he was. Suits based on failure to diagnose are more likely to be brought against other health care providers. Even when such a suit is brought, it will be successful only when the health care provider was negligent in failing to rule out certain illnesses based on the symptoms presented. Not discovering an illness when there are no symptoms of it is not negligent behavior.

Nonmedical mental health professionals should require that their clients have a recent physical examination from their physician when their emotional problems seem unexplainable on the basis of a functional disorder or when their response to an emotional problem is not what one would expect given their history and life circumstances. Psychiatrists who do not perform physical examinations or take a full medical history should do the same. Whenever a therapist believes there may be a possibility of a medical basis for the patient's behavior, the therapist is obligated to inform the client of this and to insist on a medical consultation. Additionally, non-medical mental health professionals whose clients take prescribed medication should be aware of the medication the client is taking and the expectable side effects. The therapist should work with the prescribing physician to coordinate the total care of the client as much as possible.

Many mental health professionals make psychiatric diagnoses in order to obtain third party payment for the client's care, whether the client is treated in an agency setting or in private practice. Some professionals deliberately report the listed diagnosis differently from the actual diagnosis. Increasing the "severity" of the diagnostic condition sometimes occurs to qualify the client for insurance coverage for an otherwise excluded condition. Decreasing the "severity" of the diagnosis sometimes occurs to protect the client from a stigmatizing label. In the former case, the clinician exposes himself to civil or criminal liability for insurance fraud and the loss of his professional license. The latter case may lead to inappropriate treatment, failure to refer for medical consultation, and liability to the client for a missed diagnosis. Mental health clinicians would be wise to avoid such practices.

C. Negligent Release

When a person who has been recently hospitalized harms another person, or even himself, suit may be brought against the hospital and the treatment staff for negligent release. This suit is based on the premise that, but for the release of the patient, the third party would not have been injured. In such suits, the plaintiff must prove that release was improper, or that the hospital was negligent in allowing the patient to escape. This topic is covered extensively in Chapter 8.

D. Sexual Activity with a Patient

Experienced clinicians acknowledge that it is not unusual for a therapist and a client to become sexually attracted to each other. A recent survey revealed that 87% of psychologists had been sexually attracted to their clients, at least on occasion. Surveys of psychiatrists, psychologists, and social workers have estimated that up to 14% of therapists have been involved in an overt sexual relationship with a client. Such contacts have no gender boundaries, although the vast majority involve male therapists and female clients. Such intimacies can have a devastating effect on the client and client's spouse or loved ones. The client's underlying mental condition may deteriorate. The client may also develop a new disorder, such as posttraumatic stress disorder or a depressive or adjustment disorder.

Sexual activity with a current client is considered unethical by all professional mental health associations. This ethical proscription applies to hospital-based treatment as well as community or office treatment. It includes involvement with professional staff as well as support staff, including custodians, regardless of whether the therapist or the client initiates the sexual behavior. Unethical behavior can result in sanction by any professional association in which the clinician is a member, including expulsion.

Sexual activity with a current or even a former client can additionally serve as the basis for a malpractice action, loss of professional licensure, loss of hospital staff privileges, and criminal charges. A number of states have made it a crime for a therapist to have sexual contact with an adult client or one who was a client within the preceding year. Sexual contact with a minor client is a felony in all states. Conviction on criminal charges can result in incarceration, fine, and loss of professional licensure.

In addition, a few states regulate the conduct of a therapist who subsequently treats a client who was previously sexually exploited in treatment. The second therapist may be required to inform the patient about her rights to pursue legal or administrative redress. Further, the second therapist may be permitted or even required to report the exploitation to the district attorney or state licensing board; such a report may or may not require the client's consent. Failure to make such a report could result in disciplinary or criminal action against the second therapist. Some states also interpret their professional licensure statutes or regulations to require therapists to report any unprofessional conduct of their peers. Although there have been few reported instances of failing to report another therapist's sexual exploitation, the enactment of such reporting laws reflects the seriousness with which client–therapist sexual activity is viewed by legislators.

Litigation based upon sexual activity with a client, or a client's spouse or relative, is increasing. The majority of malpractice claims against social workers insured by the National Association of Social Workers from 1965 to 1985 was based on sexual impropriety. This is considered a breach of the fiduciary duty to the client, and as a violation of the trust the client has given to the therapist. Despite the apparent consent of the client to engage in sexual activity with the therapist, most judges and juries conclude that the client's transference reactions distort the client's judgment to the extent that the consent is incompetent, not fully informed, absent, or irrelevant to the breach of the standard of care by the therapist. The violation of trust between the therapist and the client is considered so great that when such cases go to a jury, the amount of damages awarded is typically large. There are no circumstances in which "fornication therapy," as one court labeled it, is acceptable.

From the plaintiff's perspective, the initial problem in these cases is first coming forward to acknowledge the sexual experience. Despite feelings of having been exploited by the therapist, clients are often too ambivalent about the therapist to bring legal sanctions against him. The client also may not want to inform a spouse or others of the sexual activity, a usually necessary consequence of litigation. These factors combine to pit the word of the client, who will be labeled "disturbed" (otherwise why else was the client seeking treatment?), against that of the therapist. Problems of proof abound, unless the therapist has engaged in sexual relations with others, who become known to the plaintiff. In some instances the sexual contact will occur outside business hours and in other locations, so the plaintiff will be able to document the contacts.

Because of the significant jury appeal in cases of patient–therapist sexual contact, few actually go to trial. Cases in which the therapist acknowledges the sexual contact with the client are usually settled. In those which are tried, usually because there is contradictory evidence about whether the sexual contact in fact occurred, the plaintiff is more likely to be successful and the actual award large, when the client is more mentally disordered or psychotic or much younger than the therapist, or when the therapist used physical or sexual violence such as sadomasochistic activities as the sexual contact. Judges and juries are less sympathetic to the plaintiff when it can be shown that the plaintiff encouraged the sexual relationship and did not appear to have been exploited or damaged by the therapist.

Successful suits have also been brought when a therapist has engaged in sexual activity with the spouse of a client. This situation may arise when the couple are part of marital or family therapy, one spouse has ended therapy, and the therapist has sexual relations with the remaining spouse. Under these circumstances, the former client and the children may bring suit.

The courts have usually rejected the defense that the sexual contact occurred outside the office or outside the scope of the therapist–client relationship. Arguments that the sexual relations were a necessary component of the treatment process (e.g., for a sexual dysfunction, for converting a client's sexual orientation, or for providing a corrective emotional experience for the client) have been unsuccessful. Alleged damages to the plaintiffs include aggravation of the preexisting mental disorder, deprivation of the proper treatment for the presenting problem, and destruction of marital relationships (loss of consortium). Possible defendants include the individual therapist, the therapist's employer, the therapist's supervisor, and the treatment facility.

Malpractice insurance coverage for therapists charged with sexual intimacy with clients is sometimes capped or includes coverage only for the legal defense and not the ultimate judgment. In some cases, such coverage is excluded entirely under the assumption that the conduct is criminal or is outside the scope of appropriate therapeutic services. The insurance carrier will be responsible for the claim if other (i.e., nonsexual) grounds of liability are alleged. If coverage is denied, then the costs of the litigation and the judgment will become personal expenses for the therapist. Additionally, if charges are brought against the therapist by the state licensure authorities or professional society, his professional liability insurance will not cover the cost of legal representation in those proceedings.

Somewhat less clear from an ethical or legal perspective is the case in which a therapist has a personal relationship or sexual contact with a former client. Professional ethical codes are ambiguous about the acceptability of such conduct, and there is limited case law experience. In surveys, a substantial minority of mental health professionals believe that sexual contact after termination of therapy may sometimes be appropriate. The contrary view is that neither transference nor the inequality in the therapist–client relationship ends upon the termination of treatment. Questions may arise about when the treatment relationship "ended" and whether an adequate delay between the treatment and the personal relationship ensued. Should suit ultimately be brought, the specific facts of who initiated the relationship and how long it began after the therapy ended will be crucial factors in determining whether the acceptable standard of care has been breached.

E. Improper Psychotherapy

Perhaps the area which is least likely to result in successful litigation against a mental health professional is a lawsuit based on improper psychotherapy. Because there are many different schools of therapy and no universally accepted guidelines as to what approaches should be employed in specific circumstances, it would be difficult to document that the approach selected was a negligent one. It would be easier for the plaintiff to contend that the therapist negligently conducted a particular but accepted form of therapy (e.g., mishandled the transference and countertransference in psychodynamic psychotherapy). A finding of negligence would have to be combined with establishing damages and proving that the alleged harm to the plaintiff was not preexisting but was the result of the improper therapy. Successful suits in this area are only imaginable when the therapy provided is so far removed from what is customary that the approach taken would seem unacceptable to the layperson. Lawsuits due to cases of willful verbal or physical abuse during the course of, or as a component of psychotherapy, resulting in emotional and physical harm, could be successful. Generally, consultation with colleagues, and securing informed consent to treatment with the client, are the legal remedies to situations in which (1) the therapist elects to use an unorthodox or innovative form of therapy with a particular client; (2) the therapist substantially departs from the applicable practice standards for an accepted therapy; or (3) the client significantly deteriorates in treatment. Referral to another therapist, or use of an alternative form of treatment, may be the appropriate clinical, ethical, and legal approach in cases in which the treatment is demonstrably ineffective.

F. Abandonment

In a malpractice action based on abandonment, the plaintiff alleges that the therapist was providing care and then unilaterally terminated treatment without referral to another practitioner. The termination can be either intentional or negligent. The plaintiff must show that he was directly harmed by the abandonment and that the harm resulted in a compensable injury. The plaintiff must also establish that the termination was not his fault, that he kept his appointments, complied with treatment recommendations, and paid his bills. Abandonment is distinguished from the more general situation in which there is no intent to terminate care by the practitioner, but the client is denied proper care because of the clinician's delay or lack of diligence.

In nonemergencies, a mental health professional in private practice has no affirmative legal duty to accept a client into treatment. Once an agreement has been made to initiate treatment, the professional has a duty to continue the appropriate treatment as long as it is necessary. Even if still indicated, treatment can be terminated at the request of the client, or by the therapist with sufficient notice so that proper alternative treatment arrangements can be made. Generally, therapists are not legally required to treat clients they are not comfortable with for whatever reason, whether finances or the patient's problem. Nor are they required to treat clients who have threatened them or their family, offended other clients or health care personnel, damaged their office, or threatened litigation against them. Therapists in institutional settings (clinics, HMOs) have less freedom to select their clients, depending upon the presence of a contract between the client and/or institution and the funding agency. For all clinicians, there may be ethical constraints against refusing to treat a client because of race, sex, age, religion, or national origin.

Abandonment can occur only when a bona fide therapist–client relationship has been established. Serving as a consultant or evaluator does not give rise to such a treatment relationship. Analogously, a practitioner who refers his client to a specialist for continued care and treatment will not be liable for abandonment.

The availability of the therapist to clients between visits, after hours, or on weekends often presents problems for those who practice in the community. Medical practitioners have traditionally made themselves available to their patients on a continual basis either personally or through colleague backup, but nonmedical private practitioners have, at least in the past, maintained more typical business hours. As more nonmedical mental health professionals enter private practice in the community, it is likely that they will need to adopt the approach of their medical colleagues in order to avoid allegations of abandonment or deficient care. Coverage during off-hours or vacations should be provided only by other competent practitioners, and liability will attach to injuries that occur because the primary therapist fails to use reasonable professional judgment in selecting his substitute. He should also make his records available to the covering clinician should it be necessary to review them.

The patient who initiates a lawsuit against his therapist, but who wishes to remain in treatment, presents an interesting clinical and legal dilemma to the professional. Many such patients will not wish to withdraw from the treatment relationship, or the hospital facility, upon filing a lawsuit. There is little case law to guide conduct in this area, but it is likely that an additional action for abandonment, should the therapist terminate care, would fail, given appropriate notice of withdrawal and referral to another practitioner. Withdrawal from the patient's care will not usually be possible in the inpatient setting, and it is important that hospital staff not compromise the patient's treatment because of litigation against them or the institution. Transfer of the patient to another treatment unit or facility may be necessary in these cases rather than continued care of the patient.

G. Negligent Administration of Medication

A number of activities can serve as the basis for a malpractice action against a physician who prescribes psychotropic medications:

1. Absence of an adequate history, physical examination, and laboratory testing prior to treatment.
2. Prescribing a medication without demonstrated efficacy.
3. Prescribing a medication or combination of medications when they are not indicated.
4. Prescribing an incorrect dosage.
5. Prescribing a medication for the wrong time period.
6. Not recognizing or carefully monitoring side effects.
7. Failing to reduce or prevent the possibility of drug reactions and interactions.
8. Failing to consult with the necessary experts during treatment.

Physicians may also be subject to civil or criminal penalties with regard to the prescription of controlled substances. This liability is incurred by creating false treatment records, providing false information to regulatory authorities regarding controlled substances, and distributing controlled substances outside the scope of professional medical practice. Physicians have been found guilty of malpractice in causing or contributing to the addiction of a patient to controlled substances.

Tardive dyskinesia and tardive dystonia, consequences of the long-term use of antipsychotic medication, have also prompted litigation for negligent psychopharmacology. Lawsuits against general medical practitioners and psychiatrists because of a patient's tardive dyskinesia or tardive dystonia have been successful when the physician prescribed antipsychotic medication without proper indication, for inappropriately long durations, and without proper monitoring of the patient's condition. Because severe tardive dyskinesia and tardive dystonia are often irreversible, as well as disabling, damage awards in these cases have been substantial.

While the responsibility for prescribing medication and monitoring the effects of treatment is clearly that of the prescribing physician, other treatment personnel who have contact with the patient may be held responsible for failing to diagnose drug side effects, or for failing to refer the patient to the primary physician for evaluation of possible adverse results. These personnel include consulting physicians and covering physicians, as well as nonmedical personnel such as psychologists and psychiatric social workers who have had training in the use of psychotropic medication and the detection of adverse medication effects. In some clinics, for example, nonmedical personnel are routinely expected to complete drug-side-effect ratings since they have more frequent contact with the patient than the prescribing physician. In these cases, it is likely that negligent failure to detect adverse side effects will be found against both medical and nonmedical personnel.

H. Electroconvulsive Therapy

Despite the public perception of the considerable risks and misuse of ECT, there have been remarkably few lawsuits against hospitals or practitioners with regard to ECT in recent years. According to a survey of malpractice claims filed by members of the American Psychiatric Association insurance program, 17 of 711 resolved claims filed from 1972 to 1983 pertained to ECT. Patients obtained settlements in seven cases, four of which averaged $1,000. Settlements were more substantial in three wrongful death cases, averaging $110,000. Just two ECT claims were filed against the program from 1984 to 1987. Successful lawsuits based on the negligent administration of ECT have also been brought against hospitals, nurses, and hospital attendants.

Allegations of negligence-induced injuries by patients who have received ECT include inappropriate treatment for the particular condition, failure to administer the ECT properly, failure to obtain an informed consent, and failure to diagnose concurrent organic disorders. When filing a malpractice claim based on the administration of ECT, the plaintiff must establish that the standard of care was violated in prescribing the ECT, in its performance, or in monitoring the patient after ECT.

To avoid litigation in this area, or to be successful in the event of a suit, it is important for the practitioner to have followed the recommendations for clinical practice in ECT established by the American Psychiatric Association. Documentation of the informed consent to ECT should become part of the chart. In most states, if the patient is considered incompetent to consent to treatment, a guardian must be appointed to provide substituted consent. In some states, a court order is required before the ECT may be administered. When it is questionable whether the patient's consent is competent, it is advisable to have the closest family member also provide consent. Although this consent may not have legal validity, it is obtained from the person who could sue if something went wrong, thus making litigation less likely.

Claims pertaining to negligence in the prescription and use of ECT are sometimes problematic because of the difficulty in establishing the time and cause of some medical disorders. Thus, it may be difficult to determine whether an injury occurred before, during, or after ECT, or whether it was related in any way to the series of ECT treatments.

I. Negligent Psychological Evaluation

In addition to the actions detailed above, psychologists must be concerned with the administration of psychological tests. Often psychologists are called upon to perform evaluations which will have a profound effect on the examinee's life. Such evaluations may determine whether a person is employed or advanced in his career, whether the person is given the custody of his child, or whether he is convicted of a crime and sentenced to prison. In performing psychological tests in these potentially life-altering situations, the psychologist is warranting that he will use the appropriate standard of care in performing the evaluation.

To avoid liability, the psychologist must be familiar with the issues to be addressed by his diagnostic evaluation. He should be aware of any medical history as well as other psychological tests the examinee has taken and their results. The psychologist must be able to justify the choice of a certain battery of tests for the specific issue being addressed and the particular examinee. The tests must ordinarily be administered in the standard manner specified in the test manual. Any exceptions to the test manual in how the tests were administered or scored must be accounted for and reported. The psychologist must be familiar with the reliability and validity of the tests employed for the particular examinee and must use standard methods for interpreting the results. If others administer a test, the psychologist must be sure it was administered and scored properly. Informed consent to the use of the tests must be obtained from the examinee or his legal representative.

To establish malpractice liability against a psychologist for a diagnostic evaluation requires showing a deviation from the appropriate standard of care and resulting damages. Whatever tests would ordinarily be deemed appropriate in a given circumstance should be administered. If not, the psychologist must be prepared to justify why they were not given or were not given in the manner expected. As long as the appropriate standard of care was employed in selecting, administering, scoring, and interpreting the psychological tests, an erroneous diagnostic conclusion will generally not be sufficient to prove negligence. In addition to showing a deviation from the appropriate standard of care, the plaintiff must show the actual damages to him as a result of the psychologist's actions. Although malpractice suits against psychologists are infrequent, improper psychodiagnostic evaluations are one of the most prevalent causes of action against psychologists. It is thus critical for the clinician to be familiar with advances in the psychological testing literature and to perform all tests in accordance with the standards of the profession.

J. Social Worker Negligence

Though psychiatric social workers are infrequently sued, with more social workers expanding their careers to include psychotherapy in private practice, increased litigation against them is likely. The most likely areas for lawsuits against social workers relate to suicide, misdiagnosis, or sexual relations with a client. Social workers, particularly in a private practice setting, must be careful to call in medical consultants when they believe there may be a medical basis for the client's behavior, or when they are concerned about the individual's having an illness severe enough to warrant medication or hospitalization.

The other area of potential malpractice liability against social workers is the negligent investigation and assessment of a family in making decisions regarding their children. This circumstance could arise when charges of child abuse have been brought, or as part of an adoption or child custody proceeding. Although suits in this area are rare, and immunity may exist if the social worker was acting as an employee of a governmental agency, the social worker must be careful that the investigation is thorough. If it cannot be completed in the manner the social worker believes is appropriate, the report should clarify the investigation's shortcomings and should emphasize what information the recommendation is based upon. In a lawsuit against a social worker by a dissatisfied parent, liability will result only when the social worker has not done a proper evaluation and has drawn conclusions that do not relate to the information obtained. Even if these things can be proven, the plaintiff must then show how he was specifically damaged by the social worker's actions. (See Chapter 10, Section IX, "Legal Rights of Children," for a further discussion of liability issues facing social workers.)

III. PROBLEMS IN PROVING LIABILITY AGAINST MENTAL HEALTH PROFESSIONALS

Patients claiming injuries from their mental health treatment face several deterrents in bringing suit against the mental health professional. One of the major deterrents in initiating litigation is the imprecise nature and diagnosis of emotional disorders. There is considerable ongoing controversy about the definition of mental disorders, illnesses, and diseases. With some exceptions, damages from negligent mental health care are generally subjective, intangible, and poorly defined. It is often difficult to distinguish to what extent the claimed injury is really part of a preexisting emotional problem. These problems are compounded by the relatively low monetary value of the injury.

Given the limited knowledge about the causation or etiology of most psychiatric disorders, it is often difficult to establish the proximate causation of the patient's damages by negligent mental health care. A third problem is that the considerable variety of treatment approaches to mental and emotional disorders makes it difficult to establish a proper standard of care against which to measure the unsuccessful treatment provided by the clinician. It is difficult to establish that any single approach to the patient's care is the correct one. Refuting the appropriateness of the approach taken by the defendant is similarly difficult. It might therefore be difficult to find qualified experts who are willing to testify that the standard of care was breached in a particular case.

A fourth barrier to suit is the social stigma attached to having been treated for mental health problems. Many people are reluctant to publicize their emotional problems and treatment in litigation. Such suits not only are a matter of public record but may also require taking depositions from the client's family, friends, or colleagues regarding his emotional condition and ability to function.

The personal nature of the relationship between a therapist and a client is the fifth reason why litigation against a mental health professional is unlikely. Mental health professionals are trained to dispel negative therapeutic reactions in their patients. Clinical transference reactions, ambivalence, or ungratified dependency needs of the patient also reduce the likelihood that patients will find fault with the treatment or sue therapists with whom they have had a close relationship.

Finally, mental health treatment commonly occurs on an individual basis without the presence of third parties. Thus, the client who claims that a particular event occurred during treatment will have no witnesses to verify this claim. Even when the malpractice is blatant, such as the therapist's having sexual intercourse with the client, the client may be unwilling to sue because the likelihood of success is ultimately reduced to the client's word against the therapist's, and the client is likely to be considered less credible.

The stigma attached to having sought mental health care, the imprecise standards of practice, the problems of proving that an injury was caused by a violation of those standards, and the lack of measurable physical damages have made suits against mental health professionals unlikely. Although they will continue to be sued far less than other health care providers, there are other causes of liability which are not as difficult to prove as a case where negligence is alleged.

IV. OTHER CAUSES OF LIABILITY

A. Lack of Informed Consent

Every legally competent individual is entitled to decide what is done with his body. The legal doctrine of informed consent seeks to promote the patient's autonomy and self-determination regarding health care decision making. Informed consent requires that prior to treatment the patient be advised of his diagnosis, the nature and benefits of the contemplated treatment, the risks inherent in that treatment, his prognosis without treatment, and any possible alternative treatments. For the consent to be valid, the patient must be legally and clinically competent and must give the consent voluntarily. Lack of informed consent can be the basis for a negligence or even a battery action against the treatment provider. (See Chapter 5 for a discussion of informed consent and Chapter 9 for a discussion of guardianship when the patient cannot provide a valid consent to treatment.)

In many malpractice actions, a claim of lack of informed consent will be appended to a claim of negligence. An informed consent claim requires proving that the patient did not give his consent for the proposed procedure or treatment or was not advised of the risks of treatment and its alternatives. In addition, it must also be proven that the treatment was a proximate cause of the injury, and that had the therapist discussed a proposed treatment and its risks with the patient, the plaintiff would not have agreed to such a treatment approach given the information available. This is difficult for a plaintiff to prove after the fact, particularly when there was a witness to the informed consent disclosures, or when there is a notation in the chart that the therapist discussed the proposed treatment with the patient and an agreement was reached about the course of treatment.

In the mental health area, claims of lack of informed consent to treatment are most likely to arise with electroconvulsive therapy or psychotropic medication. With other therapeutic approaches, the benefits of treatment are less likely to be demonstrable, the risks of treatment are less likely to be severe or permanent, and the client's keeping appointments will provide an implied consent. In all cases, consent to treatment, along with the necessary disclosures, must be obtained from legal guardians of legally incompetent individuals (children and the severely demented or mentally retarded), except in emergencies. In cases in which multiple mental health professionals are involved in a patient's care, each professional has an obligation to obtain consent to, and to disclose the relevant information about, that form of treatment for which he is responsible. Although successful suits based on the lack of informed consent against mental health professionals are rare, the concept has the advantage of alerting therapists to the need to communicate with their patients and involve them actively in treatment decisions.

The availability of several possible treatment approaches to a particular mental health problem presents a problem for mental health practitioners with regard to informed consent. Obtaining the proper consent to treatment will generally require that the therapist review with the patient the alternative treatment methods, such as behavior therapy or psychotropic medication, and then refer the patient to the respective alternative therapists should the patient and the therapist believe such a referral to be indicated. Failure to do so, when the patient subsequently obtains successful treatment elsewhere using a different modality, is likely to prompt litigation against the first clinician. This is a common malpractice risk for the practitioner who uniformly prescribes one particular form of mental health treatment no matter what problems the patient presents.

Even a patient treated in individual psychodynamic psychotherapy in a private practice setting is entitled to participate in an informed consent dialogue, at least initially. In making the initial treatment decision with regard to this intervention, the patient will want information about the nature of this treatment process and its goals, methods, confidentiality, duration, and cost. It is often useful, both clinically and legally, for the therapist also to inform the patient that patients in psychotherapy often regress before they recover, and that transient depressions, suicidal impulses and behavior, and marital problems often occur during a long-term psychotherapy.

Finally, at this decision-making stage, patients will inquire about the therapist's qualifications, including training, experience, orientation, degrees, discipline, licensure, and board certification. At the outset of treatment, the therapist should identify his professional discipline (i.e., nursing, social work, psychology, psychiatry), specialty (i.e., school, counseling, clinical), and treatment philosophy or orientation. If the patient asks about the therapist's experience with a particular problem, then the therapist should respond forthrightly. If the therapist is a trainee, then the patient should be informed of this and that supervision will occur. The therapist need not, however, answer more personal questions. It is important for the therapist not to mislead the patient whether the issue is the therapist's qualifications or the proposed treatment itself.

Since informed consent is not a singular event but rather a process which occurs over time, the therapist has a continuing obligation to review the benefits and risks of the current treatment approach, and those of alternative treatment methods, with the patient (or guardian) during the course of treatment, particularly when the patient's condition appears to have significantly changed. Documentation of informed consent to treatment, both initially and subsequently, should be explicitly demonstrated in the patient's records. As noted later, written informed consent forms are commonly used in nonpsychiatric health care settings to document the consent process but are often avoided in mental health care settings.

B. Breach of Confidentiality

Confidentiality is the cornerstone of much of the therapeutic process in the mental health area. Society has given special recognition to this fact by enacting a variety of laws and regulations to protect confidential communications revealed to psychiatrists, psychologists, and other mental health professionals. Except when therapists are required to breach confidentiality for the protection of the patient or others, a breach of confidential information, including even the fact that someone is in treatment, is potentially actionable.

To be successful in a suit based on breach of confidentiality, the plaintiff must prove that (1) the breach of confidentiality occurred; (2) the confidential information divulged was not covered by an exception to the rules relating to confidentiality, such as civil commitment or reporting child abuse; and (3) there was tangible damage to the plaintiff as a result of the breach. The third element will be the most difficult to prove and quantify. The most likely successful scenario is the therapist's releasing information about the client to an employer without the client's consent. If this results in the client's job loss, then the damages are the lost income. (See Chapter 7 for a more thorough discussion of confidentiality.)

C. Duty to Protect Third Parties

Cases concerning the duty to protect third parties are different from ordinary malpractice cases in that the injured party has had no relationship to the treatment provider. In these cases, the injured party claims that his injury, which was inflicted by the client of the therapist, could have been prevented had the therapist warned him of potential harm from the client or taken some other action regarding the client. Holding a treatment provider liable to some third party whom he does not know and has had no contact with is a unique expansion of traditional tort law. This concept has been explicitly accepted by some states and limited by statute in several others. The potential liability for failure to protect the victims of clients has caused mental health professionals a great deal of concern. For this reason, Chapter 8 is devoted to this topic.

D. Failure to Report Child Abuse

Since 1964 all states have enacted laws requiring the reporting of suspected child abuse and neglect. Initially the laws applied only to physicians. Today they apply to a broad range of health care professionals, teachers and other school personnel, day-care-center workers, and, in some states, members of the general public. All mental health professionals have an obligation to make a report if there is a reasonable cause to suspect or believe that child abuse or neglect has occurred. Although the definitions of child abuse and neglect vary with each state, the goal of these laws is the same: to protect the child from further harm.

Both civil and criminal liability can occur as a result of not reporting suspected child abuse or neglect. Almost all states provide specific criminal penalties for not reporting. The crime is usually a misdemeanor with a fine ranging from $100 to $1,000 and a term of imprisonment varying from five days to one year. Although criminal liability against mental health professionals in this area is almost unheard of, these laws have the advantage of making clear to the professional, who may have some doubts about reporting, what his obligations are. Under the mandatory reporting provision, the clinician may not fail to report by claiming that the therapist–client relationship is more important than protection of the child. The requirements of these laws should be explained to the client at the outset of treatment or as soon as child abuse is raised in treatment.

To criminally convict someone for violation of the child-abuse-reporting statute requires establishing in most states that the person "knowingly" or "willfully" violated the law. The prosecutor must prove that (1) the person was legally required to report; (2) the person had knowledge of this legal mandate; (3) there was a conscious suspicion that the child was abused or neglected; and (4) the person failed to report. Criminal prosecution is likely when it can be shown that the person had direct knowledge of the abuse and took no action. Examples are the child telling a teacher, school counselor, or therapist of the harm he has experienced, or a parent in therapy describing the abuse, or hospital workers concluding that abuse has occurred but failing to act. All states have provisions which protect from liability individuals who make a good-faith report of suspected child abuse or neglect.

Not reporting can also serve as the basis for civil liability. In these cases, where the child is further harmed as a result of remaining in the home environment, and a professional was on notice of past abuse, the child or someone acting in his behalf can bring suit against the professional for not making a report. There have been a number of cases against physicians for not reporting child abuse. These cases have been based on the notion that it is negligence *per se* not to report as required by the statute, and also that it is professional malpractice since the physician owes a duty to the child, and the standards of his profession require following the reporting statutes. Other successful suits have been brought against school personnel. In these instances large damage awards have been rendered in favor of the plaintiff.

There is often some vagueness in the language of state statutes which creates clinical and legal problems for mental health practitioners. Depending upon the individual statute, it may be unclear whether to report suspicions of child abuse in the recent or distant past (e.g., more than a year ago), suspicions obtained thirdhand from others, cases in which reports have already been filed, sexual contact between minor siblings, or sexual contact between a child and a stranger. Further, some states mandate reporting only when the professional has had personal contact with the child, so that suspicions created from contact with a purported offender would not be sufficient to mandate reporting. These instances often require consultation with local mental health and legal experts with experience in child abuse. (See Chapter 10 for a further discussion of child-abuse-reporting obligations.)

E. Civil Rights Suits

For mental health professionals who work in agencies or hospitals owned or operated by governmental entities, there must also be concern about suits brought for violation of the patient's civil rights. These suits are usually brought as part of class action litigation seeking systematic changes in the mental health system. However, claims of civil rights violations can also occur when only an individual is bringing suit. These suits are based on Section 1983 of the United States Code, which was enacted after the Civil War to assure black persons full protection by the law. Section 1983 provides liability when it can be proven that someone acting under the authority of a governmental body has denied someone his civil rights.

For an attorney seeking to change the care provided by the mental health system, adding a claim of a violation of civil rights is a strategic move. It raises the seriousness of his claim, permits a claim for specific monetary damages, and provides further justification as to why the case should be heard in the federal courts rather than a state court. Unfortunately, the mental health professional who is sued is unaware of the strategic value of this type of claim and may be distressed and offended by a suit claiming he violated the rights of the patient. Often these cases occur in instances where the mental health professionals themselves are frustrated by the available care, because of the budgetary and staffing constraints placed on them by the state agency.

Although civil rights claims are almost uniformly added to class action lawsuits in the mental health area, holding an individual mental health professional liable for a violation of civil rights is unlikely. The courts are sympathetic to the plight of the professional who is trying to do the best he can, given budgetary and other constraints imposed by the mental health system.

V. HOSPITAL OR AGENCY LIABILITY

When the alleged injury occurred during hospitalization it is likely that the plaintiff will sue not only the primary treatment provider but the hospital and the individual staff members who provided care. Cases based on the patient's suicide or negligent release are most likely to include the facility, as well as numerous members of the staff. In these cases it is often difficult to determine who may have been responsible for the actual injury since a team approach to treatment is often used. By including all the caretakers, the plaintiff is more likely to determine who is responsible for the patient's injury. By naming the hospital in the suit, the plaintiff is in the best position to reach the "deepest pocket"; that is, the hospital is most likely to be sufficiently insured to cover the damages being sought.

No mental health treatment provider guarantees the results of the care provided. Yet each facility is expected to provide reasonable care for the health and safety of its patients. For the facility to be held liable, there must be a finding that it was at fault for the injury in question. This generally will require expert testimony. There are five generally recognized obligations of the treatment facility:

1. To provide proper medical equipment, supplies, medication, and food for the patients.
2. To exercise reasonable care in providing safe physical premises.
3. To adopt internal policies reasonably calculated to protect the safety and interests of patients.
4. To use care in deciding which employees to hire and retain, and in the granting of staff privileges.
5. To ensure that adequate patient care is being administered at the hospital.

Failure to meet any of these obligations can be the basis for suit, if the failure is accompanied by a compensable injury. Although these expectations are defined in terms of a hospital, they would apply with equal force to an outpatient facility.

An employer is responsible for the actions of its employees as long as the employee is acting within the scope of his employment. This is the doctrine of *respondeat superior*. This responsibility makes it imperative for a facility to screen its employees and staff physicians to verify that they have the qualifications they claim and the competence necessary for the job. If, for example, the facility hires an inadequately trained nurse and fails to supervise her, the facility will be liable for the damages that occur as a result of the nurse's negligent failures on the job. The duty of the facility includes hiring competent people and also ensuring that they remain capable of performing their jobs.

Facilities should have written policies or procedures to be followed regarding patient care. In many cases, these will be required by statute, regulation, reimbursement agencies, and accreditation bodies. There also should be formal periodic reviews of each employee's performance. Documentation of action taken against an employee who performs below the standard expected is critical for establishing that the facility is carefully monitoring the care provided under its auspices.

VI. SUITS AGAINST SUPERVISORY PERSONNEL

In the same way that a hospital can be held liable for the negligent acts and omissions of its employees, a supervisor, even if personally innocent of negligence, can be held vicariously liable for the acts of someone he supervises. This chain of liability includes employee, trainee, supervisor, and health care facility, as well as a college or university. The supervisor can also be directly liable to the patient when he uses the trainee to execute decisions negligently made by the supervisor.

The supervisor can be held directly liable if he did not determine the employee's or trainee's competence before assigning responsibilities. If the task is performed negligently, then both the employee-trainee and the supervisor may be liable for any resulting damage. The supervisor could also be liable if he determines that someone under his direction is unable to perform his job but takes no action to limit the person's activities. The supervisor must be familiar with the level of competence of the supervisee before delegating any responsibility. Supervisory personnel should also clarify with the facility the specific responsibilities of trainees or others being supervised.

Some unique issues are presented in settings where professional trainees provide clinical care under the supervision of clinical faculty. Here, the trainee has a responsibility to explicitly inform the patient of his professional qualifications and status; a patient has the right to refuse care by such a trainee. The clinical supervisor could be held vicariously liable for the negligent acts of the trainee (e.g., concealing information from the supervisor or failure to refer to a specialist), even if the supervisor has not been negligent. The supervisor could also be liable for the acts of the trainee which are not authorized by law (e.g., patient–therapist sexual misconduct). Supervisors should know whether their liability insurance covers improper supervision of the direct and indirect types.

In many mental health clinics and hospitals, administrative supervision is provided for fully trained clinicians. Here, the supervisor has actual or apparent control over the primary clinician, and the supervisor is likely to be held liable for the negligence of the clinician. By contrast, in other facilities, there are clinical supervisors who are given responsibility for a patient's care even if another fully trained therapist assumes primary responsibility for the treatment and the supervisor infrequently sees the patient. Limitations in resources in such settings may even minimize the contact between supervisor and therapist. Further, some physician "supervisors" who prescribe psychotropic medication to the patient often do not "supervise" or have control over the psychosocial treatment of the patient but rather are cotherapists. In these dual-treatment arrangements, courts may still see the physician as the "captain of the ship," that is, as the supervisor in charge of the treatment, even though he is responsible for only one of its components. Thus, clinical supervisors, as well as administrative supervisors, need to be cognizant of the often hidden legal risks, whether expressed or implied, which are entailed in supervisory arrangements.

Another form of clinical supervision in mental health care often occurs in noninstitutional practice when a mental health professional obtains outside consultation with a more experienced colleague, either for an individual case or for an entire caseload. In this arrangement, the independent consultant does not personally see the junior colleague's patients and has no actual control over the patient's treatment but nevertheless provides regular input into the treatment. Here the consultant is more of an outside instructor than a cotherapist or "supervisor." While it is possible for such a consultant to be named in a lawsuit against the primary therapist, the consultant would argue, perhaps successfully, that he has a duty to the therapist rather than to the patient, and thus no liability would attach.

VII. SUITS AGAINST STATE EMPLOYEES

In some jurisdictions, the decisions and activities of mental health professionals employed by the state are immune from tort liability through various provisions of state law. This immunity is referred to as *governmental immunity* or *statutory immunity*. Immunity provisions might apply to state agencies and departments, and any employees who act on behalf of these agencies. These would include the direct providers of inpatient and outpatient care. Immunity is sometimes available only to those professionals who are responsible for making decisions ("discretionary-decisional" acts), but not to the professional who is responsible for executing that decision ("ministerial-operational" acts). Thus, a physician's decision to permit a hospitalized patient to go on a supervised pass might be immune from tort liability, but the failure of the staff to properly supervise the patient on the pass leading to an escape and injury may not be immune from liability.

Public mental health facilities and their employees will be immune from liability only when the following factors occur:

1. When they are engaged in a governmental function, such as providing care.
2. When they act during the course of their employment.
3. When their actions are within the scope of their authority.

Thus, sexual activity with a patient would not be considered within the scope of the professional's employment and would not be immune under such a statute.

Immunity provisions in some states might apply to all mental health facilities and employees, rather than only to those in the public sector. Here, mental health facilities and professionals might, for example, be immunized from tort liability for professional negligence. They would, however, be liable for gross negligence or intentional torts, including criminal acts. The applicable law will also define what specific activities or treatment settings would be entitled to limited immunity.

VIII. MALPRACTICE INSURANCE

Most mental health professionals are covered by a professional liability insurance policy, either through their employer or independently. In recent years, many insurance companies have withdrawn from this particular market, leaving the clinician with fewer policies from which to choose. As is the case for any insurance policy (e.g., homeowners', automobile, or health), the clinician should be aware of the policy's terms, coverage, and limitations. Any insurance policy is a contract between the insurer and the insured, and its terms are legally binding. It is the insured's responsibility to read and understand the "fine print" before selecting a policy and accepting its limits. Even employees should be familiar with the nature and extent of the insurance coverage at the agency or facility.

Until the mid-1970s, most professional liability insurance was offered on an occurrence basis. Such a policy covers those incidents which occurred during the policy year regardless of when the incident was discovered by the plaintiff or when the lawsuit was filed. Because of the often lengthy delay between alleged malpractice and the filing of the suit, insurance companies had difficulty adjusting their premiums to the frequency and severity of litigation. In recent years, professional liability coverage has sometimes been offered on a claims-made basis. In this policy type, the insurer covers only those claims which are reported during the policy period, regardless of when the incident occurred. Thus, after the end of a claims-made policy term (through retirement, death, change in position, cancellation of coverage, or change in insurer), the professional is unprotected. The clinician must then purchase a separate "tail coverage" policy to cover incidents which occurred during the claims-made policy but were reported after it. Claims-made insurance is initially less expensive than occurrence coverage, but any reduction in premiums is short-term until the exposure period for each policy type equalizes.

Each insurance policy specifies those professional acts which are covered and those which are not. Most policies provide coverage for professional negligence (unintentional acts) and exclude intentional acts. There may be no coverage for civil rights violations, fraud, libel, slander, breach of contract, punitive damages, criminal actions, or gross negligence. Additional insurance must often be purchased to cover premises liability, administrative responsibilities, and vicarious liability for employees, trainees, and partners. Some policies will pay only for the defense of certain claims, such as sexual impropriety with patients, but not for an ultimate judgment or verdict for the plaintiff. Some policies have discounts or penalties for the insured depending upon his claims history. All policies limit the amount of judgment or verdict which will be paid by the insurer. Awards which exceed the limits of the policy are the personal responsibility of the defendant. Finally, some policies provide the defendant with a right to approve or refuse a settlement that may be offered by the plaintiff; others do not.

Given the relatively modest cost of professional liability insurance, the cost of attorneys' fees for even "nuisance" lawsuits, and the risk of a catastrophic event from even a single psychiatric patient, probably no mental health professional should "go bare." In many states, obtaining insurance coverage is a requirement of obtaining a professional license. The determination of the amount of coverage should be made in the context of the professional's practice. Independent insurance specialists are available in the community to review a policy with the clinician when necessary.

IX. RECORD KEEPING

Clinicians are often required by law to maintain contemporaneous records of the evaluation and treatment of their patients. Record keeping for mental health care is usually regulated by the treatment facility's administrative policy, state mental health regulation, or statute. Record keeping standards are also promulgated by reimbursement (state, federal, commercial), utilization review, professional licensure, and accreditation organizations. Such policies will dictate if and when records are to be maintained, the content of such records, the conditions of release of records to third parties, the patient's access to the records, and the conditions of record retention. Though clinicians customarily view health care records as clinical documents, they are legal documents as well.

Record keeping is an essential, but generally undervalued, part of the mental health professional's responsibilities. Many clinicians view record keeping as an unwelcome chore and overlook the value of this effort. Some believe it to be a clerical rather than a clinical responsibility, best delegated to secretarial staff. Thus, health care records sometimes neglect important events but highlight many unimportant ones. Some clinicians deliberately avoid documenting some events for fear of increasing their risk of liability. More principled documentation by clinicians, rather than additional documentation, is necessary to deal with these problems.

A. Record Keeping Functions

The keeping of health care records serves a variety of important clinical purposes, including:

1. Documenting the patient's condition and any changes in it.
2. Planning and facilitating treatment.
3. Communicating with other staff members about the patient, for both present and future care.
4. Recording the fact and necessity of treatment for reimbursement purposes.
5. Documenting the quality of treatment for utilization review and external accreditation.
6. Promoting education of trainees and facilitating clinical research.

Mental health care records also serve a variety of legal purposes. For example, a patient may use his records to establish a claim to various financial entitlements, to prove psychological damages in a personal injury lawsuit, or to reduce his criminal or civil responsibility. These records are also essential to the clinician who is defending against a malpractice suit brought by the patient. The record will serve as the only objective account of the client's treatment.

B. Contents of Records

The intake record on a patient should generally include the following information:

1. A relevant psychiatric, social, and medical history with pertinent positive and negative findings.
2. Interview observations and findings, and a mental status examination.
3. A differential diagnosis.
4. The treatment prescribed, and the additional tests, consultations, or procedures ordered.
5. Treatment or referral plans, as well as informed consent to treatment.
6. The clinician's discipline, title, and signature.

Once treatment has begun, progress notes should include a description of the patient's symptoms and the changes in them, a description of the patient's treatment and the changes in it, compliance with treatment, response to treatment, adverse effects of treatment, and contacts with third parties.

During treatment, record keeping is particularly valuable in documenting adverse treatment effects, significant clinical change, change in supervision (seclusion, privileges, passes, and discharge), legal events (certification for commitment, testimony at commitment hearings, and interactions with police), and the presence of suicide or violent intention or attempts.

There are two general types of mental health records. A clinic or facility will maintain the official or public record, which contains administrative documents, consent forms, history and mental status examination reports, treatment plans, progress notes, physician orders, laboratory results, and consultation reports. In addition, many clinicians maintain their own private record of their work with the patient which is protected from discovery by law in some jurisdictions. The clinician should approach these two types of records differently. The official record, for example, should be descriptive, observational, factual, objective, noneditorializing (not critical of other staff or the patient), written in the third person, and, of course, legible; it should be written contemporaneously with the events in the patient's life and the patient's treatment. The clinician should identify the source of the data (e.g., "Mrs. Smith's daughter reports that her mother has not been sleeping for two weeks"). A professional tone should be maintained throughout the record, and excessive jargon should be avoided. The therapist should be aware of the likelihood of the record's being read by the patient or others. In contrast, private (process) notes may contain sensitive material provided by the patient, such as fantasies, dreams, and sexual content, as well as the psychodynamic speculations and interpretations of the therapist. These notes may be written at a time and in a manner convenient to the clinician without regard for the need of other clinicians to review them, although such private notes are most often recorded for training or supervision. The personal notes should be kept physically separate from the official record and should not be used as a substitute for it.

From a clinical as well as a legal viewpoint, particularly in the case of treatment by more than a single clinician, it is not enough for the clinician to think about the diagnosis and treatment of the patient's condition without recording it; other clinicians will read the patient's record in the course of their own work with the patient and will be influenced by what appears therein. Courts and external review bodies view the absence of documentation in the record about an event as evidence that it never occurred, no matter what the subsequent claims of the clinicians. If, for example, there is no notation in the medical record that the clinician conducted a suicide evaluation prior to a patient's discharge from the hospital, then the clinician will be at a disadvantage when later trying to prove at trial after the patient's suicide that an evaluation was in fact performed (see Table 6.1).

Accurate and timely records enhance a defendant's credibility, which is evaluated by the jury during the testimony at deposition and trial. The medical record is the only forum for documenting that the patient received appropriate and standard care. The record must be sufficiently complete to explain the patient's condition and the treatment he received. It will be used to settle factual disputes between the plaintiff and the defendant about what actually occurred in the treatment process. At trial, the plaintiff's attorney will argue that the clinician did not do what he claims to have done if he failed to document it in the record. An inadequate record will itself be seen as evidence of substandard care, no matter what care was actually provided. In particular, the record should clearly document the rationale for changes in the patient's hospital privileges (grounds privileges, passes, and observation status) or transfer and discharge. Records are most useful when they reveal the clinician's thinking and decision making about the patient's care, rather than simply documenting that an event occurred. This is particularly important when the clinician is considering the admission or discharge of patients with a risk of suicide or violence. Generally, specific observations about the patient are more useful to those who may review the record at some future time than the clinician's impressions about the patient, which will be difficult to interpret.

When the clinician is taking a calculated risk, such as continuing or changing the treatment of a patient who has made a recent suicide attempt, particular attention should be given to recording the reasoning used by the clinician in formulating

Table 6.1. Record Keeping Pitfalls

A.	Overdocumentation
	Disparaging staff or patients
	Including extraneous or sensitive data
	Noncontemporaneous alterations
	Belief that no one will ever read the record
	Illegible handwriting
	Improper abbreviations
B.	Underdocumentation
	Forgetting that medical records are legal documents
	Failing to document decision making
	Failing to document significant events
	Failing to document information disclosures about informed consent
	Discarding records prematurely
	Failing to document telephone calls and medication refills
	Failing to obtain and review past records

the treatment plan. In such instances, the clinician should "think out loud for the record," for example:

> September 1, 1990; 9 a.m. Attending Psychiatrist progress note: Review of the nursing notes of August 31, 1990, indicates that the patient became extremely agitated last night and severely cut his neck with a sharp pencil. He required suturing and then was placed in seclusion and four-point restraints for the next six hours. Today's pass will be canceled because of the return of symptoms which prompted the patient's hospitalization. A pass will not be rescheduled until the patient has been restabilized. We will also attempt to understand why the patient regressed just prior to his expected pass today and will contact the patient's family in this regard. The patient now denies suicide intention, but suicide ideation persists, so that although restraints can be removed, I will order continued locked seclusion because of the patient's agitation. I will see him again later today.

Clinicians in solo, outpatient psychotherapy practices often do not maintain any record of the client's treatment except the appointment time, which is contained in the clinician's calendar book, or billing information. Except when controverted by law this is not considered a violation of clinical care or record keeping standards but carries some risks. It also presents a problem when the client requests that the clinician submit his records to third parties for one reason or another. Initiating a formal record will often be necessary if, however, there is an unusual event or a significant deterioration in the client's functioning. Events such as suicide attempts, interpersonal violence, use of consultations, or the prescriptions of psychotropic medications will also necessitate formal record keeping.

Outpatient clinicians often overlook the need to record telephone contact with the client and others. Such contact is often a significant part of the client's treatment or at least reflects significant events in the client's life and his response to them. Recording the date, the time, the caller, and the substance of the call on a regular basis may be useful should an untoward event later develop.

Record keeping should be contemporaneous with the clinical course of the patient. The clinician may make additional notations in the chart after earlier sessions but should properly identify the date and time of each entry, rather than modify an earlier entry. Corrections in the record may be made by drawing a single line through the erroneous writing, initialing this, and then recording the correct material with time and date. Use of eradicating fluid, crossing-out which obliterates the original writing, or removing entire pages of the record must be avoided. Generally, whoever made an incorrect entry in the record should be the one to amend it. Professional document examiners are now able to detect alterations in the record made with different pens, by different people, or at different times. Writing in the record which crowds other entries is risky in that it may raise a question of timeliness and truthfulness. The original medical record will be brought to court for any litigation. Any alterations in the record which appear to be tampering or doctoring will be detrimental to the clinician's case since they reveal a consciousness of guilt. A later alteration in the record will be readily detected when the clinician changes the record after the patient or his attorney has obtained a complete copy of the record, without the clinician's knowing. Alterations in a medical record can lead to punitive damages in a malpractice case, professional license revocation, or even criminal charges.

Mental health clinicians who function primarily in nonpsychiatric medical settings (e.g., general hospitals, health maintenance organizations, and group medical practices) are faced with particular challenges in record keeping. In these situations, non-mental health clinicians will have access to the records of the mental health clinician and may not appreciate the sensitivity with which this kind of information must be regarded. Because of this problem, some facilities maintain separate record keeping for the medical and mental health records. When an integrated system is in practice, however, the mental health professional needs to be particularly careful about what he records.

Patients in mental health care are usually entitled to access to their records, which is specified by state law. While ownership of the record is retained by the clinician or hospital, the patient "owns" the information contained in the record. Such state laws will identify the conditions under which patients may and may not review their records, whether they are entitled to copies of them or to modify the content of their records, and when and to what degree the clinician may deny patient access. Clinicians should be mindful of the fact that, while patients have a right to release such records to third parties, there can not truly be a valid consent to their release unless the patient is familiar with the content of those records.

X. MALPRACTICE PREVENTION

Malpractice risks are inherent in every clinical endeavor. Mental health professionals should be familiar with the risks inherent in their various activities, as well as specific methods to minimize such risks. Reducing the risk of a lawsuit is best ensured by practicing good clinical care. Other ways to reduce the likelihood of a lawsuit from a dissatisfied patient and family include the following.

A. Communication

The therapist must maintain open communication with the client. Lawsuits are often generated by clients in an attempt to attract needed attention, to compensate for perceived neglect by the therapist, to compel the therapist to acknowledge his error, or to identify the responsible clinician. A client who threatens a lawsuit during treatment is trying to convey something which he feels is otherwise not getting through to the therapist. Noncompliance with treatment recommendations should be addressed as it develops, including sending letters to clients who fail to keep their appointments.

B. Empathy

Maintaining respect for the client is a necessary ingredient of mental health care in any treatment setting. Taking control of a client in the context of involuntary treatment is a particular test of this clinical and legal prerequisite.

C. Limitations

When possible the clinician is advised to accept for treatment only those patients with whom he can work comfortably. Risking the emotional entanglement characteristic of mental health treatment with a client one dislikes from the outset is a setup for clinical failure. Attempting to care for a client whose clinical needs are beyond the therapist's skills invites problems. Referral to a more suitable clinician in these circumstances is the best long-term solution.

D. Informed Consent

Initiating treatment provides a natural opportunity to specify the terms of the agreement between the therapist and the client, including the terms of treatment and the circumstances when confidentiality will be breached. The initial sessions can serve to disabuse a client of unrealistic expectations about what treatment can accomplish or to better explain the pros and cons of specific treatment modalities. A patient surprised by an unexpected outcome or medication side effect is more likely to seek legal redress than one who has been prepared for it. No treatment guarantees should be offered, and adverse outcomes should be disclosed to the client. Developing an alliance with the client through the informed consent process is the best insurance against liability.

E. Fees

At the outset of therapy, the clinician should describe to the client his fee schedule and his payment expectations. Disputes over fees are a foreseeable cause of litigation in private practice when the clinician attempts to collect accumulated fees too aggressively. It is best to collect fees as they are incurred rather than allow the client to get too far behind. Failing to deal with financial issues as they develop is a disservice to both the client's clinical needs and his financial status.

F. Comprehensive Evaluation

The clinician must carefully evaluate the suicide and homicide potential of every patient. Liability is assessed only after the fact, so that a disastrous result tends to make the clinician appear negligent. Thorough history, examination, and documentation in a standard manner will minimize the chance of a verdict for the plaintiff.

G. Consultation

Mental health care is a complex field about which few are truly expert in many areas. Consultation is appropriate when the clinician suspects he is operating beyond his training and experience. Both formal and informal (e.g., telephone) consultations can be useful to the client as well as the therapist. It is also helpful to establish consultative relationships with other mental health professionals in advance of the clinical problem.

H. Continuity of Care

Mental health care for many chronically ill persons is regrettably provided in a discontinuous manner across different settings. Receiving clinicians should obtain prior treatment records and review them for indications of prior successes and failures. Referring clinicians can facilitate the transition by checking to see if the patient is eligible for other treatment services. If so, the therapist should consider setting up the appointment and promptly provide the records with the appropriate request. Clinicians should ideally maintain an "open door" policy so that terminating clients can return at any time, at least for an evaluation, if not for continuation of treatment.

I. Knowing the Relevant Law and Institutional Policies

Adhering to the clinical standard of care will not always immunize the clinician against liability. Various administrative policies, legal regulations, case law, or statutes may demand even more of the clinician. Following these policies is critical to avoid liability should litigation arise. Try to keep abreast of changes in the law. This is most easily accomplished through the newsletter of your local professional organization. A copy of the mental health code and regulations should be kept available, as well as the name of a knowledgeable consultant.

XI. RESPONDING TO A MALPRACTICE LAWSUIT

Although there may be some indication that the mental health professional is likely to be sued, either as a result of client threats or via a request for the record, the formal notice of suit will come with the arrival of the Complaint. This notifies the professional or the facility that the patient is suing, as well as the basis for the suit. Once the notice of suit arrives, the mental health professional should:

1. *Notify the insurance carrier*. The most important initial step for the clinician is to notify the insurance carrier, or one's employer. This must be done immediately since there is only a brief period of time to file an answer to the suit, and most insurance coverage contracts set a time limit for notification. Failure to notify the insurance carrier will jeopardize the insurance coverage for the claim. Failure to respond to the Complaint in a timely manner could result in a default judgment against the defendant.

2. *Write down everything about the case*. The clinician should use the receipt of the complaint as the time to jog his memory about everything related to the client and the case. He should systematically review the record without altering it or even adding to it. He should make additional notes which are separate from the record and which can assist him in preparing his defense. The record will often contain little information, but there will be a wealth of information in the clinician's memory that will not have been recorded in the chart. Comments about the client, his family, and the circumstances of treatment should be noted. These notes should not be added to the chart but should be kept separate for sharing with the clinician's attorney.

3. *Be comfortable with the attorney*. The clinician-defendant's insurance carrier will assign an attorney to the case. It is critical that the clinician have the utmost confidence in his lawyer and develop a good working relationship. He must be confident that the attorney is knowledgeable, is concerned about his case, and has the time to devote to it. The attorney must be someone with whom he can be completely honest, sharing any weaknesses in his treatment of the patient or any previous professional problems such as litigation or ethical complaints. If the clinician is uncomfortable

with his attorney, for whatever reason, he should ask to confer with another attorney. The clinician must realize that the attorney, not the therapist, must be in control of the case.

It is sometimes necessary for the therapist-defendant to independently retain an attorney to advise him on the case. This will also be necessary when the therapist has no malpractice insurance policy. Separate counsel is useful when the monetary demands of the lawsuit exceed the malpractice policy's limits, when there is a dispute about the scope of the policy's coverage, when there are multiple codefendants who are insured by the same carrier or defended by the same law firm, or when the defendant wishes to review a proposed settlement before committing himself. The expenses of this consultation will generally be paid personally by the mental health professional. However, some policies will cover consultation expenses with another attorney.

4. *Discuss the case only with the attorney*. The defendant should not discuss the details of the litigation with friends, colleagues, or the plaintiff or the plaintiff's family. He should not contact the plaintiff to "talk things over" or to try to talk him into dismissing the lawsuit. If friends of the client mention the suit, the therapist must avoid comment. The suit may involve other colleagues at the same treatment facility. Although the therapist should immediately contact the facility's administrator to notify him of the suit, he should not discuss the case further with colleagues without the advice of counsel, since his colleagues may have been joined in the litigation and may have conflicting interests. The therapist should never talk to the plaintiff's attorney without his own attorney being present. In the rare case where the news media become involved, the clinician should offer no comment. Anything said may later harm the clinician's case. The therapist should utilize his attorney to talk for him or to guide him as to when or to what extent outside comment is appropriate.

5. *Assist the defense attorney in the case preparation*. The clinician can assist his attorney in preparing the case in many ways. The clinician must initially commit himself to becoming involved in the case and must sacrifice the time and energy otherwise devoted to his clients and to personal and professional activities. The clinician will need to consult with his attorney, prepare for depositions, and, in rare instances, prepare for trial.

The clinician will need to reconstruct all information available about the case and may prepare a written summary of the case to assist him. This summary should include everything which is apparent from the record, as well as everything else known about the client, his family, and the circumstances of treatment. The client's record will further refresh the clinician's memory about the case. Obtaining the client's past treatment records, if not already available, sometimes provides important information in the defense of the claim.

The clinician should educate the attorney about the type of treatment given in the case. A search of the professional literature can demonstrate how the therapist's approach was appropriate. The therapist should provide his attorney with the literature in support of his position, as well as with literature that is contrary to his approach. It is critical for the therapist to dissect the plaintiff's complaint and point out its flaws. What is untrue? What are its weaknesses? What are the problems with the expert witnesses chosen by the plaintiff, and how can their testimony be discredited? How was the plaintiff's expert incorrect in his deposition, and how does his testimony in this case differ from that in other malpractice cases?

Though the therapist must know his own case in detail and be familiar with the relevant clinical literature and standards, it is also helpful to become familiar with legal precedents in the area. These include the applicable regulations, statutes, and case law. Knowledge of legal precedents will aid the defendant in distinguishing his own case from others.

Finally, the defense attorney may need assistance in finding expert witnesses who can testify that the standard of care was followed. These should not be colleagues of the therapist but can be people who know the clinician professionally. An ideal expert witness is one who is a practicing clinician, teaches, and is well respected in the community, with some courtroom experience, but who does not primarily serve as an expert witness. Selecting the expert witness can be a critical factor in determining the outcome of the case. The defense attorney, rather than the clinician, should initially contact any proposed experts.

6. *Prepare for testimony at deposition and trial.* Most malpractice cases are either dismissed or settled before reaching the trial stage. The clinician's pretrial testimony at the deposition is usually his only opportunity to officially present his side of the case. Thus, his presentation and credibility at the deposition may well determine the outcome of the case.

Before testifying, the therapist must be familiar with the record, without needing to memorize every detail. References to the plaintiff's records are permitted during testimony. The attorney will outline the direct examination and likely cross-examination in advance of the testimony. Those who have never testified in a court of law may find it helpful to attend trials in other cases to better appreciate the demands of the situation. Some even prefer to practice testifying using audiovisual equipment. Review Chapter 11 for further guidelines on testifying.

XII. COPING WITH A MALPRACTICE LAWSUIT

Being a party to any lawsuit normally arouses a variety of emotions. Being named as a defendant in a professional negligence lawsuit threatens one's professional esteem, identity, career, and economic well being. Though technically only the clinician's work is being challenged, it may appear, particularly during the trial, that the clinician is personally being discredited.

The clinician's reaction to a malpractice lawsuit often resembles the posttraumatic stress disorder that follows other stressful life events. This might be called a *malpractice stress syndrome* in terms of the symptoms which often develop. Unfortunately, the stressful event in this case is not a single momentary event in time but may last for several years as the litigation slowly proceeds to trial. Common to both syndromes is that the person is unprepared for the stressful event because he never expected it to happen to him, only to others.

Clinician-defendants develop a variety of signs and symptoms of their distress. These include anger, depression, anxiety, loss of interest in social activities or work, guilt, and loss of self-esteem. There also may be a loss of appetite, loss of self-control, and insomnia. The symptoms may resemble a major depressive disorder or adjustment disorder. The therapist may also become more vulnerable to physical illness. At work, the clinician may begin to distrust other clients and to become overcautious in managing their care.

The lawsuit is likely to affect relations with the clinician's family. The clinician may become withdrawn, embittered, and preoccupied with the suit and its defense. The litigation may lead to alcohol or substance abuse, and the therapist may relinquish his career responsibilities or may even change careers, because of his preoccupation.

It is important for the therapist to discuss his feelings about the suit with his spouse and close family members. In some communities there are support groups for professionals who have been sued. Assuming an active posture in the defense of the lawsuit provides emotional support as well as helps the defense. This effort requires considerable time investigating the case, learning the relevant clinical and legal issues involved, meeting with counsel, and participating in the defense. Failing to become involved in the defense of the case may leave the clinician with regret following its conclusion.

It is important to remember that it is foolish to retaliate against the plaintiff, his family, his attorney, or the plaintiff's expert witness by sending threatening communications or taking other inappropriate action. The clinician should keep in mind that all professionals face the likelihood of being sued when the results of their efforts are unsuccessful or unexpected. The majority of claims are dismissed or result in minimal settlements. Having a malpractice suit filed does not mean that the clinician violated the standard of care, only that the former client or his family was dissatisfied with the result which occurred. In the unlikely event that the case goes to trial and the clinician loses, it does not mean that he does not possess adequate clinical skills at the present time. It means only that he has been judged to be guilty of not meeting the standard of care expected of him in a given circumstance which occurred years before the final resolution of the dispute.

XIII. CONCLUSION

Concern about professional liability will continue to be an important issue for mental health professionals. Increased litigiousness is characteristic of our contemporary society in general, and the bases for liability against mental health professionals continue to expand. Professional organizations and state licensing boards are increasing the scrutiny of their licensed practitioners.

Yet a number of factors should be of solace. First, lawsuits against mental health professionals are still relatively uncommon, and are likely to continue to be so. Second, an adverse treatment result does not denote liability. The mental health professional does not guarantee a specific outcome but must provide services only in a manner which meets the standards of the profession. Thus, the best defense will always be the use of appropriate care. An error in judgment about a patient, without such a deviation from the standard, will not lead to liability. Third, in order for a case to merit filing, there must be significant or measurable damages. In the case of a claimed psychological injury, these will often be difficult to establish, except when there are economic damages such as a loss of earning capacity.

Although one should be aware of the law, and concerned to some extent with the expanding bases for liability, the best defense is to provide excellent care with benevolent intent. If the mental health professional keeps current with the field, his concern about professional liability will hopefully be of academic interest, rather than based on personal experience.

XIV. COMMONLY ASKED QUESTIONS

1. *Can a mental health professional from one discipline (e.g., psychology or nursing) testify as an expert witness in a malpractice case against a mental health professional from another discipline (e.g., psychiatry or social work)?*

A malpractice case requires proving that the professional violated the standard of care of his specialty. This ordinarily requires that the expert witness be from the same discipline as the defendant-clinician.

2. *Who is responsible for obtaining informed consent to treatment when several mental health professionals are involved in the treatment?*

Each clinician is responsible for obtaining and reviewing the informed consent to treatment, at least to the degree that he is involved with the patient in a treatment modality. However, the answer in part depends on the nature of the proposed treatment. In some cases a member of one discipline may be principally responsible for administering a particular modality and thus would be responsible for obtaining and reviewing the informed consent to treatment. A psychiatrist, for example, as the prescriber of medication, must be the one to obtain the consent for its use. When care is administered by a team, each team member should be clear about his respective role and responsibility.

3. *Is it appropriate to criticize a previous therapist's treatment strategy in the presence of the client?*

For a variety of clinical reasons, a client may attempt to engage the current therapist in a critical review of his previous treatment and/or therapist. With rare exceptions, it is inappropriate to criticize the previous treatment personnel, from either a clinical or a legal perspective. The former personnel may have had different data available at the time of the treatment, because the client had a different clinical presentation. Such discussion may unnecessarily prompt the client to initiate an inappropriate lawsuit, which will be disruptive to the current treatment plan.

4. *Is the therapist obligated to report another professional's alleged malpractice?*

A therapist's duty or obligation to report another professional's misconduct may be viewed from the legal, ethical, or clinical perspective. The ethical codes of some professional societies require that any such alleged misconduct, even if not proscribed by the criminal or civil law, be reported to ethical boards or agencies of that profession. Individual state laws may also require that a professional's alleged misconduct (sexual misconduct) be report to a licensing authority. The appropriate course for the therapist may also be influenced by whether the other professional practices within the same specialty. If not, the obligations may be different, and such reporting may complicate the present treatment.

5. How long after a patient has been discharged from care can the therapist be held responsible for the patient's subsequent suicide?

Finding a therapist liable for his patient's suicide requires establishing that the suicide was proximally caused by the negligent care of the therapist. The longer the interval between the discharge of the client and the suicide, the more difficult it will be for the plaintiff to succeed against the therapist. The greatest difficulty in establishing negligence arises in an outpatient setting where there was no specific suicide ideation or intention before discharge from treatment.

6. Can the therapist discharge the patient from care when he is noncompliant with the treatment recommendations?

The therapist is responsible for providing care until the treatment is properly terminated. The therapist can withdraw from the case when the client repeatedly fails to comply with the treatment plan, or when he refuses to pay for treatment despite his ability to do so. The therapist should properly document in the medical record the problems with the client. In some situations, the therapist may believe that treatment is no longer indicated, though the client does not want to stop treatment. In these situations, the client should receive adequate advance notice of the termination of the relationship so that alternate treatment arrangements can be made, if desired. The therapist should send the client a letter indicating that the therapist is formally terminating care and the reasons for this. If the therapist believes the person would continue to benefit from care, referral should be made to community mental health agencies or others who might provide the appropriate care. With the patient's consent, the therapist should provide a copy of the patient's records to the new treatment provider. The clinician should not be liable for subsequent injury if the relationship is properly terminated.

7. Should a therapist meet with the family of a client who has just committed suicide?

This is largely a matter of clinical judgment, depending on the nature of the relationship with family members as well as the course of treatment with the client. Expressing condolences to the family is important, and being able to share with them information which will alleviate their own guilt may have a beneficial psychological effect on them, as well as reduce the likelihood of a lawsuit. Failure to offer such comments or bereavement counseling may be misinterpreted by the survivors as guilt for the therapist's misconduct and may stir the family to initiate a lawsuit. Often a lawsuit after a suicide represents the family's attempt to fix blame on another party. Helping to alleviate the family's guilt may lessen the likelihood of a suit being filed.

From a clinical perspective, the therapist should not engage members of the family in an ongoing treatment relationship when treatment is necessary after such a loss but should refer them to other professionals. Consent for release of information about the deceased's condition and treatment should be obtained from the executor of the patient's estate, usually a close family member. Whether or not the clinician meets with the family, he may wish to attend the client's funeral.

8. Is a mental health professional in a rural community judged by the standard of care of a mental health professional in an urban community?

It was traditionally recognized that accepted methods of professional practice varied with geography. Therefore, professionals were judged by the standard of care in their community, the "locality rule." With advances in communication and the dissemination of information, most courts have rejected the locality rule for judging negligence and have adopted a national standard of care based on the specific training of the profession. Consideration is sometimes given to local standards when it can be established that local treatment resources are limited, and that transfer to a metropolitan area was difficult.

9. *Does a therapist who is not a physician have a responsibility to monitor the patient's response to medication?*

The nonphysician therapist should have taken a detailed history and be aware of the patient's medication as well as of the type and instructions regarding the prescription. The therapist should be aware of the anticipated side effects, should work in conjunction with the physician to monitor the patient's response to medication, and should alert the physician to any potential side effects. Although such a therapist will not be held to the same standard as a physician, mental health professionals are expected to refer to a physician when medications should be considered or changed. In any setting where a team approach to treatment is taken, there must be clear policies regarding which treatment personnel are responsible for which activities.

10. *Will obtaining a consultation and complying with the recommendations of the consultant absolve the therapist from malpractice liability?*

When in doubt about a course of treatment or the patient's response to it, obtain a consultation from a colleague; this may be formal, in which the consultant personally examines the patient, or informal. If you do not have confidence in the first consultation, seek a second opinion. The consultation will help establish the standard of care under the circumstances; if the consultant's advice is followed, this would greatly reduce the likelihood of malpractice liability, assuming the advice of the consultant was reasonable in the circumstances.

11. *Can a clinician detain a client in the office or emergency room contrary to the client's wishes?*

Each state's commitment law specifies under what conditions a person can be detained in emergency situations. This will require a bona fide mental disorder leading to the risk of substantial physical harm to the client or another. A petition or certificate must be completed to detain the client. Failure to detain the client in such circumstances may lead to the clinician's liability should harm come to the client or others. Different rules and procedures may apply in the case of the client already under an outpatient commitment.

12. *If a client has suffered an adverse event, such as a suicide attempt which has left him seriously injured with no hope of substantial recovery, should the therapist speak with the attorney representing the client's family?*

Since it is likely that an attorney will be calling for information to serve as the basis for litigation, it is advisable for the therapist to contact his insurance carrier and to respond only through the appointed defense attorney. The clinician should never speak directly to an attorney for the client when litigation is expected without the advice of the appointed attorney or the attorney for the facility.

13. After examination, a psychiatrist diagnoses a woman as having manic-depressive illness. He begins outpatient treatment consisting of psychotropic medication and refers her to a psychologist for psychotherapy. Two years later, she gives birth to a child with a birth defect. Shortly thereafter, she files a lawsuit against the psychiatrist and the psychologist for failing to warn her of the risk of congenital abnormality with treatment, as well as for failing to warn her of the risk that her child will also develop a major psychiatric illness. Who will be liable for the child's injury?

Liability for the patient's injury attaches only when the injury occurred because the clinician violated the standard of care. Liability could attach to both clinicians for failing to provide genetic counseling to her. Since the child has not yet developed the illness, an award may not occur for this cause of action. Liability for the psychiatrist's failure to warn her of the teratogenic effects of medication could result, if it were proven that the medication prescribed could have an effect on the developing fetus, that the doctor did not provide a warning, and that it was the standard of care to do so. Whenever a patient could become pregnant, it is important for the clinician to document that he advised the patient of the implications of her treatment on her pregnancy.

14. What is the National Practitioner Data Bank?

The Health Care Quality Improvement Act of 1989 created a national, centralized data bank which is a repository for information related to the professional conduct and competence of physicians and dentists in the United States. Any of four successful legal or administrative actions against physicians or dentists must be reported to the data bank: (1) any medical malpractice payment, whether settlement or judgment; (2) any disciplinary action by a state medical licensure board relating to a physician's professional conduct or competence; (3) any restriction in clinical privileges at a hospital or health care institution for longer than 30 days; and (4) any adverse change in membership in a professional society. This information will be available to hospitals, state licensing boards, professional societies, and physicians, but not the general public. At least every two years, hospitals must query the data bank when granting or renewing clinical privileges. The federal law provides for optional but not mandatory reporting of adverse actions taken against other health care professionals besides physicians and dentists. Some states independently require reporting of malpractice judgments and settlements against many kinds of health care professionals to their licensing agencies.

15. How long should a client's mental health records be retained?

Preferably as long as possible. State law or regulation sometimes dictates the minimum length of time that records must be kept. It is recommended that this be ten years following the last contact with the therapist. Since the statute of limitations for a malpractice action regarding a minor may be two years after the age of majority, a child's treatment records should be stored for not less than four years after reaching majority, but not less than ten years since the last treatment contact. For some causes of action such as fraud or negligent misrepresentation, the statute of limitations is tolled, or, in effect, lengthened, so that the usual minimum duration of retention is inadequate. In addition, complaints about violations of professional ethics are not limited by a statute of limitations, so records should be kept as long as feasible. Records may be stored on microfilm.

16. What is the therapist's obligation when he becomes aware that a colleague is unable to competently perform job responsibilities due to a mental disability or substance abuse?

The therapist's response to this dilemma depends upon the nature and context of the employment, and the severity of the problem. If the colleague is an employee, then any problems can be reported to the supervisor or the employer. If the problem arises in a hospital where the colleague is a member of a professional staff but not an employee, there may be an impaired professionals committee with whom to consult or report. If the colleague is in a solo private practice setting, then a report can be filed with the applicable professional society or state licensing agency. Many professional societies take the position that their members have an ethical obligation to ensue that fellow members are competently able to serve the public.

Confronting the colleague with the problem is often the initial step. Beyond that, it may be useful to obtain consultation with a senior clinician, ethicist, or attorney familiar with these issues.

17. What should a therapist do when he learns that a supervisee is having a sexual relationship with a client?

The supervisor should initially investigate the factual issues involved in the case. If sexual misconduct has been occurring, then the matter should be brought to the attention of the person who has ultimate responsibility for the treatment program. The supervisor should terminate, or have the therapist terminate, the client's treatment, and consider what steps should be taken to assist the client in terminating the treatment and making the transition to another therapist. If and when the therapist is discharged from the treatment program, then a report to the state's licensing agency, or the National Practitioner Data Bank (if the therapist is a physician), will probably be required.

18. What should a therapist do when he learns that a supervisee is having a sexual relationship with a minor client's mother?

The supervisee's conduct would still be considered improper due to the dual relationship with the client. Treatment should be transferred to another therapist, and the director of the program should be consulted. It may be necessary to secure an ethics or legal consultation to determine whether the supervisee should be terminated and reported to the responsible professional organizations and licensing agency.

XV. BIBLIOGRAPHY

A. Cases

1. *General*

Hammer v. Rosen, 165 N.E.2d 756 (N.Y. 1960).
Darling v. Charleston Community Memorial Hospital, 211 N.E.2d 253 (Ill. 1965).
McDonnell v. County of Nassau, 492 N.Y.S.2d 699 (1985).
Rudy v. Meshorer, 706 P.2d 1234 (Ariz. 1985).
Watts v. Cumberland County, 330 S.E.2d 242 (N.Carol. 1985).

2. *Psychopharmacology*

Chasse v. Banas, 399 A.2d 608 (N.H. 1979).
Naughton v. Bevilacqua, 605 F.2d 586 (1st Cir. 1979).

Speer v. U.S., 512 F.2d 670 (Tex. 1981).
Clites v. Iowa, 322 N.W.2d 917 (Iowa 1982).
Karasik v. Bird, 470 N.Y.S.2d 605 (A.D.1984).
Lundgren v. Eustermann, 370 N.W.2d 877 (Minn. 1985).
Barclay v. Campbell, 704 S.W.2d 8 (Tex. 1986).
Hyde v. University, 393 N.W.2d 847 (Mich. 1986).
Bell v. Hart, 516 So.2d 562 (Sup.Ct.Ala. 1987).
Crooks v. Greene, 736 P.2d 78 (Kan. 1987).
Hendricks v. Charity Hospital, 519 So.2d 163 (La.App. 1987).
McManus v. St. Joseph Hospital, 423 N.W.2d 217 (Mich.App. 1987).
Molkenbur v. Hart, 411 N.W.2d 249 (Minn.App. 1987).
U.S. v. Jones, 816 F.2d 1483 (10th Cir. 1987).
Whittle v. U.S., 669 F.Supp. 501 (D.D.C. 1987).
Bellardini v. Krikorian, 537 A.2d 700 (N.J.Sup. 1988).
Dooley v. Skodnek, 529 N.Y.S.2d 569 (A.D. 1988).
Bolen v. U.S., 727 F.Supp.1346 (Idaho 1989).
Leal v. Simon, 542 N.Y.S.2d 328 (A.D. 1989).
Edwards v. U.S., 749 F.Supp. 1070 (Kan. 1990).
Hardwick v. Reddy, 459 N.W.2d 13 (Mich.App. 1990).
Webb v. Jarvis, 575 N.E.2d 992 (Ind.Sup.Ct. 1991).

3. *Abandonment*

Brandt v. Grubin, 329 A.2d 82 (N.J. 1974).
Williams v. Bennett, 582 S.W.2d 577 (Tex. 1979).
Cranford Insurance Co., v. Allwest Insurance Co., 645 F.Supp. 1440 (Cal. 1986).
Clements v. Hendi, 354 S.E.2d 700 (Ga. 1987).

4. *Sexual Contact*

Roy v. Hartogs, 381 N.Y.S.2d 587 (A.D. 1976).
Mazza v. Huffaker, 300 S.E.2d 833 (N.Carol.App. 1983).
Dennis v. Allison, S.W.2d 94 (Tex.Sup.Ct. 1985).
Horak v. Biris, 474 N.E.2d 13 (Ill.App. 1985).
Thelen by Thelen v. St. Cloud Hospital, 379 N.W.2d 189 (Minn.App. 1985).
Yero v. Department of Professional Regulation, 481 So.2d 61 (Fla.App. 1985).
Atienza v. Taub, 239 Cal.Rptr. 454 (App. 1987).
Cosgrove v. Lawrence, 522 A.2d 483 (N.J.Super.A.D. 1987).
Torgeson v. Connor, 738 P.2d 994 (Or.App. 1987).
Dockweiler v. Wentzell, 425 N.W.2d 468 (Mich.App. 1988).
Noto v. St. Vincent's Hospital and Medical Center of New York, 537 N.Y.S.2d 446 (Sup. 1988).
Richard H. v. Larry D., 243 Cal.Rptr. 807 (App. 1988).
Spiess v. Johnson, 748 P.2d 1020 (Or.App. 1988).
Block v. Ambach, 540 N.Y.S.2d 6 (Ct.App. 1989).
Marlene F. v. Affiliated Psychiatric Medical Clinic, 257 Cal.Rptr. 98 (Sup.Ct. Cal. 1989).
Morris v. Board of Registration in Medicine, 539 N.E.2d 50 (Mass.Sup.Jud.Ct. 1989).
Sprague v. Whitenack, 564 A.2d 829 (Sup.Ct. N.H. 1989).
Weaver v. Union Carbide Corporation, 378 S.E.2d 105 (W.Va. 1989).
Doe. v. Samaritan Counseling Center, 791 P.2d 344 (Sup.Ct. Alaska 1990).
Faulk v. Ludwig, 732 F.Supp. 591 (W.D.Pa. 1990).
Orozco v. Sobol, 557 N.Y.S.2d 738 (A.D. 1990).
Perkins v. Dean, 570 So.2d 1217 (Ala.Sup.Ct. 1990).
St. Paul Fire & Marine Insurance Co. v. Love, 459 N.W.2d 698 (Minn.Sup.Ct. 1990).
State v. Dutton, 450 N.W.2d 189 (Minn.App. 1990).
Carmichael v. Carmichael, 597 A.2d 1326 (D.C.App. 1991).
Corgan v. Muehling, 574 N.E.2d 602 (Ill.Sup.Ct. 1991).
DiLeo v. Nugent, 592 A.2d 1126 (Md.App. 1991).
Figueiredo-Torres v. Nickel, 584 A.2d 69 (Md.App. 1991).

MacClements v. LaFone, 408 S.E.2d 878 (N.C.App. 1991).
Pundy v. Dept. of Professional Regulation, 570 N.E.2d 458 (Ill.App. 1991).
Riley v. Presnell, 565 N.E.2d 780 (Mass.Sup.Jud.Ct. 1991).
Sisson v. Seneca Mental Health Council, 404 S.E.2d 425 (Sup.Ct. W.Va. 1991).
Homer v. Long, 599 A.2d 1193 (Md.App. 1992).
St. Paul Fire & Marine Insurance Co., v. Mori, 486 N.W.2d 803 (Minn. App. 1992)
Annotation: Improper or immoral sexually related conduct toward patient as ground for disciplinary action again physician, dentist, or other licensed healer, 59 A.L.R.4th 1104.

5. *Suicide*

Fernandez v. Baruch, 244 A.2d 109 (Sup.Ct.N.J. 1968).
Bellah v. Greenson, 146 Cal.Rptr. 535 (App. 1978).
Comiskey v. New York, 418 N.Y.S.2d 233 (1979).
Abille v. U.S.A., 482 F.Supp. 703 (N.D.Cal. 1980).
Ray v. Ameri-Care Hospital, 400 So.2d 1127 (La.App. 1981).
Topel v. Long Island Jewish Medical Center, 431 N.E.2d 293 (N.Y. Ct.app. 1981).
Bell v. New York City Health and Hospitals Corporation, 456 N.Y.S.2d 787 (A.D. 1982).
Stokes v. Leung, 651 S.W.2d 704 (Tenn.App. 1983).
Speer v. State of Connecticut, 495 A.2d 733 (Conn.App. 1985).
Krapivka v. Maimonides Medical Center, 501 N.Y.S.2d 429 (A.D. 1986).
Psychiatric Institute v. Allen, 509 A.2d 619 (D.C.App. 1986).
Getty v. Abbott Laboratories, 235 Cal.Rptr. 48 (App. 1987).
Guilbault v. Department of Mental Health, 408 N.W.2d 558 (Mich.App. 1987).
Werner v. Pennsylvania, 530 A.2d 1004 (Pa.Cmwlth. 1987).
Brandvain v. Ridgeview Institute, 372 S.E.2d 265 (Ga.App. 1988).
Cowan v. Doering et al, 545 A.2d 159 (N.J.Sup.Ct. 1988).
Porter v. Maunnangi, 764 S.W.2d 699 (Mo.App. 1988).
Weathers v. Pilkinton, 754 S.W.2d 75 (Tenn.App. 1988).
Bourne v. Seventh Ward General Hospital, 546 So.2d 197 (La.App. 1989).
Clark v. Maine Medical Center, 559 A.2d 358 (Sup.Jud.Ct. Me. 1989).
DeSanchez v. Genoves-Andrews, 446 N.W.2d 538 (Mich.App. 1989).
King v. Smith, 539 So.2d 262 (Sup.Ct.Ala. 1989).
McNamara v. Honeyman, 546 N.E.2d 139 (Mass.Sup.Ct.Jud. 1989).
McNesby v. New Jersey Department of Human Services, 555 A.2d 1186 (N.J.Super.A.D. 1989).
Paddock v. Chacko, 533 So.2d 168 (Fla.Sup.Ct. 1989).
Vinchiarello v. Kathuria, 558 A.2d 262 (Conn.App. 1989).
Davitt v. State, 549 N.Y.S. 803 (A.D. 1990).
Farwell v. Un, 902 F.2d 282 (4th Cir. 1990).
Jensen v. Augusta Mental Health Institute, 574 A.2d 885 (Sup.Jud.Ct. Me. 1990).
Mahoney v. Lensink, 569 A.2d 518 (Sup.Ct. Conn. 1990).
Pelermo v. NME Hospitals, 558 So.2d 1342 (La.App. 1990).
Pessagno v. U.S., 751 F.Supp. 149 (S.D. Iowa 1990).
Tomfohr v. Mayo Foundation, 450 N.W.2d 121 (Minn.Sup.Ct. 1990).
Weeks v. Harris County Hospital District, 785 S.W.2d 169 (Tex. App. 1990).
Bloom v. Dubois Regional Medical Center, 597 A.2d 671 (Pa.Super. 1991).
Ex parte AMI West Alabama General Hospital, 582 So.2d 485 (Ala.Sup.Ct. 1991).
Peoples Bank of Bloomington v. Damera, 581 N.E.2d 426 (Ill.App. 1991).
Rogers v. Marrow by Marrow, 413 S.E.2d 344 (Va.Sup.Ct. 1992).
Annotation: Liability of doctor, psychiatrist, or psychologist for failure to take steps to prevent patient's suicide, 17 A.L.R.4th 1128.
Annotation: Liability of mental care facility for suicide of patient or former patient, 19 A.L.R.4th 7.
Annotation: Hospital's liability for mentally deranged patient's self-inflicted injuries, 36 A.L.R.4th 117.
Annotation: Hospital's liability for patient's injury or death resulting from escape or attempted escape, 37 A.L.R.4th 200.

6. *Supervision and Consultation*

Weinstock v. Ott, 444 N.E.2d 1227 (Ind. 1983).
Andrews v. U.S., 732 F.2d 366 (4th Cir. 1984).

Gitlin v. Cassell, 484 N.Y.S.2d 19 (1985).
McGhee v. Bhama, 363 N.W.2d 293 (Mich. 1985).
Sangiuolo v. Leventhal, 505 N.Y.S.2d 507 (1986).
Doe v. Samaritan Counseling Center, 791 P.2d 344 (Sup.Ct. Alaska 1990).
Hill by Burston v. Kokosky, 463 N.W.2d 265 (Mich.App. 1990).

7. *Record Keeping*

Gotkin v. Miller, 514 F.2d 125 (2nd Cir. 1975).
Pisel v. Stamford Hospital, 430 A.2d 1 (Conn. 1980).
Bondu v. Gurvich, 473 So.2d 1307 (Fla. 1984). [negligent loss of records]
Haley v. U.S.A., 739 F.2d 1502 (10th Cir. 1984). [failure to review past treatment records]
Ehredt v. Forest Hospital, 492 N.E.2d 532 (Ill. 1986).
Breesmen v. Department of Professional Regulation, 567 So.2d 469 (Fla.App. 1990).
Pharr v. Cortese, 559 N.Y.S.2d 780 (Sup.Ct. 1990). [physician falsified records]
Jimenez v. Department of Professional Regulation, 556 So.2d 1219 (Fla.App. 1990). [physician falsified records]
Suslovich v. New York State Education Department, 571 N.Y.S.2d 123 (A.D. 1991). [psychologist failed to maintain records]

8. *Electroconvulsive Therapy*

Woods v. Brumlop, 377 P.2d 520 (N.Mex 1962).
Stone v. Proctor, 131 S.E.2d 297 (N.Carol. 1963).
Collins v. Hand, 246 A.2d 398 (Pa. 1968).
Kapp v. Ballantine, 402 N.E.2d 463 (Sup.Jud.Ct.Mass. 1980).
Lillian F. v. Superior Court (Santa Clara Val. M.C.), 206 Cal.Rptr. 603 (Cal.App. 1984).
Gowan, conservator for Gowan v. U.S., 601 F.Supp. 1297 (Or. 1985).
Lojuk v. Johnson, 853 F.2d 560 (7th Cir. 1988).
Annotation: Malpractice in connection with electroshock treatment, 94 A.L.R.3d 317.

9. *Informed Consent*

See "Informed Consent" in Bibliography of Chapter 5, pp. 142–145.

10. *Breach of Confidentiality*

See "Liability for Breach of Confidentiality" in Bibliography of Chapter 7, pp. 230–231.

B. Articles and Books

1. *General*

Abraham, K. S. (1988). Medical liability reform: A conceptual framework. *Journal of the American Medical Association, 260*, 68–72.
American Medical Association. (1991). *The guide to medical professional liability insurance.* Chicago: American Medical Association.
Appelbaum, P. S., & Gutheil, T. G. (1991). *Current handbook of psychiatry and the law* (2nd ed.). Baltimore: Williams and Wilkins.
Bennett, B. E., Bryant, B. K., VandenBos, G. R., & Greenwood, A. (1990). *Professional liability and risk management.* Washington, DC: American Psychological Association.
Beresford, H. R. (1972). Professional liability of psychiatrists. *Defense Law Journal, 21*, 123–167.
Besharov, D. J. (1985). *The vulnerable social worker: Liability for serving children and families.* Silver Spring, MD: National Association of Social Workers.
Busch, K. A., & Cavanaugh, J. L. (1985). Physical examination of psychiatric outpatients: Medical and legal issues. *Hospital and Community Psychiatry, 36*, 958–961.

Charles, S. C. (1989). Stress associated with medical malpractice litigation. In A. Tasman, R. E. Hales, & A. J. Frances (Eds.), *American Psychiatric Press review of psychiatry, Vol. 8*. Washington, DC: American Psychiatric Press.
Charles, S. C., & Kennedy, E. (1985). *Defendant: A psychiatrist on trial for medical malpractice*. New York: Free Press.
Dorken, H. (1990). Malpractice claims experience for psychologists: Policy issues, cost comparisons with psychiatrists, and prescription privilege implications. *Professional Psychology: Research and Practice, 21*, 150–152.
Fish, F. M., Ehrhardt, M. E., & Fish, B. (1989). *Malpractice: Managing your defense* (2nd ed.). Oradell, NJ: Medical Economics Books.
Fishalow, S. E. (1975). The tort liability of the psychiatrist. *Bulletin of the American Academy of Psychiatry and the Law, 3*, 191–230.
Furrow, B. (1980). *Malpractice in psychotherapy*. Lexington, MA: Lexington Books.
Gutheil, T. G., Bursztajn, H. J., Brodsky, A., & Alexander, V. (Eds.)(1991). *Decision making in psychiatry and the law*. Baltimore: Williams & Wilkins.
Hampton, L. P. (1984). Malpractice in psychotherapy: Is there a relevant standard of care? *Case Western Reserve Law Review, 35*, 251–281.
Hogan, D. B. (1979). *The regulation of psychotherapists*. Cambridge, MA: Ballinger.
Johnson, K. B., Hirshfeld, E. B., Ile, M. L., Kelly, J. T., Bierig, J. R., Raskin, R. D., & Fleisher, L. D. (1990). *Legal implications of practice parameters*. Chicago: Author.
Jones, J. A., & Alcabes, A. (1989). Clients don't sue: The invulnerable social worker. *Social Casework, 70*, 414–420.
Kahn, M., & Taft, G. (1983). The application of the standard of care doctrine to psychological testing. *Behavioral Sciences and the Law, l*, 71-84.
King, J. (1986). *The law of medical malpractice* (2nd ed.) St. Paul: West.
Klerman, G. L. (1990). The psychiatric patient's right to effective treatment: Implications of *Osheroff v. Chestnut Lodge*. *American Journal of Psychiatry, 147*, 409–418.
La Puma, J., Schiedermayer, D. L., Toulmin, S., Miles, S. H., & McAtee, J. A. (1990). The standard of care: A case report and ethical analysis. *Annals of Internal Medicine, 108*, 121–124.
Malcolm, J. G. (1988). *Treatment choices and informed consent: Current controversies in psychiatric malpractice litigation*. Springfield, IL: Thomas.
Margolin, G. (1982). Ethical and legal considerations in marital and family therapy. *American Psychologist, 37*, 788–801.
Mullan, F., Politzer, R. M., Lewis, C. T., Bastacky, S., Rodak, J., & Harmon, R. G. (1992). The National Practitioner Data Bank. *Journal of the American Medical Association, 268*, 73–79.
Paquin, G. W. (1988). The malpractice of family therapy: An analysis of two "schools." *Law and Psychology Review, 12*, 21–59.
Rheingold, P. (1984). How to know a good medical malpractice case. *American Bar Association Journal, 70*, 71-74.
Shapiro, R. S., Simpson, D. E., Lawrence, S. L., Talsky, A. M., Sobocinski, K. A., & Schiedermayer, D. L. (1989). A survey of sued and nonsued physicians and suing patients. *Archives Internal Medicine, 149*, 2190–2196.
Simon, R., & Sadoff, R. L. (1992). *Psychiatric malpractice: Cases and comments for clinicians*. Washington, DC: American Psychiatric Press.
Slawson, P. F. (1979). Psychiatric malpractice: The California experience. *American Journal of Psychiatry, 136*, 651–654.
Slawson, P. F. (1984). The clinical dimension of psychiatric malpractice. *Psychiatric Annals, 14*, 358–364.
Slawson, P. F. (1989). Psychiatric malpractice: Ten years' loss experience. *Medicine and Law, 8*, 415–427.
Slawson, P. F., & Guggenheim, F. G. (1984). Psychiatric malpractice: A review of the national loss experience. *American Journal of Psychiatry, 141*, 979–981.
Smith, J. T. (1986). *Medical malpractice: Psychiatric care*. Colorado Springs: Shepard's, McGraw-Hill.
Stone, A. A. (1990). Law, science, and psychiatric malpractice: A response to Klerman's indictment of psychoanalytic psychiatry. *American Journal of Psychiatry, 147*, 419–427.
Sugarman, S. D. (1990). The need to reform personal injury law leaving scientific disputes to scientists. *Science, 248*, 823–827.
Tancredi, L. R., & Weisstub, D. N. (1986). Malpractice in American psychiatry: Toward a restructuring of the psychiatrist-patient relationship. In D. Weisstub (Ed.), *Law and mental health, Vol. 2*, pp. 83–139. New York: Pergamon Press.

Watkins, S., & Watkins, J. (1983). Malpractice in clinical social work: A perspective on civil liability in the 1980s. *Behavioral Sciences and the Law, 1,* 55–70.

Wettstein, R. M. (1989). Psychiatric malpractice. In A. Tasman, R. E. Hales, & A. J. Frances (Eds.), *American Psychiatric Press Annual Review, Vol 8.* Washington, DC: American Psychiatric Press.

Widiger, T. A., & Rorer, L. G. (1984). The responsible psychotherapist. *American Psychologist, 39,* 503–515.

Wilbert, J. R., & Fulero, S. M. (1988). Impact of malpractice litigation on professional psychology: Survey of practitioners. *Professional Psychology: Research and Practice, 19,* 379–382.

2. *Psychopharmacology*

American Psychiatric Association, Task Force. (1990). *Benzodiazepine dependence, toxicity, abuse.* Washington, DC: Author.

American Psychiatric Association, Task Force. (1992). *Tardive dyskinesia.* Washington, DC: Author.

Appelbaum, P. S., Schaffner, K., & Meisel, A. (1985). Responsibility and compensation for tardive dyskinesia. *American Journal of Psychiatry, 142,* 806–810.

Ayd, F. J. (1985). Problems with orders for medication as needed. *American Journal of Psychiatry, 142,* 939–942.

Brackins, L. W. (1985). The liability of physicians, pharmacists, and hospitals for adverse drug reactions. *Defense Law Journal, 34,* 273–344.

Brown, P., & Funk, S. C. (1986). Tardive dyskinesia: Barriers to the professional recognition of an iatrogenic disease. *Journal of Health and Social Behavior, 27,* 116–132.

Brushwood, D. B., & Simonsmeier, L. M. (1986). Drug information for patients. *Journal of Legal Medicine, 7,* 279–340.

Deveaugh-Geiss, J. (1979). Informed consent for neuroleptic therapy. *American Journal of Psychiatry, 136,* 959–962.

Drugs in litigation (1992). Charlottesville, VA: Michie.

Dukes, M. N. G., & Swartz, B. (1988). *Responsibility for drug-induced injury.* Amsterdam: Elsevier.

Gilhooley, M (1986). Learned intermediaries, prescription drugs, and patient information. *St. Louis University Law Journal, 30,* 633–702.

Howe, E. G. (1984). Legal aspects of psychopharmacology. *Psychiatric Clinics of North America, 7,* 887–900.

Junewicz, J. J. (1979). Physicians' liability for failure to anticipate and control reactions and interactions precipitated by prescribed or administered drugs. *Medical Trial Technique Quarterly, 26,* 8–41.

Kapp, M. B. (1981). Prescribing approved drugs for non-approved uses: Physicians' disclosure obligations to their patients. *Law Medicine and Health Care, 9,* 20–23.

Kleinman, I., Schachter, D., & Koritar, E. (1989). Informed consent and tardive dyskinesia. *American Journal of Psychiatry, 146,* 902–904.

Kofoed, L., Bloom, J. D., Williams, M. H., Rhyne, C., & Resnick, M. (1989). Physicians investigated for inappropriate prescribing by the Oregon Board of Medical Examiners. *Western Journal of Medicine, 150,* 597–601.

Mills, M. J., Norquist, G. S., Shelton, R. C., Gelenberg, A. J., & Van Putten, T. (1986). Consent and liability with neuroleptics: The problem of tardive dyskinesia. *International Journal of Law and Psychiatry, 8,* 243–252.

Munetz, M. R., & Benjamin, S. (1990). Who should perform the AIMS examination? *Hospital and Community Psychiatry, 41,* 912–915.

Munetz, M. R., & Roth, L. H. (1985). Informing patients about tardive dyskinesia. *Archives of General Psychiatry, 42,* 866–871.

Sovner, R., Dimascio, A., Berkowitz, D., & Randolph, P. (1978). Tardive dyskinesia and informed consent. *Psychosomatics, 19,* 172–177.

Stone, A. A. (1978). The history and future of litigation in psychopharmacologic research and treatment. In D. M. Gallant & R. Force (Eds.), *Legal and ethical issues in human research and treatment.* New York: Medical and Scientific Books.

Tancredi, L. R. (1988). Malpractice and tardive dyskinesia: A conceptual dilemma. *Journal of Clinical Psychopharmacology* (Suppl. 8), 71S-76S.

Taub, S. (1986). Tardive dyskinesia: Medical facts and legal fictions. *St. Louis University Law Journal, 30,* 833–873.

Tietz, G. F. (1986). Informed consent in the prescription drug context: The special case. *Washington Law Review, 61,* 367–417.

Tozer, F. L., & Kasik, J. E. (1967). The medical-legal aspects of adverse drug reactions. *Clinical Pharmacology and Therapeutics, 8*, 637–646.
Wettstein, R. M. (1983). Tardive dyskinesia and malpractice. *Behavioral Sciences and the Law, 1*, 85–107.
Wettstein, R. M. (1985). Legal aspects of neuroleptic-induced movement disorders. In C. H. Wecht (Ed.), *Legal medicine 1985*. New York: Praeger.
Wettstein, R. M. (1988). Informed consent and tardive dyskinesia. *Journal of Clinical Psychopharmacology, 8*, 65S-70S.

3. *Abandonment*

Hirsh, H. L. (1984). Abandonment: Actual or constructive premature termination of the physician-patient relationship. *Transactions and Studies of the College of Physicians of Philadelphia, 6*, 207–222.
Bernstein, R. M., Feldberg, C., & Brown, R. (1991). After-hours coverage in psychology training clinics. *Professional Psychology: Research and Practice, 22*, 204–208.

4. *Sexual Contact*

Akamatsu, T. J. (1988). Intimate relationships with former clients: National survey of attitudes and behavior among practitioners. *Professional Psychology: Research and Practice, 19*, 454–458.
Appelbaum, P. S., & Jorgenson, L. (1991). Psychotherapist-patient sexual contact after termination of treatment: An analysis and a proposal. *American Journal of Psychiatry, 148*, 1466–1473.
Bates, C. M., & Brodsky, A. M. (1989). *Sex in the therapy hour: A case of professional incest*. New York: Guilford Press.
Borys, D. S., & Pope, K. S. (1989). Dual relationships between therapist and client: A national survey of psychologists, psychiatrists, and social workers. *Professional Psychology: Research and Practice, 20*, 283–293.
Bouhoutsos, J., Holroyd, J., Lerman, H., et al. (1983). Sexual intimacy between psychotherapists and patients. *Professional Psychology: Research and Practice, 14*, 185–196.
Coleman, P. (1988). Sex between psychiatrist and former patient: A proposal for a "no harm, no foul" rule. *Oklahoma Law Review, 41*, 1–52.
Coleman, P. (1988). Sexual relationships between therapist and patient—Different countries, different treatment. *Journal of Psychiatry and Law, 16*, 577–623.
Committee on Women in Psychology. (1989). If sex enters into the psychotherapy relationship. *Professional Psychology: Research and Practice, 20*, 112–115.
Conte, H. R., Plutchik, R., Picard, S., & Karasu, T. B. (1989). Ethics in the practice of psychotherapy: A survey. *American Journal of Psychotherapy, 43*, 32–42.
Council on Ethical and Judicial Affairs, American Medical Association. (1991). Sexual misconduct in the practice of medicine. *Journal of the American Medical Association, 266*, 2741–2745.
Gabbard, G. O. (1989). *Sexual exploitation in professional relationships*. Washington, DC: American Psychiatric Press.
Gartrell, N., Herman, J. L., Olarte, S., Feldstein, M., & Localio, R. (1986). Psychiatrist-patient sexual contact: Results of a national survey: 1. Prevalence. *American Journal of Psychiatry, 143*, 1126–1131.
Gartrell, N., Herman, J. L., Olarte, S., Feldstein, M., & Localio, R. (1987). Reporting practices of psychiatrists who knew of sexual misconduct by colleagues. *American Journal of Orthopsychiatry, 57*, 287–295.
Gartrell, N., Herman, J. L., Olarte, S., Feldstein, M., & Localio, R. (1988). Management and rehabilitation of sexually exploitive therapists. *Hospital and Community Psychiatry, 39*, 1070–1074.
Gunnells, S. L. (1990). Patient-therapist sexual relations: Professional services rendered? *Law and Psychology Review, 14*, 87–105.
Gutheil, T. G. (1989). Borderline personality disorder, boundary violations, and patient-therapist sex: Medicolegal pitfalls. *American Journal of Psychiatry, 146*, 597–602.
Herman, J. L., Gartrell, N., Olarte, S., Feldstein, M., & Localio, R. (1987). Psychiatrist-patient sexual contact: Results of a national survey: 2. Psychiatrists' attitudes. *American Journal of Psychiatry, 144*, 164–169.
Jorgenson, L., Randles, R., & Strasburger, L. (1991). The furor over psychotherapist-patient sexual contact: New solutions to an old problem. *William and Mary Law Review, 32*, 645–732.
Kluft, R. P. (1989). Treating the patient who has been sexually exploited by a previous therapist. *Psychiatric Clinics of North America, 12*, 483–500.

Mikkelsen, E. J., Gutheil, T. G., & Emens, M. (1992). False sexual-abuse allegations by children and adolescents: Contextual factors and clinical subtypes. *American Journal of Psychotherapy, 46,* 556–570.

Pope, K. S. (1990). Therapist-patient sex as sex abuse: Six scientific, professional, and practical dilemmas in addressing victimization and rehabilitation. *Professional Psychology: Research and Practice, 21,* 227–239.

Pope, K. S., Tabachnick, B. G., & Keith-Spiegel, P. (1987). Ethics of practice: The beliefs and behaviors of psychologists as therapists. *American Psychologist, 41,* 993–1006.

Pope, K. S., Tabachnick, B. G., & Keith-Spiegel, P. (1988). Good and poor practices in psychotherapy: National survey of beliefs of psychologists. *Professional Psychology: Research and Practice, 19,* 547–552.

Schoener, G. R., Milgrom, J. H., Gonsiorek, J. C., Luepker, E. T., & Conroe, R. M. (1989). *Psychotherapists' sexual involvement with clients: Intervention and prevention.* Minneapolis: Walk-In Counseling Center.

Strasburger, L., Jorgenson, L., & Randles, R. (1991). Criminalization of psychotherapist-patient sex. *American Journal of Psychiatry, 148,* 859–863.

Williams, M. H. (1992). Exploitation and inference: Mapping the damage from therapist-patient sexual involvement. *American Psychologist, 47,* 412–421.

5. *Suicide*

Amchin, J. D., Wettstein, R. M., & Roth, L. R. (1990). Suicide, ethics, and the law. In S. J. Blumenthal & D. J. Kupfer (Eds.), *Suicide over the life cycle.* Washington, DC: American Psychiatric Press.

Benensohn, H. S., & Resnik, H. L. (1973). Guidelines for "suicide-proofing" a psychiatric unit. *American Journal of Psychotherapy, 27,* 204–212.

Berman, A. L. (1989). Case consultation: Malpractice. *Suicide and Life-Threatening Behavior, 19,* 395–402.

Bongar, B. (1991). *The suicidal patient: Clinical and legal standards of care.* Washington, DC: American Psychological Association.

Bursztajn, H., Gutheil, T. G., Brodsky, A., & Swagerty, E. L. (1988). "Magical thinking," suicide, and malpractice litigation. *Bulletin of the American Academy of Psychiatry and the Law, 16,* 369–377.

Bursztajn, H., Gutheil, T. G., Hamm, R. M., & Brodsky, A. (1983). Subjective data and suicide assessment in the light of recent developments, Part 2. *International Journal of Law and Psychiatry, 6,* 331–350.

Ebert, B. W. (1987). Guide to conducting a psychological autopsy. *Professional Psychology: Research and Practice, 18,* 52–56.

Greenberg, D. F. (1974). Involuntary psychiatric commitments to prevent suicide. *New York University Law Review, 49,* 227–269.

Gutheil, T. G., Bursztajn, H., Hamm, R. M., & Brodsky, A. (1983). Subjective data and suicide assessment in the light of recent developments, Part 1. *International Journal of Law and Psychiatry, 6,* 317–329.

Kaye, N. S., & Soreff, S. M. (1991). The psychiatrist's role, responses, and responsibilities when a patient commits suicide. *American Journal of Psychiatry, 148,* 739–743.

Litman, R. E. (1982). Hospital suicides: Lawsuits and standards. *Suicide and Life-Threatening Behavior, 12,* 212–220.

Margolis, P. M., Meyer, G. G., & Louw, J. C. (1965). Suicidal precautions: A dilemma in the therapeutic community. *Archives of General Psychiatry, 13,* 224–231.

O'Leary, W. D. (1989). Custodial suicide: Evolving liability considerations. *Psychiatric Quarterly, 60,* 31–71.

Pauker, S. L., & Cooper, A. M. (1990). Paradoxical patient reactions to psychiatric life support: Clinical and ethical considerations. *American Journal of Psychiatry, 147,* 488–491.

Rachlin, S. (1984). Double jeopardy: Suicide and malpractice. *General Hospital Psychiatry, 6,* 302–307.

Szasz, T. (1986). The case against suicide prevention. *American Psychologist, 41,* 806–812.

6. *Supervision and Consultation*

American Psychiatric Association. (1980). Guidelines for psychiatrists in consultative, supervisory, or collaborative relationships with nonmedical therapists. *American Journal of Psychiatry, 137,* 1489–1491.

American Psychiatric Association. (1989). Guidelines regarding psychiatrists' signatures. *American Journal of Psychiatry, 146,* 1390.
American Psychiatric Association. (1991). Guidelines for psychiatric practice in community mental health centers. *American Journal of Psychiatry, 148,* 965–966.
Firman, G. J. (1988). Ostensible agency: Another malpractice hazard. *American Journal of Psychiatry, 145,* 510–512.
Goldberg, R. S., Riba, M., & Tasman, A. (1991). Psychiatrists' attitudes toward prescribing medication for patients treated by nonmedical psychotherapists. Hospital and Community Psychiatry, 42, 276–280.
Harrar, W. R., VandeCreek, L., & Knapp, S. (1990). Ethical and legal aspects of clinical supervision. *Professional Psychology: Research and Practice, 21,* 37–41.
Kapp, M. (1983). Legal implications of clinical supervision of medical students and residents. *Journal of Medical Education, 58,* 293–299.
Kapp, M. (1984). Supervising professional trainees: Legal implications for mental health institutions and practitioners. *Hospital and Community Psychiatry, 35,* 143–147.
Morgan, D. (1987). Liability for medical education. *Journal of Legal Medicine, 8,* 305–338.
Oliver, R. (1986). Legal liability of students and residents in the health care setting. *Journal of Medical Education, 61,* 560–568.
Reamer, F. G. (1989). Liability issues in social work supervision. *Social Work,* 445–448.
Simpson, C. L. (1977). Misrepresentation of medical students in teaching hospitals. *Medical Trial Technique Quarterly 1977 Annual,* 233–270.
Slovenko, R. (1980). Legal issues in psychotherapy supervision. In A. K. Hess (Ed.), *Psychotherapy supervision: Theory, research and practice.* New York: Wiley.
Vasile, R. G., & Gutheil, T. G. (1979). The psychiatrist as medical backup: Ambiguity in the delegation of clinical responsibility. *American Journal of Psychiatry, 136,* 1292–1296.

7. *Record Keeping*

Albeck, J. H., & Goldman, C. (1991). Patient-therapist codocumentation. *American Journal of Orthopsychiatry, 45,* 317–334.
Beers, M. H., Munekata, M., & Storrie, M. (1990). The accuracy of medication histories in the hospital medical records of elderly persons. *Journal of the American Geriatrics Society, 38,* 1183–1187.
Fulero, S. M., & Wilbert, J. R. (1988). Record-keeping practices of clinical and counseling psychologists: A survey of practitioners. *Professional Psychology: Research and Practice, 19,* 658–660.
Gutheil, T. G. (1980). Paranoia and progress notes: A guide to forensically informed psychiatric record keeping. *Hospital and Community Psychiatry, 31,* 479–482.
Hirsh, H. L. (1987). Physicians and medical records—A necessary evil? *Medicine and Law, 6,* 1–12.
Prosser, R. L. (1992). Alteration of medical records submitted for medicolegal review. *Journal of the American Medical Association, 267,* 2630–2631.
Rappaport, R. G. (1979). The psychiatrist on trial. *Journal of Psychiatry and Law, 7,* 463–469.
Roach, W. H., Chernoff, S. N., & Esley, C. L. (1985). *Medical records and the law.* Rockville, MD: Aspen Publications.
Roth, L. H., Wolford, J., & Meisel, A. (1980). Patient access to records: Tonic or toxin? *American Journal of Psychiatry, 137,* 592–592.
Siegel, C., & Fischer, S. K. (Eds.). (1981). *Psychiatric records in mental health care.* New York: Brunner/Mazel.
Slovenko, R. (1979). On the need for record keeping in the practice of psychiatry. *Journal of Psychiatry and Law, 7,* 399–440.
Thompson, T. J., Thornhill, C. A., Realon, R. E., & Ervin, K. M. (1991). Improving accuracy in documentation of restrictive interventions by direct-care personnel. *Mental Retardation, 29,* 201–205.
Van Vort, W., & Mattson, M. R. (1989). A strategy for enhancing the clinical utility of the psychiatric record. *Hospital and Community Psychiatry, 40,* 407–409.
Wilson, S. J. (1980). *Recording: Guidelines for social workers.* New York: Free Press.

8. *Electroconvulsive Therapy*

Abrams, R. (1989). Malpractice litigation and ECT. *Convulsive Therapy, 5,* 365–367.
American Psychiatric Association, Task Force Report. (1990). *The practice of electroconvulsive therapy.* Washington, DC: Author.

Baxter, L. R., Roy-Byrne, P., Liston, E. H., & Fairbanks, L. (1986). Informing patients about electroconvulsive therapy: Effects of a videotape presentation. *Convulsive Therapy, 2,* 25–29.
Benedict, A. R., & Saks, M. J. (1987). The regulation of professional behavior: Electroconvulsive therapy in Massachusetts. *Journal of Psychiatry and Law, 15,* 247–275.
Guze, B. H., Baxter, L. R., Liston, E. H., & Roy-Byrne, P. (1988). Attorneys' perceptions of electroconvulsive therapy: Impact of instruction with an ECT videotape demonstration. *Comprehensive Psychiatry, 29,* 520–522.
Kramer, B. A. (1990). ECT use in the public sector: California. *Psychiatric Quarterly, 61,* 97–103.
Krouner, L. W. (1973). Shock therapy and psychiatric malpractice: The legal accommodation to a controversial treatment. *Forensic Science, 2,* 397–439.
Perr, I. N. (1980). Liability and electroshock therapy. *Journal of Forensic Sciences, 25,* 508–513.
Slawson, P. F. (1985). Psychiatric malpractice: The electroconvulsive therapy experience. *Convulsive Therapy, 1,* 195–203.
Slawson, P. F. (1989). Psychiatric malpractice and ECT: A review of national loss experience. *Convulsive Therapy, 5,* 126–130.
Taub, S. (1987). Electroconvulsive therapy, malpractice, and informed consent. *Journal of Psychiatry and Law, 15,* 7–54.
Whitcomb, D. (1988). The regulation of electroconvulsive therapy in California: The impact of recent constitutional interpretations. *Golden Gate University Law Review, 18,* 469–494.
Winslade, W. J., Liston, E. H., Ross, J. W., & Weber, K. D. (1984). Medical, judicial, and statutory regulation of ECT in the United States. *American Journal of Psychiatry, 141,* 1349–1355.

9. *Informed Consent*

See "Informed Consent" in Bibliography of Chapter 5, pp. 142–145.

7

Confidentiality

I. The Importance of Confidentiality • II. What Is Considered Confidential • III. Breach of Confidentiality • A. When the Therapist Can Breach Confidentiality • B. Advising Clients about Confidentiality • C. Waiver of Confidentiality by the Client • D. Disclosure to Investigative Agencies • E. Clinical and Social Erosions of Confidentiality • **IV. Privileged Communications** • A. Physician–Patient Privilege • B. Psychologist–Patient Privilege • C. Psychotherapist–Patient Privilege • D. To Whom the Privilege Belongs • **V. Exceptions to the Therapist–Patient Privilege** • A. Court-Ordered Examinations • B. Patient-Litigant Exception • **VI. Nonstatutory Protection of Confidentiality** • A. The Ethics of the Mental Health Professional • B. The Common Law • C. The Constitutional Right of Privacy • **VII. Minors' Confidentiality • VIII. Confidentiality of Drug Abuse and Alcoholism Treatment Records • IX. Acquired Immunodeficiency Syndrome • X. Group and Family Therapy • XI. Disclosure of Records** • A. Patient Access • B. Statutory Access by Others • C. The Records of Minors • D. Obligation to Patient • E. Disclosure in Publications • **XII. Responding to a Subpoena • XIII. Commonly Asked Questions • XIV. Bibliography**

In the United States, much emphasis is placed on the concepts of privacy and confidentiality, particularly in the health care setting. In this computer age, when information is stored in data banks which are readily available to many agencies, including potential employers, credit bureaus, and insurance companies, health professionals must have heightened awareness of the individual's right to confidentiality and what must be done to protect it. The stigma that still attaches to being labeled "mentally or emotionally ill" or "mentally retarded" has required an increased awareness on the part of mental health professionals to the confidentiality rights of their patient. The professional must be knowledgeable about the specific law related to confidentiality of information disclosed in the therapeutic setting and must understand under what circumstances confidentiality can or must be breached. This chapter will fully discuss these issues as well as the client's access to his record.

I. THE IMPORTANCE OF CONFIDENTIALITY

Confidentiality is considered the *sine qua non* of successful psychiatric treatment. Without the promise of confidentiality, provided primarily through the clinician's professional ethics but also the law, many individuals in need of treatment would be afraid to seek it. It is even clearer that once in treatment, clients would be affected by the absence of confidentiality. Research has shown that clients expect confidentiality in treatment and wish to be informed of its extent and limits. Every client, however well motivated, has to overcome the resistance to therapeutic exploration. These resistances seek support from every possible source, including the possibility of unwanted disclosure outside the treatment setting. At best, the possibility of disclosure will prolong treatment by reducing the client's openness with the therapist; at worst, it will preclude thorough exploration of emotional conflict and aggravate symptoms. Ideally, when one obtains psychiatric care, he lays himself bare, sharing with the therapist his dreams, his fantasies, his sins, and his shame. This makes the person feel highly vulnerable.

Many of those who recognize a need for mental health services also recognize the potentially negative career, social, and economic consequences of seeking that assistance if it became generally known. These consequences can include the inability to obtain a job or promotion; inability to obtain disability, health, and life insurance; and social ostracism. In addition, a history of having been treated for mental illness or emotional problems can have adverse consequences in litigation in which the person is a plaintiff, a defendant, or a witness. In the litigation setting, a past or present history of treatment may be used to try to impeach the credibility of the person as a witness, with hints or direct statements that his past or present mental health care is evidence of his instability or unreliability. Thus, the mental health professional has information which is potentially of significance to others, including insurance companies, employers, legal adversaries, and law enforcement agencies, but is also potentially harmful if made available to them. Disclosure of information without the client's consent is likely to erode the therapist–client relationship and impair the therapist's ability to help the individual.

The person entering into a therapeutic relationship expects that his contact and communications with the therapist will be kept in confidence. This expectation is based in part on the long-held notion that health care providers have an ethical duty to keep confidential information they learn about a client. This ethical obligation has become a basic tenet of each mental health specialty. The importance of confidentiality is further reinforced by laws and regulations which impose fines and potential loss of professional license for breaching confidentiality. In addition, the therapist is subject to a malpractice suit for breach of confidentiality (see Chapter 6).

Notwithstanding its importance, confidentiality in the mental health setting is never absolute. Under certain circumstances, the law demands that the therapist subordinate the confidentiality entrusted to him. In other instances, the needs of the client or the ethics of the therapist may require him to reveal information. The therapist may have divided loyalties or responsibilities to other individuals or organizations besides the client.

II. WHAT IS CONSIDERED CONFIDENTIAL

Any information related to the fact that an individual has sought mental health services is considered confidential. The fact that the person is, or has been, in treatment is confidential. Communications by the client during treatment, observations by the therapist, the results of psychological testing and laboratory testing, diagnosis, and prognosis are confidential. Even the fact that someone had a one-session consultation with a therapist is confidential. In contrast, statutory testimonial privileges, which govern release of information for litigation, are not so uniformly protective (see below).

III. BREACH OF CONFIDENTIALITY

A breach of confidentiality involves the release of confidential information without the client's informed consent, whether oral or written. Consent to release information can be obtained from:

1. A legally competent adult.
2. The legal guardian of an adult found legally incompetent.
3. An emancipated minor.
4. The parent of an unemancipated minor.
5. The executor or administrator of the estate of a deceased person.

At times, confidentiality must be breached in the course of the therapist's work. Under certain circumstances, the therapist will have an affirmative duty to breach confidentiality. There are also times when clinical judgment would dictate such breaches, though in many of these circumstances the client will consent to the release of information if asked. In addition, issues may arise in litigation which will compel release of information provided in the therapeutic setting.

A. When the Therapist Can Breach Confidentiality

There are several well-recognized clinical circumstances in which disclosure of information without the client's (or legal guardian's) explicit consent is legally justified: (1) during an emergency; (2) in acting to civilly commit the client for mental health care; (3) in protecting third parties from the client; (4) in conforming to child-abuse reporting requirements; (5) in conforming to other statutory reporting requirements; and (6) in discussing a case with supervisors and collaborators in the case. If possible, the therapist should attempt to obtain the client's or legal guardian's consent to release the information prior to doing so in any of these cases, but this may not be possible or the client may refuse.

1. Emergencies

When faced with an emergency which places the patient's welfare or that of others in immediate jeopardy, the therapist must act in the best interests of the patient. An emergency is often defined as any circumstance in which the patient or others are in immediate danger of serious physical harm. Disclosure of confidential information in an emergency situation may occur even if the patient refuses to give consent or cannot be located. For example, an acutely suicidal woman's husband might be contacted without her prior consent to discuss her clinical status and treatment needs. Release of information can similarly occur in emergencies or clinical situations requiring immediate action involving a patient who the clinician does not believe is functionally competent to consent to the release if close relatives or a guardian are not available. Nonconsensual disclosure of information may also occur when a patient is seeking emergency care and the medical staff is trying to determine previous diagnosis and medication history. Once the therapist verifies that the call is from the hospital, the relevant clinical information may be released.

2. *Civil Commitment*

Most hospitalizations for mental illness in the United States occur on a voluntary basis. Not infrequently, however, an individual will either not acknowledge his illness, not admit its seriousness, or refuse hospitalization. In such situations, civil commitment proceedings may be instituted. Often the person most knowledgeable about the patient's illness and his need for hospitalization will be his therapist.

Breaching confidentiality to effect treatment may be necessary if the needs of the patient are to be served. The therapist's breach of the confidential relationship in the courtroom is taken to serve, rather than undermine, the patient's best interests. Additionally, the therapist may not have to reveal many confidences from the patient at the civil commitment hearing if others (e.g., police, family, and neighbors) are there to testify about the patient's statements and behavior. Instead the therapist will be able to rely on his general observations and examination of the patient. In this way, the therapist can try to obtain for the patient the level of services he needs while still maintaining the therapeutic relationship. Of course, the patient may not always appreciate the therapist's claimed concern for his best interests and may become hostile to the therapist for the duration of the hospitalization. Nonetheless, breaching confidentiality for the purpose of involuntary treatment is justifiable in terms of the patient's medical interests, society's needs, and the therapist's professional ethics.

3. *Duty to Protect Third Parties*

The therapist may also be under an affirmative duty to breach confidentiality when there is a duty to protect a third party from potential violence caused by the patient, after therapeutic interventions have failed to adequately reduce the risk of violence. (See Chapter 8, for a discussion of this topic.) Revealing to the potential victim or the police that a person is in treatment or stating the basis of concern for the third party's safety, without the patient's consent, will be a breach of confidentiality. The therapist should document that the warning, or any attempt at warning, was given, as well as the reasons which led him to conclude such a breach was necessary.

4. *Child Abuse Reporting*

Since 1964, all states have adopted laws that require the reporting of suspected child abuse and neglect. Originally the laws were aimed at physicians and required the reporting of nonaccidental injuries or serious physical injuries. Since then these laws have been greatly expanded as to who must report and what must be reported. All states now require that health care professionals, social workers, and teachers report the maltreatment of children; in some, reports are required only when the professional has personally examined the child, as opposed to his having heard about the abuse from the offender or a third party. In many states, these reporting requirements also include child day care center workers.

Suspected cases of child physical abuse, sexual abuse, physical neglect, and sometimes emotional maltreatment mandate reporting. For child abuse reporting purposes, a child is someone under the age of 18, except in a few states which do not require reporting after the child reaches 16 years of age. In many states, the reporting requirements are extended to the age of 21 for children who are mentally disabled or physically handicapped.

The therapist must be aware that he does not need proof of the maltreatment, but that it must only be suspected. All states grant immunity to the professional from liability for the good-faith reporting of suspected child abuse or neglect. Because of the heightened awareness of child abuse and the feeling that professionals often do not intervene when it is suspected, most of the states now have criminal penalties for failure to report. The crime of failing to report suspected child abuse is usually considered a misdemeanor. In addition to criminal penalties, the professional may be subject to loss of professional licensure as well as civil suits for failing to report suspected abuse. (This topic is discussed in more detail in Chapter 6, "Professional Liability," and Chapter 10, "Legal Rights of Children.")

5. *Other Statutory Reporting Requirements*

The legally mandated reporting of specified occupational or communicable diseases such as sexually transmitted diseases also takes precedence over the patient's confidentiality. However, the reporting requirement in these circumstances falls upon the physician who diagnosed the disease, not on the therapist who later learns about it during therapy. For example, if a patient in psychotherapy reveals that he is HIV-positive, it is not the therapist's responsibility to report this to the state public health agency, but it is the responsibility of the physician who ordered the blood test and made the diagnosis.

In a growing number of states, there is a requirement of reporting abuse of the elderly (see Chapter 9). Many states have also expanded reporting requirements to cover the abuse of institutionalized adults, including the mentally ill, the developmentally disabled, and those in nursing homes. The mental health professional should familiarize himself with the specific conditions which trigger reporting in his state.

Finally, many states require that mental or physical conditions which impair a person's ability to drive a motor vehicle be reported to the state department of transportation or driver's license bureau. The clinician does not revoke the client's driver's license by reporting the disability, but this report initiates an investigation into the client's driving ability.

Clinicians who comply in good faith with any of these mandatory reporting obligations are afforded immunity from civil liability for breach of confidentiality. Of course, the client could initiate a lawsuit for the breach (e.g., claiming that he lost his job because of the report), but the applicable statute would obviate a successful suit (see Figure 7.1).

6. *Discussions with the Treatment Team*

The primary caregiver need not obtain the client's consent when he shares information with those who are directly participating in the client's care. These may include supervisors, members of the treatment team, or outside consultants. In some instances, they may include an attorney consulted by the therapist or agency. Each of these individuals is obligated to keep the information confidential. It is advisable, however, for clients to be told of the confidentiality policies and procedures of the treatment setting when treatment begins. In contrast, sharing confidential information with former or future treatment staff, even those who will receive a hospitalized patient upon discharge or transfer, generally requires obtaining the client's consent, preferably in writing.

B. Advising Clients about Confidentiality

Clients vary widely in their expectations of confidentiality. The therapist will be unable to assess the importance of confidentiality to the client unless this is explicitly discussed in the treatment. At the outset of therapy, it is advisable to establish with the client the limits placed on the therapist in terms of maintaining confidentiality. Clients should be told that there are circumstances in which, for the protection of the client or others, the therapist will be required to breach confidentiality. The client should also be informed that the therapist will attempt to obtain the client's consent to release the requested information before actually doing so. At that time, even if the client refuses to consent to revealing a confidence, but the therapist will do so anyway because it is required under the circumstances, the therapist should inform the client that he will disclose the information without the client's consent.

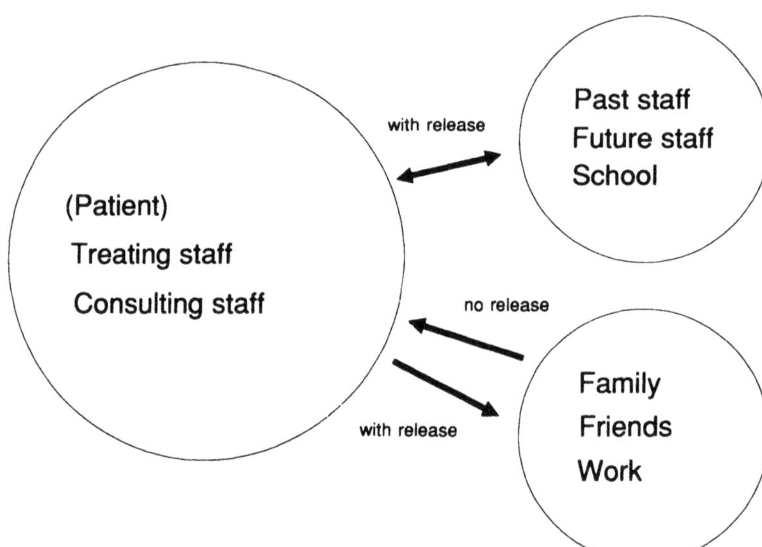

Figure 7.1. The Geography of Confidentiality. Without the patient's explicit consent, confidential information can be shared with only those mental health clinicians who are currently involved in the treatment of a patient. Explicit consent to release information, apart from legally authorized exceptions, is required to otherwise share information. Any therapist can receive information without the patient's explicit consent.

Some clinicians or facilities use a written contract or agreement, signed by the adult client, which authorizes the treatment staff to contact a designated friend or relative of the client in some future necessity. Such an agreement may be useful if the client is failing appointments and cannot be contacted directly, or when there is concern that the client is suicidal. This form of prospective consent may help ensure the safety of the client without disrupting the therapist–client alliance by a breach of confidentiality.

C. Waivers of Confidentiality by the Client

Not infrequently, an individual will waive confidentiality of his records for the purposes of obtaining health insurance benefits or for seeking a job or promotion.

1. Release in the Employment Setting

Before July 1992, it was not unusual for employers to require pre-employment physical examinations or to inquire on job applications whether the person had been treated for a mental illness. In 1990, the Americans with Disabilities Act (ADA) (42 United States Code Section 12101) was enacted. The ADA provides protection to mentally and physically disabled people against discrimination in private employment, public accommodation, public transportation, and other public services.

In the employment context, questions about a history of psychiatric treatment are now forbidden as part of the application process. Employers are also prevented from performing pre-employment physical examinations. At most, the employer can inquire whether the applicant has the ability to perform job-related functions. The job description should set forth all the qualifications necessary for the position. Once on the job, if the employee has a disability, then the employer is required to make a "reasonable accommodation" for the employee to be able to function with his disability. Employers also may not inquire about previous use of health insurance coverage. Thus, an employer could not refuse to hire an applicant with a history of psychiatric treatment for fear that the employer's health insurance rates would rise. However, the employer would be permitted to limit the scope of health insurance available to all employees.

After being hired, an employee may voluntarily request a leave of absence to receive treatment for drug and alcohol abuse or for emotional problems. The employer also can take the initiative of encouraging the employee to seek such treatment. To return to work, the individual will then often have to reveal his records or have a report submitted by his therapist. In addition, the employer may require the company's physician or psychologist to determine if the employee is emotionally able to return to his former position. This is particularly true where the employee is a public servant, such as a police officer or fire fighter, or where he is in a position of stress. In either event, the fact of treatment will be known to the employer and may affect future job assignments or promotions, although such discrimination is prohibited by the ADA.

It is a rare situation in which the fact of an employee's past treatment for a mental illness will not affect, at least subtly if not overtly, the employer–employee relationship. Consequently, some employees choose to forego making health insurance claims under a company plan for fear that their claims for reimbursement, and their mental illness, will become known to their employer.

2. *Release to Insurance Companies*

The most common consensual release of information about mental health treatment occurs when requests are made to insurance companies for reimbursement of the costs of treatment. The health insurer needs proof that the claim is a valid one and needs to know the type of service which was provided to the patient. The standard insurance reimbursement form requires the patient to authorize the therapist to release all records and other information relating to treatment. Such a request to release information may occur prospectively, that is even before the treatment has occurred; thus, the client has minimal knowledge of that which he is consenting to release. The need to release records for reimbursement may create a conflict for the therapist who wishes to keep records that are sufficiently detailed to document the treatment needs but that also contain the kind of personal information whose release to outsiders would be detrimental to the patient.

Misuse of such information by insurance companies is well documented. Knowledge of psychiatric treatment, for example, has been put to questionable use in assessing eligibility for automobile and life insurance. The therapist, in keeping records, should be aware of how records may be used for nontreatment purposes and who is likely to see them. Accordingly, the formal record should contain only sufficient information to document the need for treatment and its course. In addition, the therapist should inform the patient of the risks of submitting an insurance claim for mental health services.

D. Disclosure to Investigative Agencies

Mental health professionals are sometimes asked to release information to law enforcement agencies. Generally, state law will govern when information must be disclosed and the extent of the disclosure. The records of the patient should never be nonconsensually disclosed without a specific court order unless advice to the contrary has been provided by the professional's attorney. When there is concern about a patient's being a missing person, it is appropriate for the therapist to state that the person has been hospitalized and the dates of hospitalization. The United States Secret Service will sometimes contact the hospital or agency to determine the location or condition of a person who has made a threat against a protected person, usually the President. The law does not accord the Secret Service any authority to obtain records or interview the therapist in the absence of consent from the patient or a court order.

E. Clinical and Social Erosions of Confidentiality

Confidentiality can be strained by many clinical and social issues, apart from the erosion which has occurred through legal and economic forces (see Tables 7.1 and 7.2). In this regard, it is clinically useful to adopt a relative rather than absolute conception of confidentiality; in practice, there are typically levels or degrees of confidentiality rather than all or none of it.

Clinicians are often uncertain about the propriety of disclosing information to

Table 7.1. Confidentiality Problem Areas

Disclosures without past or present consent
Discussions in halls and elevators
Discussions with clinician's family and friends
Telephone disclosures without verification of party
Ignoring patient's confidentiality expectations
Promising absolute confidentiality
Failing to disclose limits of confidentiality in advance
Confidentiality for third-party evaluations
Group therapy
Child, family, marital treatment
Requests to keep information secret from patients

family members who provide care or supervision to a mentally disabled person in the household. A misinterpretation of confidentiality which values adherence to this principle over the best interests of the patient might result in failing to provide certain information to the family which would assist in properly caring for the patient (e.g., nature and purpose of medication, side effects of treatment, need to monitor for recurrent illness, cautions about driving or weapons). It is never a breach of confidentiality to ask the patient whether staff can discuss these matters with selected family members and, with consent, then to do so. The staff can still preserve some degree of confidentiality by agreeing what information and patient communications will and will not be shared with the family. It is much more problematic when the patient refuses to cooperate with these efforts at treatment planning, at which time the clinician needs to help the patient resolve this form of treatment refusal.

Confidentiality can be strained by social contact between the therapist and client outside of the treatment setting, either directly or through third parties. In smaller or rural communities, therapist and client might be involved in overlapping social circles of organizations, activities, friends, or relatives. Even in larger communities, one client still in treatment may refer a friend or relative to the therapist, one client may independently discover that a friend or relative is also seeing the therapist, or the therapist and client may have a colleague in common. These social contacts may make clients, as well as therapists, feel as though their privacy, if not their confidentiality, has been invaded. It is important to realize that while the therapist is bound by the confidentiality ethic, the client is free to seek or disclose information about the

Table 7.2. Pitfalls of Releasing Records

Forgetting who owns the records
Release without patient's written informed consent
Releasing more information than necessary
Patient's being unaware of record contents when consenting to release
Insertion of corrections by patients
Responding to global release requests
Responding to prospective release requests
Rereleasing another facility's records
Releasing social histories

therapist and the therapy as he wishes. In these situations, it is the therapist's responsibility to carefully manage the client's confidentiality, despite encroaches by social factors or the client himself.

Finally, confidentiality can inadvertently be breached through the physical layout of the office or clinic. The placement of the secretary's desk and telephone, waiting room, or office exit area can readily betray one or another client's confidences through their mutual presence in an area or overhearing of a secretary's conversation. Some simple protective measures can be used to enhance confidentiality but there are often limits to what realistically can be accomplished.

IV. PRIVILEGED COMMUNICATIONS

A basic principle of the American legal system is that litigation through the adversarial process will produce truth and justice. By insulating some information from disclosure no matter how relevant or even critical it may be in a given litigation setting, testimonial privilege laws conflict with this quest for truth. These laws, then, are the result of a balancing process; the legislatures have determined that the protection of certain relationships is, or is not, more important than an unbridled quest for an accurate outcome in judicial proceedings. Testimonial privilege statutes are the most common manifestations of the states' concern with protecting information revealed by the patient to the therapist. To encourage full disclosure to a therapist, these state statutes provide that what has been disclosed in the therapeutic setting cannot be revealed without the patient's consent in a court of law. However, the term *privileged communication* refers only to information that is at issue in litigation. The matter of privilege arises only when the bearer of the privileged communication is asked a question that would cause him to divulge that information. These statutes govern only disclosures of information or records in court or during the litigation process. In the litigation contest, testimonial privilege is not absolute. Each statute provides exceptions as to when information or, sometimes, records obtained as a result of the therapeutic relationship may be disclosed in the courtroom. Testimonial privilege laws do not govern access by third parties such as insurance companies outside of litigation, nor access in the clinical setting.

Testimonial privilege laws have a long history dating back to the 1500s and the development of the attorney–client privilege. This testimonial privilege is recognized in every state and is based on the concept that a lawyer cannot effectively represent his client unless he has been fully advised of all the facts, and that without a testimonial privilege available to foreclose public disclosure, the client would not be willing to divulge to his attorney all relevant information. In addition, all states have recognized the priest–penitent testimonial privilege, which is rooted in the need for secrecy in religious confessions. This privilege has been made applicable to all clergy and is based on the First Amendment constitutional right to the free exercise of religion. Additionally, all states recognize a marital privilege, which prohibits one spouse from testifying against the other except when one is suing the other or has committed a criminal act against the other. This privilege is based on the concept that open communication is essential for promoting marital harmony.

Statutory testimonial privileges are sometimes less protective of client's privacy than the confidentiality provisions of mental health professionals' codes of ethics.

Even though the fact that a person has received mental health services is protected by professional ethics, for example, testimonial privilege law could allow this information to be presented in courtroom proceedings. Further, some testimonial privilege statutes do not explicitly protect treatment records from courtroom disclosure. Testimonial privilege laws in some cases protect only the client's "communications" to the professional and not the clinician's observations, assessment, diagnosis, prognosis, or treatment plan or the records reflecting these matters. Finally, there is no statutory testimonial privilege for mental health professionals under federal law, though some protection from courtroom disclosure is offered under federal child abuse as well as drug and alcohol treatment program provisions.

Testimonial privilege statutes relevant to our discussion take one of several forms: (1) general physician–patient and psychiatrist–patient privilege, (2) psychologist–patient privilege, and (3) psychotherapist–patient privilege. In a growing number of states, there are also specific privilege statutes for rape crisis counselors, marriage and family counselors, and licensed social workers. Almost every privilege statute provides exceptions when confidentiality will not be honored in the judicial setting.

A. Physician–Patient Privilege

Initially, the Hippocratic Oath prohibited physicians from voluntarily revealing the secrets of their patients. Now, ethical obligations of physicians prohibit such disclosures except when required by law. Were a physician to be called to testify in a court proceeding, he would be required in that setting to reveal the confidences entrusted to him, the oath notwithstanding. The physician–patient privilege is the most common source of protection against courtroom disclosure of psychotherapeutic communications (and, sometimes, records) in the absence of specific privilege statutes for psychiatrists or psychotherapists. The privilege applies, however, only to communications made to physicians and not to those made to other types of mental health professionals.

The physician–patient privilege statutes, which exist in almost every jurisdiction, generally provide that a physician shall not disclose during the litigation process any of his patient's communications that were necessary to enable the physician to treat the patient. As physicians, psychiatrists are covered by such statutes. However, in a number of states there are specific privilege statutes which apply to psychiatrists.

B. Psychologist–Patient Privilege

A specific psychologist–patient testimonial privilege has been adopted in nearly every state. These privilege statutes are usually located in the psychologist licensing provisions. Typically they are qualified by exceptions for civil commitment, court-ordered examinations, and the patient-litigant exception.

C. Psychotherapist–Patient Privilege

Numerous states have testimonial privilege provisions specifically applicable to the psychotherapist–patient relationship. In most of these states, psychotherapists are defined as including psychiatrists and licensed psychologists. In many of these statutes, therapists are also defined as including licensed social workers, psychiatric nurses, and others such as marriage and family counselors and rape crisis center workers.

Even if there is no statutory privilege for a particular type of therapist (e.g., unlicensed social worker, psychology intern), if that therapist is treating the client while employed by another professional who enjoys a statutory privilege, then that privilege will sometimes apply to the therapist.

D. To Whom the Privilege Belongs

The right of privilege protects the interest of the patient and is designed to promote the seeking of mental health services rather than the quest for truth in the litigation process. Its goal is to encourage open disclosure in treatment while preventing unwanted disclosure in the courtroom. The privilege generally belongs only to the patient, who is the one to decide whether it will be exercised or waived. A fundamental legal rule is that if something is not raised as an issue in litigation, it is waived. This means that if the patient does not assert the privilege to prevent courtroom disclosure of his communications or records, then the privilege is waived, and the communications or records can be revealed in court.

It has been argued that patients are often unaware of what their records contain and thus cannot make a knowing decision about whether to assert or to waive the privilege. It is for this reason that some have suggested that the therapist, rather than the patient himself, should be the one to exercise the privilege on behalf of the patient. Illinois is one of the few jurisdictions which has thus far accepted this concept, but it is limited in that the courts will review the record to make a specific determination as to whether to prevent disclosure. For this reason, mental health professionals should immediately contact a patient or former patient and inform him that the therapist or his records have been subpoenaed. The therapist should discuss the contents of the records and advise the person to have his attorney seek to quash the subpoena if the person wishes the information not to be disclosed as part of litigation. Without the therapist's notifying the patient, the patient may be unaware of the subpoena. Confidential health care information, whether in the form of courtroom testimony or of written records, should not be released without the written consent of the patient or legal guardian, or by order of the court.

V. EXCEPTIONS TO THE THERAPIST–PATIENT PRIVILEGE

Each state that grants a testimonial privilege also specifies certain exceptions to the privilege. These exceptions arise in the context of suspected child abuse cases, when civil commitment is sought, and when the patient raises his mental condition as a claim or defense in a civil or criminal proceeding. In addition, there is no privilege when a court-ordered examination occurs, and when the courts are called upon to determine the validity of a will. Arguably, these exceptions can go so far as to practically "swallow up" the protection of a privilege. The exceptions to the privilege for court-ordered examinations and the patient-litigant exception are discussed below. The exceptions for civil commitment and child abuse are discussed in Section III above, and in Chapters 3 and 10, respectively.

A. Court-Ordered Examinations

There are many times when courts, in both civil or criminal matters, seek the expert advice of a mental health professional as to an issue raised at trial. Such instances can involve evaluations of the litigants as well as of witnesses. For example, a court may be interested in determining whether a witness is emotionally stable before deciding whether to permit his testimony. Likewise, a court may need to determine the extent of emotional damage in a personal injury claim, or the best placement for a child who is the subject of a custody dispute, or the competency of a defendant to stand trial in a criminal proceeding.

Approximately half the states specifically set forth an exception to the psychotherapist–patient privilege for court-ordered examinations. Typical wording is that of New Mexico's law, which provides:

> If the judge orders an examination of the mental or emotional condition of the patient, communications made in the course of these examinations are not privileged under this rule with respect to the particular purpose for which the examination is ordered unless the judge orders otherwise. (New Mexico Statutes Annot. Rules of Evidence 504(d)(a)(1991))

Even without a specific statutory provision, it is well accepted that the court has the authority, in certain instances, to obtain a physical or mental health examination, the results of which are not confidential.

With or without the exemption, the risk of harm from disclosure of confidential information in court-ordered examinations is limited, since these examinations typically will not be conducted by the individual's therapist. Additionally, the examiner must notify the person that the evaluation is being conducted pursuant to a court order and that statements made during the examination may be contained in the report to the court or revealed during testimony. Thus, a court-ordered examination will not usually violate a therapeutic relationship, since it is unlikely that any relationship would have been formed.

B. Patient-Litigant Exception

Introduction into litigation of a claim or defense of mental or emotional illness may subject to courtroom disclosure any previous treatment undergone by the claimant or defendant. This is termed the *patient-litigant exception* to the testimonial privilege laws. Almost half the states specifically provide for this exception. Typical is Delaware's statute, which provides:

> There is no privilege under this rule as to a communication relevant to an issue of the physical, mental or emotional condition of the patient in any proceeding in which he relies upon the condition as an element of his claim or defense, or after the patient's death in any proceeding in which any party relies upon the condition as an element of his claim or defense. (Del. Code Annot. title 16, Uniform Rules of Evidence 503(d)(3)(1991))

Even in those states that have not enacted a specific patient-litigant exception provision, the courts will usually find that an exception to privilege law exists. The court will reason that by raising the issue of his mental or emotional condition, the claimant has brought into question his mental health and therefore justice requires making all relevant facts known to the judge or jury.

The patient-litigant exception to privilege laws raises significant problems for litigants. Fear of disclosure of mental health records may cause potential litigants to avoid seeking legal redress even when they have justifiable claims, or to acquiesce to otherwise unwarranted settlements out of fear of public disclosure of their past or present treatment.

The patient-litigant exception does not necessarily require that all previous communications or records be admitted into the proceeding. The court will admit as evidence only that which is relevant or material to the case. Disclosure is required only as to the mental condition put into issue; no other aspects of the patient-litigant's mental condition or treatment will have to be revealed. However, the burden rests on the litigant to show that a given communication or finding is not directly related to the issue he has tendered to the court. He will have to reveal to the court to some extent the nature of the psychotherapeutic communications if he is to convince the court that they are not at issue in the matter before it.

When the court evaluates what should be admitted into evidence, it must try to balance the individual's right to privacy against the right to have full knowledge regarding the legal dispute before it. In some cases, the claim that the past mental health record is irrelevant is easily made, because the treatment given was provided many years before the current issue arose. However, in many cases this is not so clear-cut. In a child custody case, for example, the fact that one parent had been psychiatrically hospitalized five years before the present custody dispute might be relevant to the case. In a personal injury case in which a plaintiff claims that as a result of his injury he is suffering an exacerbation of pre-existing emotional distress which has necessitated a return to treatment, examination of the earlier treatment records would be helpful in clarifying how much of his current problem has been caused by the situation before the court, and how much was preexisting.

Five common occasions on which the patient-litigant exception comes into play are (1) child custody disputes, (2) personal injury actions, (3) malpractice suits against the therapist, (4) disability and workers' compensation claims, and (5) will contests.

1. *Child Custody Disputes*

With the high rate of divorce and the acceptance of the sex-neutral "best interest of the child" child custody standard, litigation in family court often relates to the custody of the children. Often the contest has less to do with the children and more to do with financial issues, since the child custody decision will be related to the disposal of the marital home and family income. The guiding legal principle in adjudicating these disputes is determining which parent can better meet the needs of the child; this frequently means choosing the less detrimental alternative. In making this determination, the court can and must consider a wide range of factors, including the physical and emotional health of both the parents and the child. The existence of a present mental illness or a past history of psychiatric hospitalization will be relevant to a child custody dispute. In addition, a parent may attempt to present the fact that the other parent has previously been in psychiatric treatment as evidence of that parent's instability.

Even when neither parent raises the issue of the other's mental health, the court can do so on its own motion. The court may order an evaluation of the entire family by a therapist or a social service agency attached to the court system. The evaluators will usually review the charges and countercharges and obtain sufficient information about each person's parenting skills and his or her relationship to the children so that a thoughtful recommendation can be made to the court. These evaluations may reveal a history of earlier psychiatric care, which will lead to seeking disclosure of those records or contact with the former therapist.

A therapist who is treating someone involved in a child custody dispute may be called into court to testify as to what he knows about the client. If a subpoena is received for either testimony or records, the therapist should immediately notify the client. The client should then contact his attorney, who can attempt to have the subpoena quashed. When the therapist contacts the client, he should discuss with him the contents of the record and the nature of any testimony.

Because of the public policy of encouraging people to seek mental health services under stressful circumstances such as divorce, an attorney may be successful in limiting what is disclosed. He should be able to argue that when there has been no history of psychiatric hospitalization, the mental health treatment of his client is something that is not relevant to the parenting skills of the client. However, if there are specific allegations of abnormal thinking and behavior, then mental health records will be admitted and the therapist will be forced to breach confidentiality by either revealing the records or testifying. With the increases in child custody and postdecree litigation, it is likely that at some point a clinician will become involved in a contested custody proceeding.

2. *Personal Injury Actions*

Another frequent occasion for the application of the patient-litigant exception to testimonial privilege is the personal injury suit in which a litigant raises a claim or defense of mental or emotional injury. One of the first questions that will be asked by the opposing party's attorney during discovery is whether the litigant is receiving, or has received, treatment for an emotional illness. If the answer is affirmative, the attorney will try to discover the extent of that treatment by taking the deposition of the treating therapist and by subpoenaing the records. The burden will be upon the litigant to show that his past history is not relevant and is thus beyond the proper scope of discovery.

The patient-litigant exception attempts to balance an individual's need for privacy when seeking mental health services against the need for the court to obtain information relevant to its decision. Knowledge of a person's history of treatment for emotional problems can greatly affect the assessment of the extent of the injury the plaintiff may have incurred. It may be that, for example, contrary to the plaintiff's claim that his emotional problems were caused by the defendant's negligence, his emotional problems really preceded the allegedly negligent or wrongful act.

In these situations, the confidentiality of the treatment relationship can be preserved by having a nontreating expert examine the claimant to determine the validity of his claim and then testify in court. This procedure is useful in that confidentiality is less important for an examination limited to the area of the litigation than it is for the treatment relationship. While the testimony of the treating therapist is sometimes valuable in that the therapist can provide a longitudinal perspective on the individual before the injury occurred and on any changes resulting from the injury, the testimony of the appointed expert may be adequate for the purpose of the litigation.

To minimize the breach of confidentiality and to ensure that only relevant and material matters will be opened up to scrutiny, the court can limit the scope of discovery. However, in order to effectively evaluate what is relevant and probative and cannot be obtained from any other source, the court must have some knowledge of what is being sought to be discovered. If the treatment occurred ten years in the past, then it is easier for the patient-litigant's attorney to argue that it is not relevant. However, if the person is currently in treatment and claims that the injury resulted in psychological damages, then full discovery of the records is necessary to determine how much of the psychological problem was preexisting.

3. *Malpractice Suits*

In a malpractice action, the plaintiff claims that the care he received was substandard, and that as a result of the negligence of the therapist, he was harmed. When an individual sues his therapist for malpractice, he automatically opens up the issue of his treatment with that therapist. The question before the court is whether the appropriate standard of care was provided (see Chapter 6 for further discussion). Without a detailed revelation of what occurred during treatment, there is no way to evaluate whether the therapist was negligent. When such a suit is filed against him, the therapist has the right to breach confidentiality to reveal to his attorney the facts and records of the case, and to testify about them during any depositions or the trial.

4. *Disability and Workers' Compensation Claims*

Every state has workers' compensation laws. These laws provide employees with a form of insurance for job-related injuries. Their goal is to compensate the employee without forcing him to resort to litigation for a determination of negligence and the amount of recompense. The acts are administered by workers' compensation boards, which rule on the extent of the injury or disability. The amount which can be recovered is based on a predetermined fee schedule, frequently established by the state legislature.

By applying for workers' compensation, the employee relinquishes his right to file a civil action against the employer for the injury. To succeed in a workers' compensation claim, the employee must prove that the injury was job related and that his damages were directly related to the injury. Earlier workers' compensation laws provided that employees could recover for emotional illness only if they had also been physically injured, even if the physical injury was slight. More recently, however, only a risk of physical danger, without any actual physical harm, may be sufficient to support a finding that a work-related psychological injury is compensable. For example, in many states, if a worker witnessed his coworker killed on the job, and the worker was in danger of being injured himself, he would be able to recover for the psychological damage caused by the accident. Recovery for emotional injuries which are work related is an expanding area of workers' compensation law.

When an employee claims a job-related mental or emotional illness, he places his mental condition at issue, and the patient-litigant exception will usually permit discovery of his previous or current treatment. The workers' compensation boards take the same view as the courts in personal injury actions, that is, that the information, when relevant, will be discoverable and admissible in the courtroom.

5. *Will Contests*

A will speaks only at one's death. At the time the individual executes his will, he must have testamentary capacity; that is, he must be able to understand the nature and extent of his property and identify his natural beneficiaries (e.g., family). The issue before the court is whether the testator, the author of the will, was competent at the time he wrote his will. His mental competency at the time he died is irrelevant, if it is not the same as at the time he wrote the will. (See Chapter 9 for a discussion of competency.) There is a legal presumption that unless the testator had been declared legally incompetent, he will be presumed to have been competent to write the will. Overcoming this presumption is a heavy burden for the challenger to the will. To meet this burden, the challenger may try to introduce either the testimony or the records of the therapist who treated the testator around the time the will was written.

Most courts are hesitant to set aside wills unless a bequest seems plainly irrational. In the face of a will challenge, the court will not require the release of mental health records if the information can be obtained from other sources. Challengers can accomplish their goals without having to impinge on psychotherapist–patient confidentiality by calling as witnesses laypersons who knew the testator and his mental state at the time of writing the will. A testator can help forestall breaches of confidentiality following his death by videotaping his act of affirming and then signing the will and by securing affidavits from reliable individuals as to his understanding of his actions at the time. This makes sense when an individual is bequesting his money to persons or groups other than the expected ones. For example, if a man disinherits his children and leaves his money to care for his pets, the issue of his testamentary capacity might be raised. Corroborative evidence of mental ability at the time the will was executed will provide justification for the court's refusal to breach the privilege and will also uphold the validity of the will.

VI. NONSTATUTORY PROTECTION OF CONFIDENTIALITY

In addition to privilege and licensure statutes which guarantee confidentiality, there are three other potential sources for protecting patient–therapist communications: (1) the ethics of the mental health professional, (2) the common law, and (3) the constitutional right of privacy.

A. The Ethics of the Mental Health Professional

The physician's ethical obligation to maintain the confidentiality of his patient's communications has been codified since the fourth century B.C. in the Hippocratic Oath, which states: "All that may come to my knowledge in the exercise of my profession . . . or in daily commerce with men, which ought not to be spread abroad, I will keep secret and will never reveal."

All providers of mental health care are governed by their profession's code of ethics, each of which contains a provision emphasizing the importance of confidentiality. Although not necessarily carrying the weight of law, these codes establish standards of conduct that members of the profession are expected to uphold. Breach of those ethical standards may cause the professional to lose membership in his professional society. It also could result in a suspension or loss of his professional license.

B. The Common Law

Traditionally, the only testimonial privilege which existed under the common law was the attorney–client privilege. However, both Illinois and Alaska have recognized a common law privilege for therapist–patient communications. Since almost all states have testimonial privilege statutes, a common law argument might be raised where the privilege did not apply to a specific type of therapist or type of confidence. It can be envisioned that, in some states, there might not be a privilege for psychiatric nurses, yet the nurse could argue that the common law would extend to protect the information revealed in the treatment setting for this class of treatment professional. This argument has been persuasive in some instances where there was no specific privilege for information shared with a rape crisis counselor.

C. The Constitutional Right of Privacy

Beginning in 1966, the United States Supreme Court, through a series of decisions, has enunciated a constitutionally protected right to privacy. First expressed in a case related to the access of married couples to contraceptives and continuing through the cases affirming a woman's right to have an abortion, the Court has recognized that, in certain circumstances, individual privacy is protected against governmental action which invades that privacy. Although the Supreme Court has not directly addressed the issue of confidentiality of mental health records, numerous state and federal courts have addressed this issue and upheld the right of privacy. In *Hawaii Psychiatric Society v. Ariyoshi* (1982), a federal district court struck down a Hawaiian Medicaid fraud statute that permitted the seizure and examination of the notes of therapists to determine if payment for the service was justified, holding that "the disclosure of a patient's innermost thoughts, feelings, conduct, and beliefs is, quite simply, not justified by the State's interest in verifying the necessity of performance of psychotherapeutic treatments." The court suggested that Hawaii could find another statutory scheme that would strike a more appropriate balance between preventing fraud and minimizing any violation of the individual's right to confidentiality.

Constitutional protections apply only when there is governmental action. Thus, making constitutional arguments will apply only when challenging a state statute or when the breach of confidentiality occurs in a case involving a governmental agency. This could apply when child protective agencies are involved, as well as when proceedings occur under state or federal laws. Constitutional arguments will not apply when the patient-litigant exception is raised in personal injury proceedings, for example. The concept of a constitutionally protected right of privacy, combined with privilege statutes, has not been utilized often enough to argue against disclosure of confidential information or to limit that disclosure. It can be envisioned, for example, that in child custody proceedings an attorney might be successful in arguing that certain information is not discoverable because of the constitutional right of privacy. Hopefully, in the future, attorneys will be more aggressive in setting forth constitutional arguments to prevent or limit the disclosure of information about an individual's treatment.

VII. MINORS' CONFIDENTIALITY

The confidentiality of a minor's health care raises special issues. Parents and legal guardians are generally entitled to some medical information about their child. Information which parents need to make informed decisions concerning their child's care must be provided to them. The child or teenager should be informed about the type of information which will be shared with his parents (e.g., self-destructive behavior, running away, homicide plans, or severe depression or psychosis), and that which will be kept in confidence (e.g., sexual fantasies).

As a teenager approaches majority, parental authority is less absolute. Maintenance of the adolescent's confidentiality is often a necessary condition for therapy. The older adolescent's confidentiality rights parallel those of adults, with the same recognized exceptions for harm to life. The scope of the minor patient's confidentiality rights should be thoroughly discussed at the time of accepting the case for treatment. In most situations, adolescent patients should be encouraged to inform their parents themselves about those matters that parents need to know. (Chapter 10 elaborates on this issue.)

VIII. CONFIDENTIALITY OF DRUG ABUSE AND ALCOHOLISM TREATMENT RECORDS

The United States Congress has enacted laws and regulations for the protection of records of individuals receiving treatment for drug abuse or alcoholism (42 C.F.R. Part II, 42 U.S.C. 290dd, 42 U.S.C. 290ee). These regulations apply only to federally funded programs that specialize, in whole or in part, in providing substance abuse diagnosis, referral, or treatment.

The regulations do not apply when the hospital or treatment program does not have an evaluation or treatment program specifically designed for substance abuse. Nor will the regulations apply when treatment is in conjunction with other medical problems and is not part of a specialized alcohol or substance abuse program. Federal government funding of the health care services will generally be a criterion for the regulations to apply. In most states, state-funded treatment programs are covered through state laws and regulations, which may differ from the federal regulations and whose confidentiality provisions may be more stringent than the federal rules.

These laws have been enacted in recognition of the special stigma attached to having a substance abuse disorder and receiving treatment for it. Their goal is to encourage people to seek treatment without fear that their records will haunt them. This is accomplished by greatly restricting any information that may be released.

Alcohol and substance abuse treatment records may be released:

1. With the written consent of the patient.
2. Without the patient's consent to meet a bona fide medical emergency.
3. When used for research purposes, but without patient identifying data.

SAMPLE NOTICE REGARDING CONFIDENTIALITY

The confidentiality of alcohol and drug abuse patient records maintained by this program is protected by federal law and regulations. Generally, the program may not say to a person outside the program that a patient attends the program and may not disclose any information identifying a patient as an alcohol or drug abuser UNLESS:

1. The patient consents in writing.
2. The disclosure is allowed by a court order.
3. The disclosure is made to medical personnel in a medical emergency or to qualified personnel for research, audit, or program evaluation.

Violation of the federal law and regulations by a program is a crime. Suspected violations may be reported to appropriate authorities in accordance with federal regulations.

Federal law and regulations do not protect any information about suspected child abuse or neglect from being reported under state law to appropriate state or local authorities.

4. To law enforcement personnel when the patient commits a crime on program premises or against program personnel or threatens to do so.

A court order is required for the therapist to release records in any other circumstance, including when the patient is under investigation for criminal activity. The court may authorize disclosure of confidential communications only when:

1. Disclosure is necessary to protect against an existing threat to life or threat of serious bodily injury of another person.
2. Disclosure is necessary to investigate or prosecute an extremely serious crime.
3. The patient brings the matter up in any legal proceeding.

Viewed as model confidentiality provisions which could be utilized for other health care records, the regulations restrict the disclosure of any information, whether written or oral, that would identify a patient as an alcohol or drug abuser. They also prohibit the patient's records from being used to initiate or substantiate any criminal charges against the patient or to conduct any investigation of the patient, except as authorized by a court order.

Substance abuse treatment records can be disclosed with the written release of the patient. The consent form must be specific as to the person or organization to whom records will be released, the nature of the requested information, and the purpose of or need for the disclosure. The consent form must state that the release can be revoked by the patient, and it must be signed and dated. Blanket consent forms are unacceptable.

When information is requested and there is a valid release or a court order, only information which is relevant to the present purposes can be released. The treatment program personnel are not otherwise permitted to reveal any information about a person, including whether he is in the treatment program. When queried, treatment personnel should provide a copy of the federal confidentiality regulations to the person who asks for the information. In addition, patients must be told about the regulations and must be provided a written summary of them.

Because of these regulations, medical records administrators will not release these records without a special release form designed to comply with the federal regulations for substance abuse treatment records. These provisions attempt to carefully protect the right of the individual to confidentiality and provide for release only in justified or authorized circumstances.

IX. ACQUIRED IMMUNODEFICIENCY SYNDROME

Acquired immunodeficiency syndrome (AIDS) is one of the leading health problems of the 1990s. Persons diagnosed with AIDS, and those who are infected with the AIDS virus (i.e., who are HIV-positive) face great stigma. Many states have recognized this stigma and have provided protection against discrimination in employment or housing. For the health care professional, treating an AIDS or HIV-infected patient often raises complicated clinical, legal, and ethical issues. These are compounded by the specific laws in each state which try to address the AIDS crisis.

Every state now mandates reporting of persons who have AIDS. Some also mandate reporting those who are HIV-positive but who do not yet have AIDS. The reporting obligation falls to the health care provider who ordered the test of the person and made the diagnosis. For the mental health professional, questions arise as to whether and when the confidentiality of an HIV-infected client should be breached. This may arise because of concern for the risk to public safety from an HIV-infected person.

Generally, a hospital or other health care provider can be held liable for breaching confidentiality and revealing that someone has AIDS or is HIV-positive without the patient's consent. Yet this right is not absolute. It is appropriate to share this information with health care providers who may be in a situation where the knowledge will affect their care of the patient or the precautions they take when caring for the person. In addition, it may be legally and ethically appropriate to notify a sexual partner when the patient refuses to share this information with the partner, when the therapist believes the partner is unlikely to be aware of the patient's condition, and when the patient refuses to take action which would protect the partner. It is not, however, appropriate to generally share this information with other family members or employers.

Some state laws or regulations specifically regulate HIV-related patient information differently from other medical or mental health patient information. There may be specific release of information procedures or consent forms for HIV-testing results. HIV results are sometimes segregated from the remainder of the patient's medical record, and their access limited to certain health care workers. Since there are frequent legal developments in this area, a therapist confronted with a clinical-legal question about HIV or AIDS should seek the advice of counsel.

X. GROUP AND FAMILY THERAPY

Traditionally, statements made in the presence of third parties are not protected by testimonial privilege statutes. Group and family therapy are special examples of communications in the presence of third parties. Unless a testimonial privilege statute explicitly grants a privilege to group treatment situations, it should be assumed that testimony concerning the content of the group's sessions can be compelled from any group member. This may not be the case for family therapy, since there may be statutory protection against court testimony by family members against each other. Apart from privilege, patients participating in groups should be informed of their general (but obviously not professional) responsibility to respect the confidences of the group as well as the limitations of confidentiality in the group setting. In this sense, the group members should act like cotherapists rather than patients. When keeping notes concerning group sessions in individual clients' charts, the therapist should not make identifying references to other group members. To record group interactions, the clinician may choose to keep separate notes not included in individual charts.

Secrets present any therapist with confidentiality and clinical dilemmas, especially if unwarned. They are most likely to occur in family or group therapy, during a patient's hospitalization (information withheld from some members of the treatment team), or by a family member's involvement in a client's individual outpatient therapy. While it is advisable for the therapist to immediately interrupt the offering of a secret to forestall any problems, this is often not possible. In resolving the burden of secrets, it is helpful for clinicians to formulate and communicate to patients and others the relevant "rules" about such information, hopefully in advance of the problem. These might include clarification of the identity of the agency to whom the therapist is primarily responsible (e.g., individual patient, marriage couple, family, institution), risks of secrets to all involved, and the unwillingness of the therapist to collude in those dangers.

XI. DISCLOSURE OF RECORDS

Third-party payments and computerization by insurance carriers, health providers, and governmental agencies have made the handling of personal medical information a complex matter. Problems arise as to whether the information recorded is accurate and how it is to be used. The possibilities of professional and clerical errors, of substantive mistakes in information obtained from the patient, and of misfiling and illegibility compound the potential damage that may be caused by use of medical records for purposes other than treatment.

As in the case of the testimonial privilege, it is difficult to balance the individual's control over disclosure of personal information with society's need for the data on which to base decisions about individual situations. Almost all state jurisdictions have enacted statutes to protect the confidentiality of patient records. Most of these statutes are specifically concerned with records relating to the identification, commitment, and treatment of patients in state mental hospitals. This section will review the issues which arise related to disclosure of records (See Chapter 6 for additional discussion of record keeping.)

A. Patient Access

The vast majority of states have enacted statutes covering the patient's access to his records. Typically, these laws do not offer unrestricted access to the records. Rather, most make access conditional on the patient's mental health status and the nature of the material. The patient's right to review his records is foreclosed if the information would be significantly detrimental to his mental health or its disclosure to him would not be in his best interests. Furthermore, some statutes provide that the patient must show good cause in order to see his records. Other statutes provide that the patient shall have "reasonable access." In almost half the states, the patient does not have a specific right to review his records, even though other persons or agencies do have such a right.

Several arguments support patient access to records. By being able to review his record, the patient has the opportunity to verify its accuracy. Patient access also can enhance continuity of care when the patient moves and seeks a new treatment provider. Perhaps most significantly, the patient's access serves to protect his privacy interests by enabling him to make an adequately informed decision before he permits disclosure of his records to others.

Patients often request to review their own records. The clinician is advised to initially explore with the patient the reason for the request so that both can better understand the issues and fantasies involved in the request. This initial discussion will also permit the clinician to assess if disclosure would have a harmful impact upon the mental health of the patient. Some states permit mental health professionals to partially or completely restrict the access of records that would have a negative impact upon the patient's health or well-being, although the records must still be released to others of the patient's own choosing. Other states permit the professional to prepare a written summary of the patient's treatment and share this with the patient, rather than the original record itself. A joint review of the records by the patient and the therapist is recommended when access is permitted.

In many jurisdictions, patients who have a right to review their records also have a right to a copy of them. The original record belongs to the treatment provider (not the patient's individual therapist but the hospital or clinic), and under no circumstances should it be given to a patient or shown to him without direct supervision, since he could modify or destroy it. In some states, the patient has a right to amend his record by adding a statement to it when he believes the record is inaccurate. The therapist should not remove the portion of the record to which the patient objects. Only the written statement of the patient, which is signed and dated, should be added to the record.

B. Statutory Access by Others

The statutes designed to ensure the confidentiality of mental health records usually provide for certain exceptions. In most states, these statutes apply only to public health facilities, agencies, or practitioners. In the private setting, the release of records is usually governed by statutes relating to medical records in general or by other broader confidentiality provisions, including the testimonial privilege statutes discussed earlier.

C. The Records of Minors

The issue of the confidentiality of minors' records is especially complex. To develop a therapeutic relationship, the therapist needs to obtain the confidence of the child, and this may be possible only if he promises not to disclose information to the parents. But the parents usually will want to know what the child is doing in treatment and what they can do to help. Since the child is their responsibility, they may feel they have a right to review the records of the therapy.

It is possible for the child's therapist to reach a compromise without breaching any expectations of confidentiality. At the beginning of treatment, the therapist should make clear to both the child and the parents what access to records he will give to each, thereby enabling all concerned to know what to expect.

To release records of minors, the consent of either parent is adequate except in cases of divorce or third-party custody. In those instances, consent is required from the custodial parent or the agency. In joint custody, either parent may consent to treatment or release of treatment records. When there is a question, the therapist can ask for a copy of the divorce decree or parenting agreement. If questions remain, the professional should consult an attorney. When releasing data concerning an adolescent, it is desirable to obtain the formal written consent of both the parent and the client. Clients of all ages should be informed of the limitations of confidentiality during any particular assessment.

In keeping records on minors, it is important for the therapist to assume that eventually the parent will have access to the records. Thus, the therapist should be careful to not record information which, if revealed, may damage the child's relationship with his parents.

D. Obligation to Patient

Mental health professionals should become familiar with the relevant statutes in their jurisdiction related to consent to release records. The professional should discuss with the client the benefits and risks of disclosing information prior to actual release. The client should also be informed of what is in his record so he may determine if he wishes the information released. The clinician should release information limited to the particular purpose of the disclosure request. Records in the clinician's possession from other health care providers should not be released unless they are specifically requested by the release and their rerelease is not otherwise prohibited. Similarly, release of written social histories which have been provided by third parties generally should not occur without the informed consent of the client as well as the collateral; alternatively, the section of the social history which was provided in confidence to the treatment team can be deleted from that which is released.

E. Disclosure in Publications

All material used for publishing case reports or as part of research should be edited to carefully remove identifying information about the patient or subject. If there is some reason to use identifying information, or if audio or video recordings will be used for educational purposes, then a written authorization from the patient is typically required. The authorization should be specific about the intended use of the information or recordings and should explain that the patient can withdraw his consent at any time. The clinician should be confident that the client has adequate capacity to consent to the taping. Videotapes depicting patients should be treated with the same care as medical records themselves; in some cases, they will be considered part of the record (e.g, videotaped consent to treatment). The clinician should be aware that he has been entrusted with sensitive information about a person, and that its revelation in an identifiable manner could cause the patient significant harm.

Grand rounds or teaching conferences in which a patient is formally presented should be held only after obtaining a patient's consent. During the presentation, care must be taken to conceal the patient's identity, and to avoid revealing sensitive or embarrassing material especially if it is not directly related to the presentation.

XII. RESPONDING TO A SUBPOENA

A subpoena is an order, under court protection, issued by an attorney for a therapist to appear and testify or to produce records. It is not a direct order of the court, however. Receiving a subpoena does not compel a therapist to testify, only to appear in court or produce the records. A subpoena does not represent an authorization to release information or records from the patient. A subpoena differs from a court order, which is signed by a judge, which orders the records released or the therapist's testimony.

Upon receiving a subpoena, the clinician should contact the patient or the patient's attorney to determine if the patient will consent to the release of the information to the party that subpoenaed the clinician. If the patient consents, a written consent should be obtained from him. If the patient refuses to consent to the release, then the clinician has three alternatives: (1) to contact the attorney who issued the subpoena and explain why the clinician will not comply without the specific written authorization of the patient; (2) to consult with an attorney to file a motion to quash the subpoena on the basis that the requested information is confidential or privileged as a matter of law (it may be worth trying to convince the patient's attorney to file this motion); or (3) to attend the deposition or trial as specified with the requested documents, but to refuse to answer any questions or to release documents while asserting the therapist–patient confidentiality or the specific statutory testimonial privilege. In each instance, it is for the judge to decide whether the testimony or records in question are subject to a claim of privilege.

If a motion to quash the subpoena is presented or the therapist refuses to testify, there will be a hearing to determine the relevance of the testimony or records to the issue before the court. The judge may hold an *in camera* (in chambers) inspection of the records to determine their relevance and the probative value of the issues in the trial. If there are other ways of obtaining the information, the court is unlikely to order the information revealed or the records disclosed.

XIII. COMMONLY ASKED QUESTIONS

1. Should the therapist notify the client at the beginning of treatment about the limits of confidentiality?

Absolute confidentiality in mental health care does not exist. The therapist may be required to breach confidentiality to protect the client from harming himself or others or to comply with legal reporting requirements. Clients should be told in advance that the therapist will attempt to keep communications confidential, but that if the client poses a harm to himself or others, confidentiality may need to be breached for the client's protection or that of others. The client may need to be reminded of the earlier warning if the issue of harm later arises during treatment. Clients should also be informed of the consequences of their filing insurance claims for the costs of their mental health treatment, including possible difficulty in obtaining health, life, or disability insurance in the future.

2. *How should a therapist respond to a consent form which requires release of all records about the client?*

Generally, the therapist should tell the client the nature of the information in the record and then verify that the client wishes such information to be released. The therapist should avoid releasing the entire record; rather, the therapist should attempt to learn the purpose of the consent and reveal only that information which is necessary to accomplish the goals of the release.

3. *If a client tells a therapist that her boyfriend is abusing her preschool child, does the therapist have an obligation to report such abuse to the child welfare agency, if the therapist has not evaluated or treated the child?*

In every state, a therapist has an obligation to report any suspected child abuse or neglect, even if the client is working on the child abuse issues in therapy. In some states, however, there is no obligation to report the alleged abuse unless the therapist has personally evaluated or treated the child. In those jurisdictions, the clinician is permitted to file a child abuse report with the responsible agency, but is not required to do so. Immunity from liability will apply for a report made in good faith.

4. *How are confidentiality issues managed in family therapy?*

When beginning family therapy, it is prudent to have all involved family members review the need for confidentiality and reach an agreement about access to the chart and release of information. It may be useful to have everyone sign a statement which details their rights and responsibilities. Particular care must be taken not to improperly release information if a separation or divorce occurs or a child reaches majority.

5. *When a minor is in treatment, and the parents are divorced, which parent can consent to release of the minor's records?*

The custodial parent will generally have the right to consent to the release of the child's record. This is the parent who has the legal authority to consent to the treatment in the first place. When there is a "joint custody" agreement, then either parent can consent to the release. If the parents are disputing the child's care, the therapist should avoid being caught in the middle. The therapist should request a copy of the court order awarding custody to determine which parent can make treatment decisions, including the ability to consent to the release of information. In many states, irrespective of who has custody, both parents are entitled to see their child's health and school records.

6. *If an adolescent is in treatment, and the school seeks information, can it be released to the school?*

To release any information about an adolescent, it is necessary to have the consent of the parent and, in many cases, the consent of the adolescent client as well. Exceptions are made when the adolescent is in treatment as part of an educational program which is funded by the school system.

7. When the police seek information on a client or former client, how much must be revealed?

The information to be revealed will be governed by state law. Generally, the police are not any more entitled to confidential information about the client than any other party. In particular, they should not have access to the client's record without a court order. Even without a court order, the police are entitled to know whether the person is or is not in treatment and the date of discharge. It is important for therapists not to reveal information which may be used against the client without having consent from the client or a court order, even if it is the police who are making the request.

8. How should the process notes of trainees be managed?

After such notes have been used for supervision, they should be destroyed. Prior to their use, they should be kept separate from the official chart because of the sensitive material they may contain.

9. A client who is HIV-positive refuses to control behavior that is likely to transmit the disease. What is the therapist's obligation in this matter?

Confidentiality is not absolute. The law has long recognized an exception for disclosure without the patient's consent when he poses an imminent danger to others. Disclosure to third parties without the patient's consent should be viewed as a last resort after therapeutic efforts have failed. Disclosure should be limited to identifiable third parties currently at risk of continued exposure, if this is permitted under the law of the state. The therapist should familiarize himself with the specifics of his state's law and seek legal advice when these issues arise.

10. Do the client's records remain confidential after his death?

Yes. The therapist's legal and ethical obligations to maintain the confidentiality of a client's treatment do not end upon his death. States permit access to records after the death of a client by the representative or executor of the estate. Release of records should occur only upon proper documentation that a person has been appointed by the court to serve as the representative or executor. The content of the information released should be limited to that necessary for the purpose requested.

11. If someone is receiving treatment for a substance abuse problem which is federally funded, can a law enforcement officer see the records without the client's consent?

No. A court order must first be obtained.

12. May a therapist ignore a subpoena when he believes that information disclosure would be detrimental to his client?

No. The therapist should never ignore a subpoena, whether for courtroom testimony or for records. This could result in being held in contempt of court with a fine or jail term. The therapist should contact the client to determine how he wishes the therapist to proceed. If the client does not wish the information released, his attorney should attempt to quash the subpoena. If the therapist believes that release of the information would be detrimental to the client, he can go to court and explain why, under the legal and ethical principles of confidentiality, or under the therapist–patient testimonial privilege, he believes the information should not be released. The therapist should obtain a written, rather than oral, release from the client or a court order before testifying.

13. *If someone is involved in personal injury litigation, will his history of treatment for a mental illness be revealed?*

When an individual raises as part of his claim or defense some type of psychological illness or suffering, then the parties are justified in exploring the bases for the claim. In those circumstances, it is likely that the person's treatment will be revealed if it is close in time to the claim or appears to be relevant. Both treatment records and the courtroom testimony of the therapist could be compelled by the defendant's attorney. To preserve the treatment relationship, it is preferable for an independent evaluator to testify about the plaintiff's mental condition in the litigation, rather than the therapist.

14. *Can the therapist of the client in question #13 refuse to be interviewed by the defendant's attorney apart from testimony at deposition or trial?*

Many states prohibit such *ex parte* (one party only) contact between the therapist and the defendant's attorney. Where this is permitted, the therapist is not obligated to meet with the opposing side's attorney, but may do so. However, it would be wise for the therapist to first obtain the written consent of the client, and contact the client's attorney about the request. When possible, treatment records should be released to the opposing side's attorney by the client's attorney, not by the therapist.

15. *If a patient refuses to allow the therapist to reveal any confidential information to another party, does this prevent the therapist from speaking with that person?*

No. The therapist is free to listen to anyone, whether by telephone or in person, even without the patient's consent. He may not, however, reveal even the fact that the patient is in treatment without proper consent from the patient, absent an emergency situation.

16. *If a client reports that a previous therapist has engaged in a sexual relationship with the client, is the new therapist obligated to report the previous therapist?*

In the majority of states, there is no legal obligation to report the allegations concerning the previous therapist. However, a few states do impose an affirmative legal duty to report colleagues who engage in such behavior. Ideally, the client should be the one to report the previous therapist to the state licensing agency or the local professional society. Generally, when a therapist reports the misconduct of another therapist, it will be breaching the confidences of the client, unless the client has provided consent to do so.

17. *If the clinician learns through other sources or the news media that the client is wanted for a crime, is he obligated to contact the police?*

Generally, the clinician is not obligated to contact the police to report a client's past crime or to turn him over to the authorities. However, if the client were accused of a serious crime, and the clinician were concerned about his posing a risk to others of a violent act, the clinician would have an obligation to protect endangered third parties. This duty may be discharged by a variety of clinical interventions, as well as contacting the police or potential identifiable victims.

18. A client is asked to sign a consent form which releases all past and future mental health records to his employer. How should the therapist proceed?

A written consent to release health care records or confidential communications should be only retrospective in time. The therapist should advise the client that, since he does not know what will appear in the records in the future, no consent to release that information should be authorized. At a later time, that information could be released to the employer, but only when specifically requested for that period.

19. How should facility incident reports be completed?

Incident reports should be considered confidential documents which may be protected from discovery by the attorney–client privilege. They should not be inserted into the patient's record and are often stored with quality assurance records. The content of the report should be restricted to the facts of the incident and should avoid assigning responsibility or blame for what happened.

20. What risks to confidentiality are presented by fax machines?

Health care records (discharge summaries, physician orders, laboratory reports) are now commonly communicated by fax, especially in hospitals. Faxed communications can be accidentally misdirected, sent by unauthorized parties, or received by personnel untrained in confidentiality practice. For these reasons, faxed clinical information should be sent with a cover page indicating the sender and intended recipient, the need to return it to the sender if missent, and the fact that it is confidential information. Fax machines in clinical facilities should be attended only by those who are properly trained in confidentiality. Fax thermal paper deteriorates rapidly and medical documents which are to be retained should be permanently photocopied.

21. Is oral consent sufficient to release mental health records?

In many but not all states, the release of mental health records must be authorized in writing. In those states which do not have such a requirement, the releasing clinician or agency may proceed on the basis of the client's oral consent; the clinician, though, should be certain that the requester is who he says he is and has the authority to release the records. Thus, if a client telephones the clinician or agency and asks that the records be released to his attorney, the clinician should verify the caller's identity. Written authorization, even if not required by law, protects the releasing party from subsequent claims that the release was unauthorized or otherwise improper. Whenever information has been released, the clinician should appropriately document that fact in the medical record, indicating the date of release, the information released, and the recipient.

22. Can the therapist release mental health records on the basis of a simple letter but without the proper authorization form?

Many states prohibit the release of confidential mental health information in the absence of an authorization which strictly follows the law. Valid authorizations typically specify the names or functions of the persons involved in the request (patient, source, and recipient), the specific type of information requested, the specific uses of the requested information, the limitations on the use of the requested information by the recipient, and the duration of the consent if prospective.

XIV. BIBLIOGRAPHY

I. Confidentiality and Privilege

A. *Cases: General*

Allred v. State, 554 P.2d 411 (Sup.Ct. Alaska 1976).
In re Lifschutz, 467 P.2d 557 (Sup.Ct. Cal. 1970).
Caesar v. Mountanos, 542 F.2d 1064 (9th Cir. 1976).
In re B, 394 A.2d 419 (Sup.Ct. Pa. 1978).
State v. Martin, 274 N.W.2d 893 (Sup.Ct.S.D. 1979).
State of Florida v. Tsavaris, 382 So.2d 56 (Fla.App. 1980).
People v. Gomez, 185 Cal.Rptr. 155 (Cal.App. 1982).
Myers v. State, 310 S.E.2d 504 (Sup.Ct.Ga. 1984).
Novak v. Rathnam, 478 N.E.2d 1334 (Sup.Ct. Ill. 1985).
People v. Wilkins, 490 N.Y.S.2d 759 (Ct.App. 1985).
State v. Miller, 709 P.2d 225 (Sup.Ct. Or. 1985).
Matter of New York News, 494 N.E.2d 1379 (Ct.App. 1986).
State v. Gullekson, 383 N.W.2d 338 (Ct.App. Minn. 1986).
U.S. v. Crews, 781 F.2d 826 (10th Cir. 1986).
Karsten v. McCray, 509 N.E.2d 1376 (Ill.App. 1987).
Commonwealth v. Clancy, 524 N.E.2d 395 (Sup.Jud.Ct. Mass. 1988).
In the matter of rules adoption regarding inmate–therapist confidentiality, 540 A.2d 212 (N.J.Super.A.D. 1988).
People v. Reidout, 530 N.Y.S.2d 938 (Sup.Ct. 1988).
Porter v. Michigan Osteopathic Hospital Association, 428 N.W.2d 719 (Mich.App. 1988).
Tumlinson v. Texas, 757 S.W.2d 440 (Tex.App. 1988).
In re Grand Jury Proceedings, 867 F.2d 562 (9th Cir. 1989).
In re Kevin F., 261 Cal.Rptr.413 (Cal.App. 1989).
Peisach v. Antuna, 539 So.2d 544 (Fla.App. 1989).
State v. Beatty, 770 S.W.2d 387 (Mo.Ct.App. 1989).
Dixon v. City of Lawton, 898 F.2d 1443 (10th Cir. 1990).
In the Matter of Guardianship of Atkins, 790 P.2d 210 (Wash.App. 1990).
Cabrera v. Cabrera, 580 A.2d 1227 (Conn.App. 1990).
Nelson v. Ferguson, 399 S.E.2d 909 (W.Va.Sup.Ct. 1990).
People v. Clark, 789 P.2d 127 (Cal.Sup.Ct. 1990).
People v. Wharton, 280 Cal. Rptr. 631 (Cal.Sup.Ct. 1991).
People v. Superior Court, 282 Cal.Rptr.418 (Cal.App. 1991).
Jorgensen v. State, 574 N.E.2d 915 (Ind.Sup.Ct. 1991).
Kalenevitch. v. Finger, 595 A.2d 1224 (Pa.Super. 1991).
Menendez v. Superior Court, 279 Cal.Rptr. 521 (Cal.App. 1991).
People v. Doe, 570 N.E.2d 733 (Ill.App. 1991).
State ex rel. Juvenile Department v. Ashley, 818 P.2d 1270 (Or.Sup.Ct. 1991).
Annotation: Physician–patient privilege as extending to patient's medical or hospital records, 10 A.L.R.4th 552.
Annotation: Privilege, in judicial or quasi-judicial proceedings, arising from relationship between psychiatrist or psychologist and patient, 44 A.L.R.3d 24.

B. *Cases: Liability for Breach of Confidentiality*

Clark v. Geraci, 208 N.Y.S.2d 564 (A.D. 1960).
Doe v. Roe and Poe, 400 N.Y.S.2d 668 (A.D. 1977).

Hopewell v. Adibempe, No. GD78–28756, Civil Division, Court of Common Pleas of Allegheny County, Pennsylvania, June 1, 1981.
Martino v. Family Service Agency of Adams County, 445 N.E.2d 6 (Ill.App. 1983).
Alberts v. Devine, 479 N.E.2d 113 (Sup.Jud.Ct. Mass. 1985).
Levias v. United Airlines, 500 N.E.2d 370 (Ohio App. 1985).
Watts v. Cumberland County Hospital System et al., 330 S.E.2d 242 (N.C.App. 1985).
Prince v. St. Francis-St. George Hospital, 484 N.E.2d 265 (Ohio App. 1985).
Bratt v. International Business Machines, 785 F.2d 352 (1st Cir. 1986).
Johnson v. Lincoln Christian College, 501 N.E.2d 1380 (Ill.App. 1986).
Rea v. Pardo, 507 N.Y.S. 361 (Sup.Ct. 1986).
Leigh v. Parker, 740 S.W.2d 101 (Tex.App. 1987).
State Board of Psychologists v. Hosford, 508 So.2d 1049 (Sup.Ct. Miss. 1987).
Allen v. Smith, 368 S.E.2d 924 (W.Va. 1988).
Bryson v. Tillinghast, 749 P.2d 110 (Sup.Ct. Okla. 1988).
Inabnit v. Berkson, 245 Cal.Rptr. 525 (Cal.App. 1988).
Zim v. Benezra, 545 N.Y.S.2d 893 (Sup. 1989).
Doe v. Portland Health Centers, 782 P.2d 446 (Or.App. 1989).
O'Donnell v. U.S., 891 F.2d 1079 (3rd.Cir. 1989).
Neal v. Corning Glass Works Corp., 745 F.Supp. 1294 (Ohio 1989).
Oringer v. Rotkin, 556 N.Y.S.2d 67 (A.D. 1990).
Susan A. v. County of Sonoma, 3 Cal.Rptr.2d 27 (Cal.App. 1991).
Saur v. Probes, 476 N.W.2d 496 (Mich.App. 1991).
Ms. B. v. Montgomery County Emergency Service, Inc., 799 F.Supp. 534 (E.D. Pa. 1992).
Annotation: Physician's tort liability, apart from defamation, for unauthorized disclosure of confidential information about patient, 20 A.L.R.3d 1109.
Annotation: Physician's tort liability for unauthorized disclosure of confidential information about patient, 48 A.L.R.4th 668.

C. Articles and Books

American Psychiatric Association. (1987). Guidelines on confidentiality. *American Journal of Psychiatry, 144,* 1522–1526.
Baird, K. A., & Rupert, P. A. (1987). Clinical management of confidentiality: A survey of psychologists in seven states. *Professional Psychology: Research and Practice, 18,* 347–352.
Bernard, J. L., & O'Laughlin, D. L. (1990). Confidentiality: Do training clinics take it seriously? *Law and Psychology Review, 14,* 59–69.
Bruce, J. A. C. (1988). *Privacy and confidentiality of health care information* (2nd ed.). Chicago: American Hospital Publishing.
Chorba, T. L., Berkelman, R. L., Safford, S. K., Gibbs, N. P., & Hull, H. F. (1989). Mandatory reporting of infectious diseases by clinicians. *Journal of the American Medical Association, 262,* 3018–3026.
Churgin, M. J. (1986). Psychotherapist-patient privilege: A search for identity. In D. N. Weisstub (Ed.), *Law and mental health, Vol. 2,* pp. 215–264. New York: Pergamon Press.
Developments in the law: Privileged communications. (1985). *Harvard Law Review, 98,* 1450–1666.
Everstine, L., Everstine, D. S., Heymann, G. M., True, R. H., Frey, D. H., Johnson, H. G., & Seiden, R. H. (1980). Privacy and confidentiality in psychotherapy. *American Psychologist, 35,* 828–840.
Farber, N. J., Weiner, J. L., Boyer, E. G., & Robinson, E. J. (1989). Residents' decisions to breach confidentiality. *Journal of General Internal Medicine, 4,* 31–33.
Faustman, W. O., & Miller, D. J. (1987). Considerations in prewarning clients of the limitations of confidentiality. *Psychological Reports, 60,* 195–198.
Freund, E., Seligman, P. J., Chorba, T. L., Safford, S. K., Drachman, J. G., & Hull, H. F. (1989). Mandatory reporting of occupational diseases by clinicians. *Journal of the American Medical Association, 262,* 3041–3044.
Gellman, R. M. (1986). Divided loyalties: A physician's responsibilities in an information age. *Social Science and Medicine, 23,* 817–826.
Griffith, E. Z., Zonana, H., Pinsince, A. J., & Adams, A. K. (1988). Institutional response to inpatients' threats against the President. *Hospital and Community Psychiatry, 39,* 1166–1171.
Gumper, L. L., & Sprenkle, D. H. (1981). Privileged communication in therapy: Special problems for the family and couples therapist. *Family Process, 20,* 11–23.
Gustafson, K. E., & McNama, J. R. (1987). Confidentiality with minor clients: Issues and guidelines for therapists. *Professional Psychology: Research and Practice, 18,* 503–508.

Huber, G. A., & Roth, L. H. (1988). Preserving the confidentiality of medical record information regarding nonpatients. *Virginia Law Review, 66*, 583–596.
Kelly, R. J. (1987). Limited confidentiality and the pedophile. *Hospital and Community Psychiatry, 38*, 1046–1048.
Knapp, S., & VandeCreek, L. (1987). *Privileged communication in the mental health professions*. New York: Van Nostrand Reinhold.
Knapp, S., VandeCreek, L., & Zirkel, P. A. (1987). Privileged communications for psychotherapists in Pennsylvania: A time for statutory reform. *Temple Law Quarterly, 60*, 267–292.
Kraft, P. (1985). The parent-child testimonial privilege: Who's minding the kids? *Family Law Quarterly, 18*, 505–543.
Lindenthal, J. J., & Thomas, C. S. (1982). Psychiatrists, the public, and confidentiality. *Journal of Nervous and Mental Disease, 170*, 319–323.
Lindenthal, J. J., Jordan, T. J., Lentz, J. D., & Thomas, C. S. (1988). Social workers' management of confidentiality. *Social Work, 33*, 157–158.
Mayo, D. J. (1984). Confidentiality in crisis counseling: A philosophical perspective. *Suicide and Life-Threatening Behavior, 14*, 96–112.
Meyer, R. G., & Smith, S. R. (1977). A crisis in group therapy. *American Psychologist, 32*, 638–643.
Miller, D. J., & Thelen, M. H. (1986). Knowledge and beliefs about confidentiality in psychotherapy. *Professional Psychology: Research and Practice, 17*, 15–19.
Petrila, J. P., & Sadoff, R. L. (1992). Confidentiality and the family as caregiver. *Hospital and Community Psychiatry, 43*, 136–139.
Roach, W. H., Chernoff, S. N., & Esley, C. L. (1985). *Medical records and the law*. Rockville, MD: Aspen.
Rubanowitz, D. E. (1987). Public attitudes toward psychotherapist-client confidentiality. *Professional Psychology: Research and Practice, 18*, 613–618.
Schuchman, H., Foster, L., & Nye, S. (1982). *Confidentiality of health records*. New York: Gardner Press.
Sherlock, R., & Murphy, W. (1984). Confidentiality and therapy: An agency privilege. *Comprehensive Psychiatry, 25*, 88–95.
Shuman, D. W., & Weiner, M. F. (1987). *Psychotherapist-patient privilege*. Springfield, IL: Thomas.
Siegler, M. (1982). Confidentiality in medicine—A decrepit concept. *New England Journal of Medicine, 307*, 1518–1521.
Sloan, J. B., & Hall, B. (1984). Confidentiality of psychotherapeutic records. *Journal of Legal Medicine, 5*, 435–467.
Slovenko, R. (1966). *Psychotherapy, confidentiality, and privileged communication*. Springfield, IL: Thomas.
Smith, S. R. (1980). Constitutional privacy in psychotherapy. *George Washington Law Review, 49*, 1–60.
Smith, S. R. (1986–1987). Medical and psychotherapy privileges and confidentiality: On giving with one hand and removing with the other. *Kentucky Law Journal, 75*, 473–557.
Spiegel, P. B. (1990). Confidentiality endangered under some circumstances without special management. *Psychotherapy, 27*, 636–643.
Stanton, A. M. (1982). Child–parent privilege for confidential communications: An examination and proposal. *Family Law Quarterly, 16*, 1–67.
Taube, D. O., & Elwork, A. (1990). Researching the effects of confidentiality law on patients' self-disclosures. *Professional Psychology: Research and Practice, 21*, 72–75.
Taylor, L., & Adelman, H. S. (1989). Reframing the confidentiality dilemma to work in children's best interests. *Professional Psychology: Research and Practice, 20*, 79–83.
Turkington, R. C. (1987). Legal protection for the confidentiality of health care information in Pennsylvania: Patient and client access; testimonial privileges; damage recovery for unauthorized extra-legal disclosure. *Villanova Law Review, 32*, 259–400.
VandeCreek, L., Knapp, S., & Herzog, C. (1988). Privileged communications for social workers. *Social Casework, 69*, 28–34.
Vickery, A. B. (1982). Note: Breach of confidence: An emerging tort. *Columbia Law Review, 82*, 1426–1468.
Watkins, S. A. (1989). Confidentiality and privileged communications: Legal dilemmas for family therapists. *Social Work, 34*, 133–136.
Watts, W. M. (1987) The parent–child privileges: Hardly a new or revolutionary concept. *William and Mary Law Review, 28*, 583–631.
Weihofen, H. (1972). Confidentiality. In A. Beigel & A. I. Levenson (Eds.), *The community mental health center*, pp. 124–135. New York: Basic Books.
Weiner, B. A. (1985). Provider-patient relations: Confidentiality and liability. In J. S. Brakel, J. Parry, &

B. A. Weiner (Eds.), *The mentally disabled and the law* (3rd ed.), pp. 559–605. Chicago: American Bar Foundation.
Weiner, M. F., & Shuman, D. W. (1983). The privilege study. *Archives of General Psychiatry, 40,* 1027–1030.
Weiss, B. D. (1982). Confidentiality expectations of patients, physicians, and medical students. *Journal of the American Medical Association, 247,* 2695–2697.
Weiss, B. D., Senf, J. H., Carter, J. Z., & Rothe, T. C. (1986). Confidentiality expectations of patients in teaching hospital clinics versus private practice offices. *Social Science and Medicine, 23,* 387–391.
Wilson, S. J. (1978). *Confidentiality in social work: Issues and principles.* New York: Free Press.
Winslade, W. J., & Ross, J. W. (1985). Privacy, confidentiality, and autonomy in psychotherapy. *Nebraska Law Review, 64,* 578–636.

II. Rape Victim Counseling

A. *Cases*

Matter of Pittsburgh Action Against Rape, 428 A.2d 126 (Sup.Ct. Pa. 1981).
Advisory Opinion to the House of Representatives, 469 A.2d 1161 (Sup.Ct. R.I. 1983).
People v. Denver, 719 P.2d 722 (Sup.Ct. Colo. 1986).
People v. Reber, 223 Cal.Rptr. 139 (Cal.App. 1986).
State v. Pierson, 514 A.2d 724 (Sup.Ct. Conn. 1986).
Commonwealth v. Lloyd, 567 A.2d 1357 (Sup.Ct. Pa. 1989).
State v. Donnelly, 798 P.2d 89 (Mont.Sup.Ct. 1990).
Commonwealth v. Stockhammer, 570 N.E.2d 992 (Mass.Sup.Jud.Ct. 1991).

B. *Articles*

Appelbaum, P. S., & Roth, L. H. (1981). In the Matter of Paar: Rape counseling and problems of confidentiality. *Hospital and Community Psychiatry, 32,* 461–462.
Laurence, M. (1984). Rape victim-crisis counselor communications: An argument for an absolute privilege. *University of California Davis Law Review, 17,* 1213–1245.
McCafferty, B. M. (1990–1991). The existing confidentiality privileges as applied to rape victims. *Journal of Law and Health, 5,* 101–142.
Scarmeas, C. J. (1982). Rape victim-rape crisis counselor communications: A new testimonial privilege. *Dickinson Law Review, 86,* 539–564.

III. Governmental Investigations of Practitioners

A. *Cases*

Hawaii Psychiatric Society v. Ariyoshi, 481 F.Supp. 1028 (D. Hawaii 1979); No. CV79–0113 (D. Hawaii December 27, 1982).
Reynaud v. Superior Court, Santa Clara County, 187 Cal.Rptr. 660 (Cal.App. 1982).
In re Subpoena Served upon Zuniga, 714 F.2d 632 (6th Cir. 1983).
Commonwealth v. Kobrin, 479 N.E.2d 674 (Sup.Jud.Ct. Mass. 1985).
Wood v. Superior Court, 212 Cal.Rptr. 811 (Cal.App. 1985).
Grand Jury v. Kuriansky, 505 N.E.2d 925 (Ct.App. N.Y. 1987).
In the Matter of A-85–04–38, 525 N.Y.S.2d 479 (Sup.Ct. 1988).
Lieb v. Department of Health Services, 542 A.2d 741 (Conn.App. 1988).
Scull v. Superior Court, Santa Barbara County, 254 Cal.Rptr. 24 (Cal.App. 1988).
U.S. v. Wettstein, 733 F.Supp. 1212 (Ill. 1990).

B. *Articles*

Khajezadeh, D. (1987). Patient confidentiality statutes in Medicare and Medicaid fraud investigations. *American Journal of Law and Medicine, 12,* 105–137.
Note: Behind closed doors: The confidentiality of psychotherapeutic records in Medicaid fraud investigations. (1986). *Pace Law Review, 6,* 441–494.

Shwed, H. J., Kuvin, S. F., & Baliga, R. K. (1979). Medicaid audit: Crisis in confidentiality and the patient-psychiatrist relationship. *American Journal of Psychiatry, 136,* 447–450.
Taranto, R. G. (1986). The psychiatrist-patient privilege and third-party payers. *Law, Medicine and Health Care, 14,* 25–29.

IV. AIDS and Confidentiality

A. Cases

Doe v. Borough of Barrington, 729 F.Supp. 376 (N.J. 1990).
Behringer Estate v. Princeton Medical Center, 592 A.2d 1251 (N.J.Super. 1991).
In re Application of Milton S. Hershey Medical Center, 595 A.2d 1290 (Pa.Super. 1991).
Hillman v. Columbia County, 474 N.W.2d 913 (Wis.App. 1991).
McBarnette v. Feldman, 582 N.Y.S.2d 900 (Sup. 1992).

B. Articles and Books

American Bar Association. (1989). *AIDS and persons with developmental disabilities: The legal perspective.* Washington, DC: American Bar Association.
American Psychiatric Association. (1988). AIDS policy: Confidentiality and disclosure. *American Journal of Psychiatry, 145,* 541.
Annas, G. J. (1988). Not saints but healers: The legal duties of health care professionals in the AIDS epidemic. *American Journal of Public Health, 78,* 844–849.
Carlson, G. A., Greeman, M., & McClellan, T. A. (1989). Management of HIV-positive psychiatric patients who fail to reduce high-risk behaviors. *Hospital and Community Psychiatry, 40,* 511–514.
Dickens, B. M. (1988). Legal limits of AIDS confidentiality. *Journal of the American Medical Association, 259,* 3449–3451.
Gostin, L., & Curran, W. J. (1987). AIDS screening, confidentiality, and the duty to warn. *American Journal of Public Health, 77,* 361–365.
Knapp, S., & VandeCreek, L. (1990). Application of the duty to protect to HIV-positive patients. *Professional Psychology: Research and Practice, 21,* 161–166.
Lamb, D. H., Clark, C., Drumheller, P., Frizzell, K., & Surrey, L. (1989). Applying *Tarasoff* to AIDS-related psychotherapy issues. *Professional Psychology: Research and Practice, 20,* 37–43.
Landis, S. E., Schoenbach, V. J., Weber, D. J., Mittal, M., Krishan, B., Lewis, K., & Koch, G. G. (1992). Results of a randomized trial of partner notification in cases of HIV infection in North Carolina. *New England Journal of Medicine, 326,* 101–106.
McDonald, B. A. (1989). Ethical problems for physicians raised by AIDS and HIV infection: Conflicting legal obligations of confidentiality and disclosure. *University of California, Davis Law Review, 22,* 557–592.
Melton, G. B. (1988). Ethical and legal issues in AIDS-related practice. *American Psychologist, 43,* 941–947.
Perry, S. (1989). Warning third parties at risk of AIDS: APA's policy is a barrier to treatment. *Hospital and Community Psychiatry, 40,* 158–161.
Perry, S., Ryan, J., Fogel, F., Fishman, B., & Jacobsberg, L. (1990). Voluntarily informing others of positive HIV test results: Patterns of notification by infected gay men. *Hospital and Community Psychiatry, 41,* 549–551.
Potterat, J. J., Spencer, N. E., Woodhouse, D. E., & Muth, J. B. (1989). Partner notification in the control of human immunodeficiency virus infection. *American Journal of Public Health, 79,* 874–876.
Price, D. P. T. (1990). Between Scylla and Charybdis: Charting a course to reconcile the duty of confidentiality and the duty to warn in the AIDS context. *Dickinson Law Review, 94,* 435–487.
Rennert, S. (1991). *AIDS/HIV and confidentiality: Model policy and procedures.* Washington, DC: American Bar Association.
Ryan, C. C., & Rowe, M. J. (1988). AIDS: Legal and ethical issues. *Social Casework, 69,* 324–333.
Schwartzbaum, J. A., Wheat, J. R., & Norton, R. W. (1990). Physician breach of patient confidentiality among individuals with human immunodeficiency virus (HIV) infection: Patterns of decision. *American Journal of Public Health, 80,* 829–834.
Totten, G., Lamb, D. H., & Reeder, G.D. (1990). *Tarasoff* and confidentiality in AIDS-related psychotherapy. *Professional Psychology: Research and Practice, 21,* 155–160.

Turkington, R. C. (1989). Confidentiality policy for HIV-related information: An analytical framework for sorting out hard and easy cases. *Villanova Law Review, 34,* 871–908.
Zonana, H. (1989). Warning third parties at risk of AIDS: APA's policy is a reasonable approach. *Hospital and Community Psychiatry, 40,* 162–164.

III. Child Abuse Reporting

See "Child Abuse and Sexual Abuse" in Bibliography of Chapter 10, pp. 343–345.

8

The Duty to Protect Third Parties and Negligent Release

I. The Duty to Protect Third Parties • A. Legal Theory • B. The *Tarasoff* Decisions • C. Post-*Tarasoff* Decisions • D. Meaning of *Tarasoff* for Mental Health Professionals • E. When There Is a Duty to Protect Third Parties • F. Methods of Discharging the Duty to Protect • G. Problems Presented by the Duty to Protect • H. Avoiding Liability • I. Duty to Protect Statutes • J. Conclusion • **II. Negligent Release** • A. Negligent Release Cases: Plaintiff Verdict • B. Negligent Release Cases: Defense Verdict • C. When Liability Is Likely • D. Avoiding Liability • E. Conclusion • **III. Liability for Motor Vehicle Accidents** • **IV. Managed Care** • **V. Commonly Asked Questions** • Appendix: American Psychiatric Association's Model Statute on the Physician's Duty to Take Precaution against Patient Violence • **VI. Bibliography** • Table of Cases

The California Supreme Court rendered two decisions (*Tarasoff* I, 1974, and *Tarasoff* II, 1976) in *Tarasoff v. Regents of the University of California* whose repercussions are far-reaching. Until that time, mental health professionals did not much concern themselves with the potential liability from the harm inflicted on others by their outpatients. The *Tarasoff* decisions and numerous subsequent cases have made the duty to protect members of the public a realistic concern for all practitioners, one they must fully understand.

In addition to concerns about the danger caused by outpatients, there is also potential liability for the release of inpatients who then harm others after discharge. These cases are called *negligent release* cases. In both duty to protect and negligent-release cases, the harm is caused to someone who has no relationship with the therapist. These two types of cases are similar in that the therapist is expected to control the behavior of someone in treatment to prevent harm to some third party. In both, there have been large awards for plaintiffs through settlements and jury verdicts, sometimes in the multimillion-dollar range. In others, plaintiffs have not prevailed because they were unable to establish that a legal duty was owed to them, or that the clinicians deviated from the standard of care in treating the patient.

Duty to protect cases involve a person in outpatient treatment, and the only control the therapist has is the control he exerts as a result of the therapy and his option to hospitalize the client. In contrast, in negligent release cases the patient is hospitalized and the therapist decides when he will be released on pass or discharged. Duty to protect cases are based on the therapist's inaction, such as failure to hospitalize, failure to call the police, or failure to warn the intended victim. Negligent release cases are based on the concept that the action of the therapist and facility staff in releasing the patient was the proximate cause of the harm to the third party.

Although these concepts represent a type of malpractice discussed in Chapter 6, the fears they raise for the mental health professional, the attention they have generated in the literature, and the increasing number of cases in this area merit a separate chapter.

I. THE DUTY TO PROTECT THIRD PARTIES

The notion that a therapist may have a duty to one who is not his patient has for many therapists changed the way they practice their profession. Concepts such as absolute confidentiality have had to be set aside. More mental health professionals are concerned about when they must act to prevent their patient from harming others. This section will discuss how the duty to protect third parties evolved, with a description of the *Tarasoff* decisions and subsequent cases. This chapter will provide practical guidelines for the clinician about what to do when concerned about a patient's harming someone. The goal of the chapter is to provide sufficient understanding of the developing law and clinical practice related to a duty to protect so that the clinician will become more comfortable with potentially violent clients.

A. The Legal Theory

It is a well-recognized American legal principle that, in the absence of a specific statutory provision to the contrary, there is no affirmative duty to control the behavior of another person or to warn a person of another's threat; thus, there is no liability for failure to do so. There have always been two exceptions to this principle. The first is when there is a "custodial relationship" which places the custodian in a position to control or limit the actions of another. A typical example is the responsibility of a mental health facility to keep hospitalized someone who is civilly committed because of potential violence. If the individual escapes because of inadequate security by the facility and then harms someone, the facility could be held liable for the injury to the third party. The notion is that the hospitalized person is under the legal authority of the facility and that the facility staff can in fact control his actions. It is partly based on this duty that negligent release suits are brought.

The second exception of when a person who does not cause the harm may be liable for it is when the person undertakes a responsibility to the injured party but does so inadequately. One example is the individual who stops at the scene of an automobile accident, claims he is a physician, waves on others who want to stop, offers assistance, and then abandons the accident victims. He could be held liable for the consequential injuries to the injured persons because he deterred others from intervening to help the victims.

In the two decisions in *Tarasoff v. Regents of the University of California* ("*Tarasoff* I," "*Tarasoff* II"), the California Supreme Court enunciated a new common law duty to warn or protect endangered third parties, applicable to mental health professionals whose patients constitute a threat to third parties, even when the patient is being seen on an outpatient basis and there is no true custodial relationship. The reasoning that led the court in *Tarasoff* to extend this duty to mental health professionals was that, when balancing the tension between the patient's right to confidentiality and the possibility of protecting someone from harm, confidentiality had to "yield to the extent to which disclosure is essential to avert danger to others." The court reasoned:

> In this risk-infested society, we can hardly tolerate the further exposure to danger that would result from a concealed knowledge of the therapist that his patient was lethal. If the exercise of reasonable care to protect the threatened victim requires the therapist to warn the endangered party or those who can reasonably be expected to notify him, we see no sufficient society interest that would protect and justify concealment.

B. The *Tarasoff* Decisions

In October 1969, Prosenjit Poddar, a graduate student at the University of California, fatally shot and stabbed Tatiana Tarasoff, a student who earlier had spurned his romantic overtures. Following her rejection of him, Tarasoff had left the country. During Tarasoff's absence, Poddar saw two therapists, a psychiatrist and a psychologist, on nine occasions at the University of California's Student Health Service in Berkeley. Both therapists diagnosed Poddar as an acute paranoid schizophrenic. During his last therapy session Poddar alluded to his intention to kill Tarasoff. His therapist requested Poddar's assurance that he would not take any such action; the therapist implied that he would take steps to prevent Poddar from doing any harm to the woman. Poddar then angrily left the session and did not subsequently return for treatment. The therapist notified the campus police for the purpose of initiating commitment proceedings. The police investigated the matter and received Poddar's promise that he would stay away from Tarasoff and then concluded that civil commitment proceedings were not justified. A few weeks later, Ms. Tarasoff returned from abroad. Poddar attempted to contact her daily but she refused to see him; ultimately he killed her.

At Poddar's criminal trial, the jury concluded that Poddar had been legally sane at the time of the killing and that he had not been suffering from diminished capacity. His murder conviction later was reversed on technical grounds relating to jury instructions. As a result of information revealed during the course of the criminal trial, Tarasoff's family filed suit against the University of California, the two therapists, and the campus police, seeking damages based on the theory that Tarasoff had been due a warning as to Poddar's danger to her and that the failure to so warn her constituted actionable negligence.

Initially the trial and intermediate appellate courts ruled that the Tarasoff family had failed to state a cause of action, and the case was dismissed. However, on appeal, the California Supreme Court in *Tarasoff* I reversed, holding that a cause of action could be maintained against the therapists and the police for failing to warn the victim. The case was subsequently reargued, and in *Tarasoff* II the court excluded the police from liability. The court reaffirmed its *Tarasoff* I reasoning that there is a special relationship between a psychotherapist and his patient which engenders affirmative duties to third persons who are endangered by the patient, and that failure to take action may expose the therapist to liability. The court held:

> When a therapist determines, or pursuant to the standards of his profession should determine, that his patient presents a serious danger of violence to another, he incurs an obligation to use reasonable care to protect the intended victim against such danger. The discharge of this duty may require the therapist to take one or more of various steps, depending upon the nature of the case. Thus, it may call for him to warn the intended victim or others likely to apprise the victim of the danger, to notify the police, or to take whatever steps are reasonably necessary under the circumstances.

The court went on to make clear that the standard of care used in malpractice suits would apply to the assessment of the patient's dangerousness:

> Obviously we do not require that the therapist, in making that determination, render a perfect performance; the therapist need only exercise that reasonable degree of skill, knowledge, and care ordinarily possessed and exercised by members of [that professional specialty] under similar circumstances. Within the broad range of reasonable practice and treatment in which professional opinion and judgment may differ, the therapist is free to exercise his or her own best judgment without liability; proof, aided by hindsight, that he or she judged wrongly is insufficient to establish negligence.

The court summarized its holding by stating that "the therapist owes a legal duty not only to his patient, but also to his patient's would-be victim and is subject in both respects to scrutiny by judge and jury." Subsequently, the University of California reached a settlement with the Tarasoff family for an undisclosed amount, making unnecessary a final determination of whether the therapist had in fact failed to meet the standard of care set by the California Supreme Court.

C. Post-*Tarasoff* Decisions

In the cases which have been brought in the United States based on a duty to protect, the decision turns on the facts of the specific case and a determination of whether there is some common law or statutory duty to protect third parties. The case usually begins with a dispute as to whether the legal duty to a third party exists, with the defendants asking for dismissal of the case. On appeal to the state's appellate and supreme courts, a decision is made as to whether the duty to protect applies. In those states in which the court has recognized the existence of this duty, the case then returns to the trial court for a trial as to whether the therapist met the standard of his profession by his actions. The issues are whether the therapist did determine, or should have determined, the client likely to be violent; whether there was an identifiable victim or class of victims; and whether the therapist did take, or should have taken, some action which would have prevented harm to the third party.

The trend in these cases is to follow the *Tarasoff* rationale and impose on therapists a duty to take some action to prevent foreseeable harm to a third party injured by their client. Most, but not all, states which have addressed this issue require that there be an identifiable victim before the therapist may be said to have a legal duty to protect him. This is a person whom the client has actually identified as a potential victim, and therefore the therapist has had knowledge of whom to protect. A few courts have extended this logic to a readily identifiable victim, which is any person who could foreseeably be harmed by the client, even though not specifically named by the client; here, the therapist need only have asked the client about the identity of the potential victim. A few cases will illustrate some of these rulings.

In *McIntosh v. Milano* (1979), a New Jersey Superior Court adopted the *Tarasoff* reasoning in holding that a psychiatrist had a legal duty to protect an ex-girlfriend who was fatally shot by her ex-boyfriend, the psychiatrist's outpatient. Dr. Milano had treated his 17-year-old patient for two years for an adjustment reaction of adolescence and substance use. During the treatment, the patient discussed with the psychiatrist his feelings of jealousy, ambivalence, and retaliation about his 20-year-old girlfriend and her dating other men, and he had once shot a BB gun at a car (her car or a boyfriend's). Though the patient had never directly threatened to injure the girl, the plaintiff alleged that the psychiatrist should have known that his patient posed a threat to the victim. After the court ruled that the victim's family could bring suit, in his trial the defendant psychiatrist was determined not to have breached his duty to protect the victim.

In *Thompson v. County of Alameda* (1980), the California Supreme Court again considered the duty to protect a third party but narrowed the duty to a foreseeable victim of a patient rather than to the public at large. The court held that there is "no affirmative duty to warn of the release of an inmate with a violent history who has made nonspecific threats of harm directed at nonspecific victims." Though the case involved the release of a juvenile delinquent from custody, rather than from a mental health facility or clinic, the court ruling is applicable to a mental health setting as well.

In contrast to *Thompson*, a Nebraska federal court in *Lipari v. Sears, Roebuck & Co. and United States* (1980) expanded the duty to protect beyond those victims who are specifically identified or readily identifiable. The victims in this case were shot in a crowded nightclub by an ex-patient of the Veterans Administration. The court held that there was a duty to protect members of the public who were foreseeably endangered even when no specific victim had been threatened by the therapist's patient. The case was later settled out of court by the parties.

A similar result to *Lipari* was obtained in *Hamman v. County of Maricopa* (1989), in which a schizophrenic son brutally attacked his stepfather two days after having been evaluated at a psychiatric emergency center. The evaluating psychiatrist allegedly failed to review the boy's psychiatric records, reassured the parents that he was "harmless," and refused to admit the patient to the hospital, even though the parents repeatedly asked him to do so. Though the boy had not threatened to injure his stepfather, with whom he lived, the Arizona Supreme Court formulated the rule that: "The psychiatrist has a duty to exercise reasonable care to protect the foreseeable victim of that danger. The foreseeable victim is one who is said to be within the zone of danger, that is, subject to probable risk of the patient's violent conduct." According to the court, proposed alternatives to simply releasing the patient included providing instructions to the parents if the patient deteriorates, arranging for outpatient treatment, or warning the parents of the potential danger to them.

With similar facts, the Pennsylvania Superior Court in *Dunkle v. Food Service East* (1990) reached a different result. In this case, a man treated as an outpatient for a schizophreniform disorder unexpectedly strangled his live-in girlfriend in a store's bathroom, believing her to be a "Russian agent." He had never previously threatened her or attempted to injure her. The court held that the therapists did not have a legal duty to protect her since the patient had never before made a specific violent threat or attempted violence against the victim. Thus, she was not a specified or readily identifiable victim.

Finally, the Florida Appellate Court, in an *en banc* decision in *Boynton v. Burglass* (1991), refused to recognize a clinician's duty to warn or protect third parties. In this case, a psychiatric outpatient shot and killed the male victim, possibly because of a jealous rage over a woman they both knew. The appellate court affirmed the trial court's dismissal of the plaintiff's malpractice complaint on the grounds that the psychiatrist had no ability or right to control a voluntary outpatient. The appellate court reasoned that imposing a duty to warn victims of voluntary psychiatric outpatients is "neither reasonable nor workable and is potentially fatal to effective patient-therapist relationships." Noting that "Because psychiatry is, at best, an inexact science, courts should be reluctant to impose liability upon psychiatrists," the appellate court concluded that "psychiatrists cannot be charged with accurately making . . . [predictions of dangerousness] and with sharing those predictions with others." The case was not appealed to the Florida Supreme Court since the defendant psychiatrist declared bankruptcy.

D. Meaning of *Tarasoff* for Mental Health Professionals

The effect of *Tarasoff* on mental health professionals is difficult to discern. As a result of *Tarasoff*, as well as the increase in litigiousness of society, mental health professionals have a heightened concern about the danger their patients might cause to others. *Tarasoff* may have led some therapists to refuse to treat those with a history of violent behavior. Perhaps other therapists have refused to manage hospitalized patients or have restricted their practice to voluntary patients. In addition, the fear of *Tarasoff* liability has made some therapists unduly defensive in their practice; that is, they have become more likely to breach confidentiality or seek civil commitment, rather than rely on continued outpatient treatment, when the threat of violence seems likely. In some cases, therapists have begun to warn at the outset of therapy that confidentiality may be breached if and when the patient becomes potentially violent to others.

E. When There Is a Duty to Protect Third Parties

Even though the courts in every state have not ruled on or affirmed *Tarasoff*-like liability, every mental health clinician is advised to proceed as if third-party liability could occur should an outpatient seriously injure another person. Of course, case law and statutory law differ significantly across jurisdictions, so there may be wide state-to-state discrepancies about whether, in a given factual situation, the duty to protect is invoked. Although the law is often vague as well as changing in this area, the therapist should uniformly consider the four parameters of danger to others in assessing a patient's risk of interpersonal violence. These include the type of harm, the seriousness of harm, the imminence of harm, and the likelihood of harm. The therapist must evaluate patient-related variables as well as those which pertain to the context or situations in which the patient interacts.

A duty to protect third parties is typically applicable when interpersonal violence rather than property damage is at issue. Damage inflicted by arson may represent a potential personal injury, so that a patient who threatens to bomb or burn property can be said to invoke the duty to protect. In only a few states does property damage by itself trigger the duty to protect.

The therapist must also consider the severity of the harm that the patient threatens to inflict on his victim. The duty to protect will be invoked only when serious harm (as judged by potential bodily injury or deformity) could occur.

The therapist must also judge that the violence is reasonably likely to occur, rather than merely possible, before the duty to protect would be invoked.

Finally, the therapist must also judge that the violence will occur in the near or imminent future rather than at some distant point in time (e.g., five years hence).

As noted earlier, the presence of an identified or readily identifiable third party may be necessary before the duty to protect is invoked, but this remains an uncertain issue in many states.

F. Methods of Discharging the Duty to Protect

1. *Assessment of Violence Potential*

If, during the course of evaluation or treatment, the client makes specific threats of violence, then the therapist must investigate these. This means that the therapist must shift from the role of therapist to that of an evaluator or investigator. Few threats of violence actually result in overt violence, so the therapist must attempt to determine which are likely to be realized, and which may be discounted. Often, the lines between violent ideation (fantasies), general plans for violence, and specific intentions to activate those plans are indistinct and variable over time. Since a past history of violence is the most likely predictor of future violence, the therapist will need to familiarize himself, if he has not already done so, with any violence in the client's past. This includes the details of when, where, why, and how. Consideration should also be given to the client's level of impulsivity, his ability to resist violent impulses, his reaction to his own violence, his motivation to maintain self-control, and the contribution of alcohol and drugs to impulse dyscontrol. Review of current and past mental health or medical records may help to confirm or elaborate some of the relevant history, which clients often fail to report. Corroborating data can and sometimes should be obtained from those familiar with the client such as family members.

The therapist must also assess the client's intent and his ability to carry out the threat. It is important to determine whether there is a detailed plan to injure the potential victim, whether the client knows the location of the potential victim, and whether he has the means to find and then injure the victim, whether with a weapon or otherwise.

2. *Risk Management and Implementation*

Once the therapist concludes that the client presents a significant risk of serious physical violence to a third party, he must make a decision about how to discharge his legal duty. He must consider the various options available under the circumstances and then implement one or more of these.

Although the 1976 *Tarasoff* decision resulted in the requirement that the therapist protect someone from impending danger from the client, the court specifically recognized that actions other than warning the potential victim could be taken. In general, such options include changing the treatment program for the client, requesting that the patient voluntarily hospitalize himself, initiating civil commitment, warning the potential victim, warning others who would be likely to notify the victim, or contacting the police in the area of the victim or the client. The action taken should be one which is likely to be effective in reducing the risk of violence, rather than counterproductive.

Reasonable changes in the treatment program for a potentially violent client include a change in the type of psychiatric treatment, such as starting psychotropic medication, beginning behavioral treatment designed to facilitate impulse control, initiating family therapy, involving others in the treatment program to assist in monitoring or supervising the client, implementing a therapy which involves the potential victim if he is emotionally close to the patient, referring the patient for more intensive treatment such as partial hospitalization, or offering voluntary hospitalization. The frequency of outpatient therapy can also be increased to deal with related issues such as the client's fear of loss of impulse control and maintaining the trust of the treatment relationship. Making social or environmental changes in the client's immediate situation may be particularly useful since many forms of interpersonal violence (e.g., domestic violence) are interactive in origin.

Civil commitment offers the best protection against a lawsuit when the therapist believes that the client will harm someone because of a mental illness. However, much threatened violence is not a product of mental illness but of intense anger or revenge, or of conflict within an intimate relationship, so that commitment will not be a reasonable alternative. When the therapist is able to seek civil commitment, the therapist acknowledges that the patient is a potential risk to others. If commitment is granted, the therapist has discharged the immediate obligation to protect the third party. If commitment is not ordered, the therapist has documented that he tried to fulfill his obligations to the public.

Tarasoff suggested that the therapist could discharge his duty to the public by notifying the police. In any large community, however, without some overt criminal action by the client, notifying the police is unlikely to be a productive strategy. The police can become involved when the therapist seeks to have the client detained to begin civil commitment proceedings. Without a criminal incident, though, the police are likely to refuse to provide protection to the endangered third party. The police may be useful, though, in the surrender or confiscation of the client's weapons, which the therapist can initiate. Notifying the police of the potential threat or intention to harm will provide documentation that the therapist has assessed the client as potentially violent and has taken some action to protect the potential victim. Another problem is identifying which police agency to contact. This is an issue when the client, the therapist, and the potential victim are in different jurisdictions.

It is somewhat unfortunate, and a source of confusion among therapists, that the major thrust of some duty to protect cases (e.g., *Tarasoff* I) is that the therapist should warn the potential victim rather than provide reasonable care to the patient. It is questionable whether such notification will truly protect the person from harm, especially when the potential victim is already aware of the risk of harm from the client (from either a previous threat, an actual injury, or violence to another person). Though it may not be therapeutic, warning a potential victim is likely to relieve the therapist from liability for a subsequent injury unless it can be shown that warning was contrary to the therapist's clinical judgment, warning was an inadequate response to the client's threat, and the therapist should have moved for civil commitment. The form the warning should take, the extent of the information about the client which should be revealed to the potential victim, and the advice given to the potential victim will vary with the circumstances of the case. Warnings should be made by telephone or in person, rather than by letter.

Finally, to discharge his duty, the therapist could also notify someone who is likely to apprise the potential victim of the potential harm, perhaps a relative, employer, or friend of the potential victim. Any of these, or the police, may be better able to locate the potential victim than the therapist. Again, it is uncertain whether this is a productive strategy, but it may be useful when the therapist cannot reach the client himself.

Discharging the legal duty to protect in one or more of the above strategies not only may protect the therapist from liability but may also result in some therapeutic benefit to the patient. Modifying or intensifying the treatment program or bringing family members or the potential victim into the treatment may result in a reduction of symptoms or interpersonal conflict which is unexpected. A therapist who confronts his client with the seriousness of the potential violence also provides limit setting and reality testing to the client, which may provide an objective perspective on the problem and thus diffuse the client's intense feelings.

G. Problems Presented by the Duty to Protect

1. *Disrupting the Therapeutic Alliance and Relationship*

Once the client has been informed of the potential need to breach the confidentiality of the relationship, the client may no longer be able to trust the therapist to continue the therapy. In particular, clients may no longer disclose, or may spuriously deny, their violent thoughts and impulses to therapists for fear that these thoughts and impulses will be reported. The relationship may become overtly disrupted when the therapist decides that the duty to protect must be invoked and the client refuses to cooperate. Also, the treatment relationship can be compromised by an unsuccessful civil commitment attempt which increases the risk of violence.

Warning third parties is ideally accomplished with the consent of the client, with the participation of the client, by the client, and in the client's presence. The client can be asked to sign a written consent to release confidential information before the therapist discusses the case with the potential victim. As much as possible, the client should be involved in the decision making about the need to protect third parties, since the client is ultimately responsible for controlling his impulses. A therapist who is forced to do the warning for the client potentially presents a therapeutic dilemma in that the client may be manipulating the therapist or the warning may inappropriately gratify the client's needs to express his angry feelings. Premature or inappropriate warnings can be unproductive not only in failing to protect the public but also in damaging the treatment process.

2. *Precipitating Violence by Warning*

Contrary to intuitive expectations, informing a third party that the client has threatened to, or intends to, injure that party may invite retaliation by the potential victim to protect himself and may thus precipitate a confrontation between the client and the third party. This potential result is understandable in that some people conceal their fear by anger, and that interpersonal violence is often precipitated by the victim. In addition, the act of warning of violence is itself a threat or a discharge of an aggressive impulse from the client. A therapist who is contemplating warning a potential victim, even with the consent of the client, should also consider the possibility that warning the identified victim may paradoxically increase the risk to the victim or may actually create a risk to the patient.

3. *Stigmatizing the Client*

Warning a family member, lover, coworker, supervisor, or other potential victim of the client's potential violence may prompt him to reject or avoid the client. This could result in a loss of job or place of residence for the client. If the police are warned, they may provoke or antagonize the client, whom they now identify as vulnerable.

4. *Changing Clinical Practice Patterns*

An important legal duty such as the duty to protect the public, as well as the fear of liability for failing to do so, has no doubt prompted much change in clinicians' practices. Therapists attend more to potential violence and tend to overpredict its occurrence, focus on less serious violence or threats, and respond sooner to a lower threshold of violence. As noted, some clinicians now avoid dealing with violent clients or deny or fail to acknowledge potential violence by clients, while others defensively overtreat, unnecessarily hospitalize, or excessively seek commitment, none of which may serve the interests of the client. An increase in the therapist's anxiety when dealing with potential violence may impair the therapist's judgment and decision making about the client.

5. *Dual Agency*

As a result of the therapist's legal duty to protect members of the public, there is a shift in the structure of the treatment relationship from one exclusively devoted to helping the client to one more focused on a social perspective. This shift can be variously seen as advantageous or detrimental to the client and to society.

H. Avoiding Liability

Although actual case law is limited in many jurisdictions, the therapist should know how to proceed when facing potential liability as a result of the client's behavior. Unless the client is prosecuted criminally for his behavior and raises an insanity defense to that prosecution, or the client is well known to the victim, it is unlikely that any victim will even be aware of the client's treatment and therefore will not know to sue the clinician. However, the key to successfully forestalling such a lawsuit is to act in conformity with clinical standards, to consult with colleagues, and to carefully and contemporaneously document one's risk assessment, clinical decision making, and discharge of the legal duty.

It is often useful to consult with a colleague familiar with the assessment and management of violent patients whenever there is doubt about what action to take or disagreement among the staff caring for the client. If the primary therapist is not a psychiatrist, he may want to consult with a psychiatrist who has experience in dealing with violent patients, since this consultation may facilitate starting medication, hospitalization, or civil commitment. The consultant may wish to interview the client or may proceed to offer a recommendation on the basis of the data provided by the therapist. In either case, the therapist should provide the consultant as much information as possible about the client and the present problem. It is hoped that the consultation will clarify what action to take. If either the therapist or the consultant has any legal questions, then an attorney knowledgeable in this area of expertise should be consulted.

Whether or not a consultation has been obtained, the therapist needs to document what he has learned about the client's history and current risk of violence. Direct quotations from the client can be recorded verbatim. The record should detail the content of the client's violent ideation, intention, plans, and relevant clinical issues such as command hallucinations. The record should also include a discussion of the therapist's thinking process, or decision making rationale, for whatever course of action is selected. It should also include a detailed description of the therapist's actions to protect any third party, including third-party notification or police reports, and when these occurred.

I. Duty to Protect Statutes

In response to the developing case law holding mental health professionals liable for the acts of their patients, almost half the states have enacted statutes which attempt to limit the liability of mental health professionals to third parties. Such statutes have arisen because of the concern of mental health professionals and their professional organizations that state courts have excessively expanded the duty to protect third parties, that they have done so in an unpredictable manner, and that there is much variation across the states.

By design, these statutes provide immunity from suit from injured third parties or the patient himself if the professional discharges his legal duty as defined by the law. They typically apply to the outpatient duty to protect cases, rather than third-party injuries resulting from negligent release or escape of a patient from a hospital (see below). They also provide legal immunity for breach of confidentiality or invasion of privacy for the necessary and good-faith disclosures of the risk of violence to police and victims. Statutory immunity may not be available for the therapist's breach of confidentiality when there has not been an explicit threat, that is, when the therapist voluntarily elected to invoke the duty outside the requirements of the statute.

Nearly every statute requires a specific threat to an identified or readily identifiable person before the duty, or the immunity provision, applies. This provision excludes liability to the general public.

Given that the case law which has prompted the enactment of these statutes has focused on the risk of interpersonal violence, rather than property damage, by the patient, most of the statutes omit mention of potential liability or immunity for property damage. This omission leaves open possible liability for property damage.

Though there are many similarities, the statutes differ in several respects:

1. The types of mental health professional covered by these laws varies across the statutes. These include physicians, psychiatrists, psychologists, social workers, nurses (registered, psychiatric, and practical), and counselors. Some statutes cover not only persons but institutions: mental health centers, hospitals, substance abuse rehabilitation programs, and health care professional corporations. There may be a requirement that the covered persons be licensed by the state before immunity can apply. Those trainees or others working under the covered professionals could also be covered.

2. Most of the statutes require an explicit threat before the legal duty to protect, or the immunity, applies. A few do not require a specific threat but require that the patient be imminently dangerous and have a known history of violence. Importantly, the requirement that there be an overt threat immunizes the therapist against a claim that the therapist "should have known" of the patient's potential violence to others even though the therapist did not in fact know of it.

3. Some statutes require not only that the patient threaten violence but also that the patient have the intent and the ability to carry out the threat. This provision is more in keeping with the intent of the duty to protect case law, rather than invoking the duty to protect whenever a patient makes any threat, no matter how credible.

4. The statutes provide that the therapist can discharge the legal duty to protect third parties by any of several mechanisms, either alone or in combination: attempts to voluntarily hospitalize the patient, seeking to or actually committing the patient to the hospital, attempts to warn or actually warning the victim, and attempts to warn or actually warning of appropriate police agencies (with regard to the victim, the patient, or both). Some statutes provide an exclusive list of options for the clinician, in effect limiting liability only if those options are implemented. Others provide immunity for taking any other reasonable precautions to prevent the threatened violence.

Since these statutes emphasize that the therapist who warns potential victims or the police about the potential violence of their patient will be immunized should violence occur anyway, there is a risk that therapists will indiscriminately report or notify third parties. This is particularly a concern when the patient verbalizes violent ideation or intention but the therapist assesses the risk of violence as insignificant. Warning a third party or calling the police in such a case may protect the therapist against the risk of third-party liability but is likely to be clinically countertherapeutic. Such a therapist inappropriately advances his own interests over those of the patient. Even though a duty to protect statute has been enacted in a state, therapists need to continue to use their clinical judgment about the benefits and risks of notifying third parties about their patient before actually breaching confidentiality. Therapists should also continue to help the client do the necessary work in therapy even though the duty to protect has been adequately discharged by a third-party warning or a police report.

Because of the range in scope of these statutes, clinicians should be familiar with their state's statute and should know its specific coverage and exclusions. Practice in one state may significantly differ from that in another because of the applicable law.

Since these statutes are so recent, it is unclear what effect they will have on clinical practice, new case law, or malpractice insurance premiums. Clinicians in states without such laws may wish to seek enactment of immunity provisions in their own states. For this purpose, the American Psychiatric Association has published a model statute on the duty to protect third parties (see the chapter appendix).

J. Conclusion

Mental health professionals should assume that the duty to protect the public from violent clients is now a reality, even if there is no specific case law or statute on the subject in every state. Though the number of these cases is expanding, the likelihood of success depends on establishing that the therapist breached the standard of his profession in the action he took or failed to take, and the interpretation of case law and statutory law in the jurisdiction. As in any area of difficult clinical practice, familiarity with legal requirements, thorough risk evaluation, independent consultation, and documentation of decision making will be the best defense against a lawsuit in this area.

II. Negligent Release

The negligent release or discharge of a hospitalized patient can be grounds for finding liability against the clinicians and the hospital. Cases involving this claim typically arise when a discharged psychiatric patient seriously injures or kills someone within a few weeks or months after release from the hospital. In the ensuing lawsuit, the plaintiff must prove:

1. The standard of care of psychiatric practice in determining the release of a hospitalized patient under similar circumstances (i.e., evaluation, testing, and procedures) and the existence of a legal duty of care to the victim.
2. Deviation from the standard of care by the physician or hospital staff (i.e., that the facility was aware of the danger that the patient posed to the victim, but that the facility improperly or prematurely released the patient or that the facility should have been aware of the danger that the patient posed to the victim, even though it was not).
3. Injury to the plaintiff.
4. The patient's discharge as the proximate cause of the harm to the victim.

Negligent release cases were litigated in the United States years before *Tarasoff*. They are different from outpatient duty to protect cases in two important respects. First, in negligent release cases, mental health professionals either have the legal authority to control the person or had actual control over the person who inflicted the harm. Second, the plaintiff in negligent release cases alleges that the affirmative act of releasing the patient on pass or discharge was the proximate cause of the harm to the victim.

In negligent release cases, in contrast to most outpatient duty to protect cases, it may or may not be necessary for the plaintiff to show that that particular victim, or the group of which he was a member, was identifiably at risk from the patient. Given the fact of a deceased or seriously injured plaintiff, jurors can often be persuaded in hindsight that the hospital's behavior was negligent and that an alternate course of action should have been pursued. Nevertheless, the law does not expect health care providers or their institutions to guarantee the public's safety from their released patients.

In practice, many cases involving injuries inflicted on third parties by released patients are litigated on one or more of the following grounds: (1) a duty to protect or warn the third party; (2) malpractice of the practitioner during the postdischarge period; (3) negligent release from the facility. Thus, it is often difficult to separate the outpatient duty to protect cases from the inpatient negligent release cases. However, some states do not litigate cases of third-party injuries as medical malpractice cases.

A. Negligent Release Cases: Plaintiff Verdict

While many negligent discharge cases have been brought against public institutions, particularly state hospitals and Veterans Administration hospitals, private psychiatric facilities have also been held liable. In many cases, the victim is a family member, perhaps a spouse or ex-spouse, and in many of these cases, the family member was aware of the risk posed by the patient. In many but not all cases, the patient was involuntarily hospitalized prior to the release. A few vignettes will illustrate some of the issues in this area.

Merchants National Bank and Trust Company v. United States (1967) involved a male patient who was involuntarily hospitalized at a Veterans Administration hospital because of marked psychosis, accusations of his wife's infidelity, threats to kill her, and an episode of choking her. After six months of hospitalization, the hospital temporarily released the patient to live and work on a ranch. The owners of the ranch were given no information regarding his mental condition or his need for supervision or restrictions. On a Friday night 13 days after his release from the hospital, the patient left the ranch, obtained a car, attempted to run his wife down, and then shot and killed her. The court concluded that the Veterans Administration had been negligent in releasing the patient, and that the release was the proximate cause of his wife's death. The court held that the attending psychiatrist had ignored reports of other staff members about the patient's disorder and his risk of harming his wife, had ignored his wife's fears of the patient, and had claimed that the patient was not in fact delusional but was "exaggerating." It also held that the chief of staff had failed to investigate the wife's concerns about the patient and had failed to follow through after receiving a consultant's recommendation not to discharge the patient.

In *Hicks v. United States* (1975), a patient was hospitalized on criminal charges for an evaluation of his competency to stand trial after assaulting his wife. The hospital reported to the criminal court that he had recovered and was competent to stand trial. The charges were dropped when the wife failed to appear in court, and the patient was released. Within two months following his discharge, he killed his wife. In the ensuing civil suit, the court ruled that the hospital had failed to report to the criminal court that the patient had a chronic organic brain syndrome and had not completely recovered; this negligence was found to be a proximate cause of the wife's death.

In *Williams v. United States* (1978), a man with a long history of violence and several psychiatric disorders was transferred to a hospital from a jail along with instructions to notify the police upon discharge so that the patient could be prosecuted. Instead, the hospital discharged the patient, who killed a stranger the next day. The court ruled that the hospital had failed to exercise reasonable care in its treatment of the patient since the staff failed to notify the authorities who were to detain the patient.

In *Semler v. Psychiatric Institute of Washington, D.C.* (1976), a man was hospitalized as a condition of his probation after conviction on charges of abducting a young girl.

After a lengthy hospitalization, he was transferred to a partial hospital program with court approval. Subsequently, the psychiatrist discharged the patient to outpatient status without notification of or approval by the referring court. The patient killed the plaintiff shortly thereafter. In the civil suit, the court ruled that the hospital had breached its duty to protect the public by failing to obtain court approval prior to releasing the patient from supervised status.

An expansive court interpretation of negligent release liability came in *Petersen v. State of Washington* (1983). In this case, the Washington State Supreme Court held that a physician at a state hospital had a duty to protect anyone who might foreseeably be endangered by a former patient's drug-related behavior. Five days after his discharge from a state hospital, the former patient, driving at an inappropriate rate of speed, caused an automobile accident, injuring the plaintiff.

Known to have a history of drug abuse and on probation for a burglary conviction, the patient had cut out his left testicle with a knife after taking "angel dust" four days prior to admission. The psychiatrist concluded that the patient's behavior was due to a schizophrenic-like reaction to illicit drugs and prescribed antipsychotic medication in the hospital. On the day before the expiration of his commitment, the patient drove his car erratically on the hospital grounds while out on a pass. Upon discharge, the patient was considered to have recovered from his drug-induced psychosis.

The plaintiff brought suit against the state, arguing that the failure to seek to extend the commitment, or to notify the probation officer of the hospitalization, was the proximate cause of her injuries. The Washington Supreme Court, affirming the $250,000 verdict, accepted this argument and held that the psychiatrist had incurred a duty to take reasonable precautions to protect anyone who might foreseeably be endangered by the patient's drug-related mental problems. In essence, the court held the psychiatrist liable for failure to seek further civil commitment. Although the expansiveness of this decision has important implications for mental health professionals, the facts of the case must be kept in mind. The staff had been aware that the patient was engaged in erratic behavior the night before his discharge, and they also had not made sure that he had taken his medication. At trial, it was learned that the patient had not in fact taken his medication.

Nevertheless, the *Petersen* case is alarming because it requires that a therapist try to control or prevent drug-induced behavior outside the hospital. While street drug use and its consequences in the hospital setting can be controlled or at least monitored, once someone is discharged there is little the therapist can do to prevent further ingestion of drugs short of continuous supervision. Whether other courts will follow the reasoning of the Washington court remains to be seen.

A similar verdict to *Petersen* was obtained in *Naidu v. Laird* (1988). A chronically ill man with multiple state psychiatric hospitalizations at the same facility discontinued his medication upon discharge from a voluntary hospitalization and, five months later, deliberately drove into the victim's vehicle, killing the plaintiff. The patient had a history of medication noncompliance, multiple suicide attempts, commitments for dangerousness to self and others, and deliberate automobile accidents. The Delaware Supreme Court upheld the jury's award of $1.4 million to the plaintiff, ruling that the hospital psychiatrist had been grossly negligent in his evaluation, treatment, and release of the patient. The absence of a specified victim in the case did not bar recovery.

B. Negligent Release Cases: Defense Verdict

While many plaintiffs have prevailed in negligent release cases, judges and juries have found many defendants not to be negligent in their decision to release a patient on pass or discharge. The court decision in *Taig v. State of New York* (1963), 30 years ago, finding no negligence in the release of a teenage patient who subsequently assaulted another teenager, is representative of the viewpoint that release decision making involves a professional medical judgment:

> The prediction of the future course of a mental illness is a professional judgment of high responsibility and in some instances it involves a measure of calculated risk. If a liability were imposed on the physician or the State each time the prediction of future course of mental disease was wrong, few releases would ever be made and the hope of recovery and rehabilitation of a vast number of patients would be impeded and frustrated. This is one of the medical and public risks which must be taken on balance, even though it may sometimes result in injury to the patient or others (pp. 496–497).

In *Eanes v. United States* (1969), the court found no negligence in the release of a voluntary patient who attacked his wife on a home visit. It reviewed the value of trial visits as part of a treatment program but cautioned: "But we do suggest that great care and caution should be taken to provide reasonable assurances that the risks involved will not ultimately prove to have been underestimated or miscalculated."

In another early case, the court in *St. George v. State of New York* (1954) held that an "honest error of professional judgment," rather than negligence, which leads to the release of the patient and the subsequent injury of the plaintiff, would not be negligence.

More recently, in *Littleton v. Good Samaritan Hospital* (1988), the Ohio Supreme Court adopted a "professional judgment" rule to determine whether a hospital's clinicians are liable for a patient's injuring another after release. This judgment involves a determination whether the clinician thoroughly evaluated the patient's risk of violence and made a "good-faith decision" that the patient was not at risk, or if the patient was at risk, whether the clinician formulated a good-faith treatment plan which balanced the benefits of release from treatment and the risks of release to the public.

In other cases, plaintiffs have been unsuccessful because they could not prove that their injury was proximately caused by the negligence of the hospital in releasing the patient. In *Doyle v. United States* (1982), a psychiatrist who discharged a patient who killed a security guard was not held to be liable since the killing occurred one month after discharge and 1,000 miles away. In *Harris v. State of Ohio* (1976), the assault of the victim occurred two years after the patient's discharge, and the court ruled that the State Department of Mental Health was not responsible for it.

By statute, many states provide absolute or qualified immunity from suit for negligent release. This is especially likely when the hospital is a state or public hospital, or when the patient is involuntarily hospitalized. For statutory immunity to apply, the defendants must be acting within the scope of their official duties. There may also be a statutory requirement that the decisions made by the clinician to assess the patient's potential violence and to release the patient were "discretionary" rather than "ministerial" in nature. This means that such decisions involved a professional judgment, rather than simply following a discrete rule or regulation which does not involve a professional judgment (e.g., complying with the physician's order to escort the patient). Courts will usually hold that the decisions regarding the assessment and management of violent patients by the senior members of the treatment teams (i.e., physicians and psychologists) are discretionary rather than ministerial. The immunity provisions may apply differently to line staff, professional staff such as physicians, the hospital superintendent, or the state itself. Immunity may not be available if the defendant's acts were considered intentional, wanton, or reckless.

C. When Liability Is Likely

Hospital staff ordinarily emphasize the diagnosis and treatment of psychiatric symptoms in their management of a patient. Staff often prefer to avoid hospitalizing or treating violent patients, especially when the violence appears to be criminal or to be related to a personality disorder or to substance use. Staff may see such patients as untreatable, antisocial, manipulative, frightening, and difficult. Regrettably, this often means that clinicians avoid spending the necessary time with the patient to properly assess his violence potential. It may also mean that clinicians avoid such patients entirely because of the absence of formal or treatable psychiatric symptoms. Many hospital staff view patient violence not as a mental health problem but as a concern for the criminal justice system. Others simply deny the presence or risk of violence and fail to inquire about it. Shunning such patients once they have been admitted to the hospital or failing to take the patient's violence history and potential seriously can set the stage for repeated violence in or out of the hospital and a lawsuit against the hospital staff.

Although mental health professionals are not expected to predict the future behavior of their patients, they are expected to apply the contemporary standard of mental health care in the assessment and management of dangerous individuals. Hospital staff cannot ignore:

1. A patient's repeated and specific threats of violence against an identified or readily identifiable person.
2. A patient's intense anger or rage in the absence of specific threats of violence to another.
3. A patient's violence in the hospital setting.
4. A patient's treatment refractory psychosis with hostility and agitation.
5. A past history of serious violence directed at other persons, whether strangers or intimates.
6. Reports from family members about their fears of the patient's violence.
7. Any combination of these elements in a patient.

Granting passes, home visits, conditional discharge, or absolute discharge to such patients without a careful clinical assessment of their violence potential is inherently risky, even given the remission of other psychiatric symptoms.

D. Avoiding Liability

Staff have many opportunities to reduce the likelihood of patient violence and a subsequent lawsuit for negligent release of a subsequently violent patient. In general, discharge planning begins when the patient is admitted to the hospital. Formulating the discharge plan occurs throughout the patient's hospitalization and is a collaborative effort by a multidisciplinary treatment team, where available. A follow-up appointment is made prior to the patient's discharge when the patient is provided with the clinic or therapist's name and the location, date, and time of the appointment. Ideally, hospital staff then request confirmation of the patient's attendance at the initial appointment or disposition. The extent to which the hospital staff should pursue a released patient who is noncompliant with outpatient treatment varies with the nature and severity of the patient's risk of violence. In cases in which outpatient noncompliance is anticipated, outpatient civil commitment can be considered.

When taking the patient's history both on admission and subsequently, the clinician must determine whether there have been any specific threats or acts of violence in the recent or distant past. Staff must ask the patient directly about this. If the patient has been violent in the past, the clinician must try to ascertain the details of this violence, including its victims, precipitants, methods, context, egosyntonicity or dystonicity, substance use, and relationship to psychiatric symptoms. This information must become known to the treating staff, particularly the people in charge of decision making regarding passes or release. It should not become buried in the chart among the rest of the clinical, administrative, and financial data. There must be a way of bringing this information to the consciousness of the treatment staff and keeping it there.

When there is a documented history of threatened or overt violence, the patient has been violent in the hospital, or the staff has been notified that someone fears harm from the patient, then staff must carefully assess and reassess the risk of the patient's future violence prior to making a decision about a pass or discharge. Repeated interviews with the patient are more likely to result in an accurate evaluation of the patient's potential for violence than a single interview. Such interviews can also focus on the patient's therapeutic alliance with staff in being able to describe his self-control and the factors which impinge on it in either direction. Interviews with others (e.g., family) who have observed the patient on a regular basis outside the structured setting of the hospital are also likely to be valuable. An interdisciplinary treatment staff meeting provides an opportunity to share the views of the various treatment team members about the patient's violence potential and impulsivity, the likelihood of benefit from continued hospitalization, and the patient's anticipated compliance with outpatient treatment. The treating psychiatrist must pay particular attention to the unit staff, who will have the most contact with the patient and may be more likely to know of any ideas, plans, concealments, or manipulations by the patient.

With the easy accessibility to guns in the United States, the clinician must ascertain whether the patient owns or has access to guns and ammunition, threatens to use them in the future, has used them in the past, and is familiar with their use. Even a one-hour pass from a hospital may provide enough opportunity to permit a patient to purchase and use a gun, which of course could be used against an identified victim, the patient, or someone else. In this context, it is sometimes helpful to inform patients that it is a violation of federal law for any person who has been "committed to a mental institution" to possess a firearm or ammunition (18 U.S.C. section 922).

In cases where a court reviews the discharge of a patient, the court must become aware of the relevant data and assessment procedures. Incidents of threatened or overt violence during the hospitalization should be reviewed in the court hearing. In cases where the hospital has the authority to discharge after a certain period but questions remain about the individual's need for treatment, the clinicians can be cautious and seek an extension of the civil commitment. Even if commitment is not ordered, the responsibility for the patient's subsequent behavior can be shifted to the court, provided that the relevant concerns were raised at the hearing.

Consultation with a colleague is as useful in deciding whether to release a potentially violent inpatient as it is in the outpatient duty to protect cases. When uncertain about whether a patient should be given a pass or discharged, the clinician can consult a colleague who is not involved in the case. Here, too, the best consultant is a senior clinician who is experienced with the assessment and management of violent patients. If a formal consultation is to be secured, then the patient should be informed that the staff would like to obtain a consultation from an expert in this area, and the staff should then obtain the patient's consent to the interview. The patient's confidentiality is not breached by sharing the patient's medical record with the consultant under this procedure. The consultant should have the relevant information available through records, social histories, and an interview with the patient. A written consultation report should be obtained which deals specifically with the patient's risk of future violence, the conditions under which it is expected to occur, the available options for the staff, and a recommendation. The value of input from an independent person should not be underestimated.

When the staff decide to authorize any type of release, the reasons for doing so should be specified in the patient's official record. The record should reflect the staff's knowledge of the patient's past violence and his potential for future violence. The record should reflect the reasons the staff consider the likelihood of harm to others to be minimal or nonexistent. These can include the patient's no longer being angry with a potential victim, the absence of violent intention regarding others, the patient's not knowing where the potential victim lives, the inaccessibility of the potential victim, the disposal of weapons, the remission of psychotic symptoms thought to be causally related to past violence, the planned supervision of medication compliance, and the imposition of restrictions on the patient's substance use. When a hospital issues a pass for a patient, the staff should document the purpose and rationale for the pass, where and how the patient will spend his time on the pass, the length of the pass, who will be with the patient during the pass, the need for medication during the pass, and any restrictions (e.g., on place, persons, activities, or substance use).

From the hospital's perspective, it is useful to have a specific hospital policy and procedure regarding the management and release of potentially violent patients. Such a policy would help to ensure that such patients will be treated in a uniform and appropriate manner in accordance with the standard of care. The policy would specify the need for an independent consultation and the manner of obtaining one and would dictate the data base necessary prior to making release decisions. In some situations, or with certain patient populations, it may be useful to require videotaped exit interviews with the patient, to document for posterity the safety of the patient's release.

E. Conclusion

Suits can be brought for negligent release in circumstances when the patient harms himself, another person, or both, after release from a hospital on pass or discharge. The likelihood of success of these lawsuits depends on the extent of the clinician's negligence, the identifiability of the potential victim, the time interval between discharge and harm, the relationship between the discharge and the subsequent injury, and the applicable law of immunity. In its defense of such suits, the hospital needs to be able to show that the patient's progress in treatment, his right to be treated in the least restrictive setting, or his noncommitability mandated his release. Further, hospital staff will need to show that the patient concealed from them his intended injuries to a specific victim, or that they applied the standard of care (i.e., careful clinical judgment) when they assessed the patient's specific threats of harm and risk of future violence prior to giving a pass or discharge. Though the problems faced by therapists in releasing potentially violent patients are similar to those faced when patients are potentially suicidal, the courts appear less likely to be sympathetic to clinicians in the case of the violent patient. In contrast to the outpatient duty to protect cases, the trend in negligent release case law is to not require specific threats against identifiable victims for liability to attach. In addition, the courts are now more likely to challenge medical judgment as a defense against liability and thus to rule in favor of the plaintiffs in negligent release cases than they were in the past, though each case is judged on its merits.

III. LIABILITY FOR MOTOR VEHICLE ACCIDENTS

Motor vehicle accidents are among the most common causes of serious injuries to people and property in our society. Many of our civil courts are occupied with litigating personal injury cases resulting from automobile accidents. It should not be surprising, therefore, that health care professionals have also become defendants when their patients injure third parties in motor vehicle accidents. Of interest here are the accidental, rather than intentional, injuries inflicted by outpatients. Some of these cases of accidental injuries from motor vehicles are litigated on other grounds, such as negligent release from a hospital (e.g., *Petersen v. State of Washington*, 1983). Most litigation against health care professionals in this regard involves institutions and physicians rather than nonphysician clinicians. Such suits are actionable only when the health care professional has a legal duty to a third party.

A variety of situations have presented opportunities for litigation in this area. Suits finding that third party liability could be established include:

1. A physician's negligent failure to perform an adequate physical examination on a truck driver (*Wharton Transport Corporation v. Bridges*, 1980).
2. A physician's negligent failure to diagnose a patient's epilepsy (*Freese v. Lemmon*, 1973, 1978).
3. A physician's negligent failure to warn a bus driver of the side effects of medication (*Kaiser v. Suburban Transportation System*, 1965).
4. A physician's negligent failure to advise an epileptic patient not to operate a motor vehicle (*Duvall v. Goldin*, 1984).
5. A physician's negligent failure to warn a patient about the side effects of a medication which could interfere with the patient's driving (*Schuster v. Altenberg*, 1988).
6. A physician's negligent failure to warn a patient about the side effects of a medication administered in the office (*Wilschinsky v. Medina*, 1989).

A further question in the litigation of these cases is the extent of the health care professional's liability to the general public, as opposed to the liability to a foreseeably injured person. In these cases, there is no identified or identifiable victim, only a member of the general public who is unknown to the professional's patient.

Though the courts in the above cases ruled that the defendant owed a duty to the plaintiff as a member of the general public, other courts have held that there is no such duty of care to a third party, whether specifically identified or not (*Kirk v. Michael Reese Hospital*, 1987; *Purdy v. Public Administrator County of Westchester*, 1988; and *Rebollal v. Payne*, 1988). As in the outpatient duty to protect cases, these courts have reasoned that creation of such a duty would unduly burden health care professionals and add to the "malpractice crisis" faced by society. It would also impose a legal duty to control those in the community whom the professional had no right or ability to control.

In the absence of case law in their state, clinicians will never know whether their state courts will rule in one direction or another with regard to their liability for their patients' motor vehicle accidents. Clinicians' liability in this area may continue to slowly or sporadically expand. Clinicians need to be cognizant that their patients will drive motor vehicles, with or without a driver's license. Clinicians also need to remind themselves that patients become involved in motor vehicle accidents just as the rest of the community does, but that health care professionals are now seen as potential defendants should third-party injuries result. Patients who are commercial truck or bus drivers present special risks in this regard. Bringing a consciousness about such accidents to patient care should be the first step in attempting to limit one's liability in this area. Such attempts should include developing a system for warning patients and families about driving during an acute episode of mental illness, after a diagnosis of some organic mental disorders has been made (e.g., epilepsy or dementia), while on psychotropic medication, or while using medication and alcohol. Referral for formal driving evaluations by rehabilitation institutions or other staff may also be useful in some cases.

Clinicians, especially physicians, should be aware of the mandatory and elective procedures for reporting mental and physical disorders to their state driver's license authority. Some patients refuse to relinquish driving, and risk endangering themselves or others. This risk is evidenced by past automobile accidents attributable to mental or physical disorders, and the likely recurrence of such disorders. Reporting such individuals to the state's licensing authority initiates an investigation into their medical problems and any resulting driving impairment. The state agency, not the clinician, then makes the decision about whether and under what conditions the patient may drive. Immunity to the physician for good-faith reporting of patients to the state agency also obtains. As with any other mandatory reporting situation, the clinician should discuss the need to do so with the patient, and perhaps his family.

IV. MANAGED CARE

A growing percentage of the American public receives health care services through some type of managed health care organization. Managed care refers to those procedures or systems of care used by third-party payors or their fourth-party agents which affect access to, or control, payment for health care. Managed care seeks to provide quality health care while containing its costs. It consists of (1) financial incentives and disincentives to patients (and providers) to use (and provide) a particular system of care; (2) utilization review (prospective, concurrent, retrospective); or (3) case management (e.g., use of gatekeepers to control access to care, or health benefits managers to reduce costs of high service users).

Each participant in managed care has differing perspectives on managed care; this in turn has important liability implications. Clinicians commonly view managed care requirements as intrusions on the therapist–patient relationship and a sacrifice of patients' best health care interests. They fear liability exposure if, for example, continued hospital care is denied by the reviewing agency, and the patient must be discharged prematurely, injuring himself or others. Managed care professionals, on the other hand, argue that peer review improves the quality of health care services, and lowers the risk of liability for adverse outcomes. Patients are often unaware of the need for utilization review of their care, and the standards and procedures by which such review is obtained. Some hospitalized patients have exacerbations when informed of the uncertainty about future care, and the staff's difficulties in attempting to secure it.

In the era of managed care, therapists have legal duties which were nonexistent in the traditional system of fee-for-service health care delivery. Therapists are responsible for providing otherwise confidential information about the patient's diagnosis and treatment to the third-party payor and its agents which is necessary for financial decisions. This could include communicating with the reviewing agency's health care professionals, or providing a complete copy of the patient's mental health records. Therapists, or the institutions where the care is provided, are also responsible for informing patients about the need for such disclosures to occur, as well as any denials of care which ensue. Therapists then need to discuss the available alternatives, including the health care consequences of each, with the patient and family. This process, sometimes referred to as "fiscal informed consent," should be thoroughly documented in the patient's record. Finally, therapists need to assist the patient in securing necessary health care services by, for example, obtaining prior authorization for proposed care, and appealing claims denied for lack of medical necessity. Such appeals may be burdensome and time-consuming to the therapist; absent an appeal, however, a court could conclude that it was the therapist's failure to protest the denial, rather than the denial itself, which was the cause of the subsequent injury to the patient. Therapists will not be able to shift the responsibility for alleged malpractice to the managed care system that denied care which was recommended but not pursued by the treatment staff.

V. COMMONLY ASKED QUESTIONS

1. A patient was involuntarily admitted to the hospital because of a major depressive illness with suicide and homicide threats to his wife. Must the hospital staff warn his wife of his threats to her?

A breach of a hospitalized patient's confidentiality (i.e., a warning without his explicit consent) in such a circumstance is not legally required and may be clinically counterproductive. The hospitalization itself, rather than a warning, here serves as the means to discharge the duty to protect the wife. Of course, in many hospitals, family members are intimately involved in the patient's treatment but the patient may be entitled to refuse this involvement, even if committed. In particular, nothing is accomplished by warning third parties when the patient will be hospitalized for a lengthy period of time and the third party will not be involved in the patient's treatment. In addition, staff are not required to warn family members of the patient's suicide ideation or intent, and patients may refuse staff's request to meet with the wife. Upon the expiration of the initial commitment, if the patient's depression has improved to the point where it is difficult to justify further commitment but homicidal intent persists, then a petition to extend the commitment can be filed with the applicable authority to decide the matter. If the court denies the petition and the patient must be discharged, then a warning to the wife should be contemplated.

2. *A patient who presents to a psychiatric emergency room revealed homicide ideation to the nurse-specialist. Is the nurse required to warn the potential victim?*

A therapist is never specifically required to warn a potential victim about a dangerous patient, but only to protect that victim. The nurse-clinician must first evaluate the patient's risk of violence by assessing the extent, intensity, duration, target, and intent of the homicide ideation. This evaluation includes obtaining a history of prior violence and ascertaining the availability of the victim as well as weapons. Homicide ideation without intent and ability to harm another, or homicide ideation without a significant past history of violence, should not invoke any duty to protect the public. Warning a potential victim in the absence of a significant likelihood of substantial violence is likely to discourage or interfere with ongoing psychiatric treatment, as well as frighten the potential victim.

3. *Is there still a duty to protect third parties when the victim knows the patient and is familiar with the risks of harm, as in a case of family violence?*

Even though a potential victim of a therapist's patient is aware of the risk of violence, whether through a previous violent episode or a prior threat of violence, the therapist may still be obligated to attempt to protect the potential victim. If the patient, for example, presents with an imminent plan to seriously injure the family member, then hospitalization may well be necessary to restrain the patient. If the potential victim has obtained a restraining order or a protection from abuse order against the patient, the police or court could become involved since the patient could be violating that order. Plaintiffs injured by chronically or intermittently violent outpatients have sometimes argued that they were unaware of the most recent exacerbation in the patient's mental condition, or that they would take the threat seriously only if the therapist informed them of it.

4. *A hospital patient tells another patient of his homicide intent once he is discharged, and the second patient so informs the first patient's therapist. What should the therapist do?*

The therapist should directly address this matter with the first patient and assess his risk of violence. The patient may deny it, knowing that he may not be discharged as planned. Continued hospitalization or transfer may be necessary to manage the patient's homicide intent.

5. *An epidemiologist conducting research in a substance abuse clinic learns in a research interview that a husband who found out about his wife's affair has made detailed plans to injure her. The researcher questions whether he has an obligation to the wife.*

Whether a researcher has a legal duty to protect the public from his research subject is an uncertain area of the law. A researcher who has never had personal contact with the subject, or one who has no clinical training, would probably not be expected to do any more than any ordinary person in such a situation. Such intervention might include suggesting that the husband discuss his feelings with his therapist at the clinic. On the other hand, a researcher with clinical training, or one who has had extensive contact with the subject, would be more likely to be expected to have a similar duty to the public as would a therapist for that person. Thus, he would be obligated to protect the wife, using his clinical skills and experience and the usual means used by therapists to protect third parties.

6. *An outpatient informs his therapist that he has killed a woman (a stranger) since the last session. The therapist, hearing of such a homicide from the news media, wonders whether he can or should inform the police about his patient's claim.*

There is typically no legal duty to report the patient's confession to the police, whether it involves a crime of violence or a property crime (e.g., burglary or theft). If the patient refuses to turn himself in to the police and instructs the clinician not to do so under penalty of lawsuit, reporting him to the police will terminate the therapeutic relationship. The therapist needs to assess the patient's risk of continuing danger to society and to hospitalize him if necessary, since the duty to protect potential victims is prospective rather than retrospective in time.

7. *Is a school guidance counselor obligated to protect third parties from his counselees?*

The range of mental health professionals obligated to protect endangered third parties from their clients is broad. Unless there is a state statute which defines what categories of therapists are obligated to protect the public, one can assume that any mental health professional, whether licensed by the state or not, will have this legal duty. There will always be cases at the borderline, such as an unlicensed school counselor without clinical training or experience, which will make new law on the subject if litigated.

8. *A patient reports that a colleague at work has threatened to kill him. What can the therapist do?*

The therapist has no legal duty to protect his client from the world's violence. He might offer practical advice from a psychological perspective about dealing with potentially violent individuals, help the client understand what he may have done to prompt the threat, or suggest the patient contact the police or the employer.

9. *Does the duty to protect third parties apply to those clients who are non-mentally ill such as organized criminal gang members?*

If a person is evaluated and treated by a mental health professional, regardless of the psychiatric diagnosis, then the therapist should assume that the legal duty to protect applies. The strategies for discharging the duty will vary depending upon the diagnosis, since medication or hospitalization will not be appropriate in some cases. As always, there will be questions about whether an identified or identifiable victim is a prerequisite to activating the duty.

10. *A patient threatens to blow up his work supervisor's home. Is the therapist obligated to protect the home?*

The case law is uncertain about the therapist's obligation to protect property.

While there has been litigation regarding property damage from arson, these cases arguably presented a risk to persons as well as property. A court might well find that bombing an individual's house presents a risk to persons, rather than just property, and thus rule that the therapist should have attempted to protect the victim and his family. Though few homicidal threats are ever actualized, the therapist must assess the credibility of the threat and the patient's risk of violence. If the therapist views the threat as significant, then he must take some action.

11. *A therapist at a substance abuse clinic learns that his patient is a school bus driver who continues to drink alcohol despite his participation in the program. What obligations does the therapist have?*

The therapist must assess the patient's risk of an automobile accident through obtaining a detailed history of the patient's alcohol use, his driving record, his driving habits, his insight into his drinking problem and the risks it presents to others, and his therapeutic alliance with the program. If the therapist is satisfied that there is in fact a serious risk of a bus accident with injuries to others, then he is obligated to attempt to prevent it. Some of the options include one or more of the following: involving the patient's family in his treatment, changing the treatment program, terminating him from the program with a referral, informing the school board or the bus company, or reporting his substance abuse disorder to the state driver's licensing bureau. Federal drug regulations may bar a breach of confidentiality (i.e., disclosure without the patient's consent) if the patient is still participating in the program. It may be argued, however, that such a breach of confidentiality is necessary under a public policy argument.

12. *After being refused cafeteria privileges, a voluntarily hospitalized patient threatens to disfigure a nurse on a different shift who is not in the hospital at the time; the patient also demands to be discharged from the hospital immediately. The staff would be happy to be rid of him but are not sure how to proceed.*

Many state mental health codes provide that the staff can temporarily detain a voluntarily hospitalized patient to evaluate the appropriateness of discharge. Even if this course is not legally available, the staff could proceed to convert the patient to an involuntary status on an emergency basis. Staff should attempt to defuse the crisis, evaluate the patient's need for seclusion or medication, and assess his risk of harm to the staff or others. It is not a breach of the patient's confidentiality to inform another member of the staff of the threat, even if the patient did not threaten that person personally. The staff responsible for authorizing passes and discharge should also be made aware of the threat.

13. *An HIV-infected client comes to the emergency room because of depression and angrily adds that he plans to infect the world. What is the therapist's obligation in this matter?*

Confidentiality of health care information is not absolute, even though clients frequently believe it to be so. Mental health law has long recognized an exception for disclosure of confidential information without the patient's consent when he poses an imminent danger to others. Disclosure of HIV-related information may be regulated by a specific state law rather than the mental health code. Generally, disclosure of the risk of violence or injury to third parties should be viewed as a last resort after clinical means of managing the client (e.g., talking down the patient's anger, civil commitment, medication, and referral for outpatient treatment) have been exhausted. Disclosure should be limited to identifiable third parties currently at risk of continued exposure, if any. It may also be possible to notify a public health official charged with the responsibility of controlling infectious disease in the community.

14. An outpatient tells her therapist that her husband is threatening to kill the child protective service worker and testifying physician who had their son removed from their custody due to child abuse. How should the therapist respond?

If only the wife and not the husband is in treatment, then there is no therapist–patient relationship between the therapist and the husband. The therapist would have no legal duty to protect the intended victims from the patient's husband, but only a legal duty to respect the confidentiality of the patient's treatment. The therapist should at least assess the seriousness of the risk of violence by reviewing the issues with the wife and encouraging the wife to respond to the problem (e.g., dissuading him from his threats, referring her husband for treatment, contacting the victims or the police). If the therapist, at the wife's request, becomes involved in directly managing the situation then she could be construed as the husband's therapist and her legal responsibilities to the victims would flow from there.

APPENDIX: AMERICAN PSYCHIATRIC ASSOCIATION'S MODEL STATUTE ON THE PHYSICIAN'S DUTY TO TAKE PRECAUTIONS AGAINST PATIENT VIOLENCE*

Developed by the Council on Psychiatry and Law and approved by the Board of Trustees in June 1987, this resource document does not represent official APA policy but rather is offered as a guide to district branches in those states in which case law has expanded the potential duty to protect liability of psychiatrists.

Duty of [Physicians] to Take Precautions against Patient Violence

1. Scope of cause of action. Except as provided in paragraph 5, no cause of action shall lie against a [physician], nor shall legal liability be imposed, for breaching a duty to prevent harm to person or property caused by a patient unless (a) the patient has communicated to the [physician] an explicit threat to kill or seriously injure a clearly identified or reasonably identifiable victim or victims, or to destroy property under circumstances likely to lead to serious personal injury or death, and the patient has the apparent intent and ability to carry out the threat; and (b) the [physician] fails to take such reasonable precautions to prevent the threatened harm as would be taken by a reasonably prudent [physician] under the same circumstances. Reasonable precautions include, but are not limited to, those specified in paragraph 2.

2. Legally sufficient precautions. Any duty owed by a [physician] to take reasonable precautions to prevent harm threatened by a patient is discharged, as a matter of law, if the [physician] either (a) communicates the threat to any identified

*Statutory approaches to limiting psychiatrists' liability for their patients' violent acts. (1990). *American Journal of Psychiatry, 146*, 821–828. In enacting such a provision, the terms "therapist" or "mental health professional" should be substituted for "physician."

victim or victims; or (b) notifies a law enforcement agency in the vicinity where the patient or any potential victim resides; or (c) arranges for the patient to be hospitalized voluntarily; or (d) takes legally appropriate steps to initiate proceedings for involuntary hospitalization.

3. Immunity for disclosure. Whenever a patient has explicitly threatened to cause serious harm to person or property, or a [physician] otherwise concludes that a patient is likely to do so, and the [physician], for the purpose of reducing the risk of harm, discloses any confidential communications made by or relating to the patient, no cause of action shall lie against the [physician] for making such disclosure.

4. Definitions.

a. For purposes of this [section], "patient" means any person with whom a [physician] has established a [physician]-patient relationship.

b. For purposes of this [section], ["physician"] means a person licensed to practice medicine in this state.

5. Limited applicability of this section. This section does not modify any duty to take precautions or prevent harm by a patient that may arise if the patient is within the custodial responsibility of a hospital or other facility or is being discharged therefrom.

VI. BIBLIOGRAPHY

A. Cases

1. *Outpatient Duty to Protect*

Tarasoff v. Regents of University of California ("Tarasoff I"), 529 P.2d 553 (Cal.Sup.Ct. 1974); ("Tarasoff II"), 551 P.2d 334 (Cal.Sup.Ct. 1976).
McIntosh v. Milano, 403 A.2d 500 (N.J.Super. 1979).
Lipari v. Sears, Roebuck & Co., and United States, 497 F.Supp. 185 (D.Neb. 1980).
Mavroudis v. Superior Court for San Mateo County, 162 Cal.Rptr. 724 (App. 1980).
Shaw v. Glickman, 415 A.2d 625 (Md.App. 1980).
Thompson v. County of Alameda, 614 P.2d 728 (Cal.Sup.Ct. 1980).
Case v. United States, 523 F.Supp. 317 (S.D.Ohio 1981).
Hopewell v. Adebimpe, No. GD78–28756, Civil Division, Court of Common Pleas of Allegheny County, Pennsylvania, June 1, 1981. Reported in Pittsburgh Legal Journal 130:107–109, 1982.
Cairl v. State, 323 N.W.2d 20 (Minn.Sup.Ct. 1982).
Hedlund v. Superior Court of Orange County, 669 P.2d 41 (Cal.Sup.Ct. 1983).
Jablonski by Pahls v. United States, 712 F.2d 391 (9th Cir. 1983).
Brady v. Hopper, 751 F.2d 329 (10th Cir. 1984).
Clark v. State, 472 N.Y.S.2d 170 (A.D. 1984).
Edwards v. Clinton Valley Center, 360 N.W.2d 606 (Mich.App. 1984).
Bauer v. Southwest Denver Mental Health Center, 701 P.2d 114 (Colo.App. 1985).
Peck v. Counseling Service of Addison County, 499 A.2d 422 (Sup.Ct.Vt. 1985).
Bardoni v. Kim, 390 N.W.2d 218 (Mich.App. 1986).
Karash v. County of San Diego, 228 Cal.Rptr. 139 (App. 1986).
McGrady v. United States, 650 F.Supp. 379 (S.C. 1986).
Cooke v. Berlin, 735 P.2d 830 (Ariz.App. 1987).
Hewett v. Kennebec Valley Mental Health Association, 529 A.2d 802 (Sup.Jud.Ct.Me. 1987).
Hinkelman v. Borgess Medical Center, 403 N.W.2d 547 (Mich.App. 1987).
Jackson v. New Center Community Mental Health Services, 404 N.W.2d 688 (Mich.App. 1987).
Paul v. Plymouth General Hospital, 408 N.W.2d 492 (Mich.App. 1987).
Wood on Behalf of Doe v. Astleford, 412 N.W.2d 753 (Minn.App. 1987).
Cantrell v. United States, 735 F.Supp 670 (E.D.N.C. 1988).

Lindsey v. United States, 693 F.Supp. 1012 (W.D.Okl. 1988).
McHale v. Cole, 547 A.2d 485 (Pa.Cmwlth. 1988).
Schuster v. Altenberg, 424 N.W.2d 159 (Sup.Ct.Wis. 1988).
Armijo v. Department of Health and Human Environment, 775 P.2d 1333 (N.M.App. 1989).
Eckhardt v. Kirts, 534 N.E.2d 1339 (Ill.App. 1989).
Hamman v. County of Maricopa, 775 P.2d 1122 (Sup.Ct.Ariz. 1989).
Jenks v. City of West Carrollton, 567 N.E.2d 1338 (Ohio App. 1989).
King v. Smith, 539 So.2d 262 (Sup.Ct.Ala. 1989).
Rogers v. South Carolina Department of Mental Health, 377 S.E.2d 125 (S.C.App. 1989).
Wagshall v. Wagshall, 538 N.Y.S.2d 597 (A.D. 1989).
Barry v. Turek, 267 Cal.Rptr. 553 (Cal.App. 1990).
Dunkel v. Food Service East, Inc. 582 A.2d 1342 (Pa.Super. 1990).
Moye v. United States, 735 F.Supp. 179 (E.D.N.C. 1990).
Onofrio v. Department of Mental Health, 562 N.E.2d 1341 (Mass.Sup.Jud.Ct. 1990).
Boynton v. Burglass, 590 So.2d 446 (Fla.App. 1991).
Smith v. Fishkill Health-Related Center, 572 N.Y.S.2d 762 (A.D. 1991).
Santa Cruz v. Northwest Dade Community Health Center, 590 So.2d 444 (Fla.App. 1991).
Webb v. Jarvis, 575 N.E.2d 922 (Ind.Sup.Ct. 1991).
Ms. B. v. Montgomery County Emergency Service, Inc, 799 F. Supp. 534 (E.D. Pa. 1992).
In re Stilinovich, 479 N.W.2d 731 (Minn.App. 1992). [commitment of HIV-infected man]
Annotation: Liability of one treating mentally afflicted patient for failure to warn or protect third persons threatened by patient, 83 A.L.R.3d 1201.

2. *Negligent Release*

St. George v. State of New York, 127 N.Y.S.2d 147 (A.D. 1954).
Fair v. United States, 234 F.2d 288 (5th Cir. 1956).
Taig v. State of New York, 241 N.Y.S.2d 495 (A.D. 1963).
Underwood v. United States, 356 F.2d 92 (5th Cir. 1966).
Merchants National Bank and Trust Company v. United States, 272 F.Supp. 409 (D.N.D. 1967).
Eanes v. United States, 407 F.2d 823 (4th Cir. 1969).
Greenberg v. Barbour, 322 F.Supp. 745 (E.D.Pa. 1971).
Hicks v. United States, 511 F.2d 407 (D.D.C. 1975).
Homere v. State of New York, 370 N.Y.S.2d 246 (A.D. 1975).
Harris v. State of Ohio, 358 N.E.2d 639 (Ohio 1976).
Semler v. Psychiatric Institute of Washington, D.C., 538 F.2d 121 (4th Cir. 1976).
Ellis v. United States, 484 F.Supp. 4 (D.S.C. 1978).
Johnson v. United States, 576 F.2d 606 (5th Cir. 1978).
Leverett v. State, 399 N.E.2d 106 (Ohio App. 1978).
Williams v. United States, 450 F.Supp. 1040 (D.S.D. 1978).
Burroughs v. Board of Trustees, 377 So.2d 801 (Fla.App. 1979).
Januszko v. State, 391 N.E.2d 297 (Ct.App.N.Y. 1979).
Bellavance v. State, 390 So.2d 422 (Fla.App. 1980).
Knight v. State, 297 N.W.2d 889 (Mich.App. 1980).
Ross v. Central Louisiana State Hospital, 392 So.2d 698 (La.App. 1980).
Thompson v. County of Alameda, 614 P.2d 728 (Cal.Sup.Ct. 1980).
Estate of Mathes v. Ireland, 419 N.E.2d 782 (Ind.App. 1981).
Fuhrmann v. Hattaway, 311 N.W.2d 379 (Mich.App. 1981).
Leedy v. Hartnett, 510 F.Supp. 1125 (M.D.Pa. 1981).
State of Indiana, Department of Mental Health v. Allen, 427 N.E.2d 2 (Ind.App. 1981).
Bowers v. DeVito, 686 F.2d 616 (7th Cir. 1982).
Bradley Center v. Wessner, 296 S.E.2d 693 (Sup.Ct.Ga. 1982).
Cairl v. State, 323 N.W.2d 20 (Minn.Sup.Ct. 1982).
Doyle v. United States, 530 F.Supp. 1278 (C.D.Cal. 1982).
Holmes v. Wampler, 546 F.Supp. 500 (E.D.Va. 1982).
Chrite v. United States, 564 F.Supp. 341 (E.D.Mich. 1983).
Durflinger v. Artiles, 673 P.2d 86 (Sup.Ct.Kan. 1983).
Furr v. Spring Grove State Hospital, 454 A.2d 414 (Md.App. 1983).
Petersen v. State, 671 P.2d 230 (Sup.Ct.Wash. 1983).
Sherrill v. Wilson, 653 S.W.2d 661 (Mo.Sup.Ct. 1983).

Larkins v. Department of Mental Health, 358 N.W.2d 7 (Mich.App. 1984).
Sharpe v. South Carolina Department of Mental Health, 315 S.E.2d 112 (S.C.Sup.Ct. 1984).
Allentown State Hospital v. Gill, 488 A.2d 1211 (Pa.Cmwlth. 1985).
Pangburn v. Saad, 326 S.E.2d 365 (N.C.App. 1985).
Roberts v. Grigsby, 339 S.E.2d 633 (Ga.App. 1985).
Schrempf v. State, 487 N.E.2d 883 (N.Y.Ct.App. 1985).
Bader v. State, 716 P.2d 925 (Wash.App. 1986).
Phillips v. Roy, 494 So.2d 1342 (La.App. 1986).
Soutear v. United States, 646 F.Supp. 524 (E.D.Mich. 1986).
Sanchez v. State of Louisiana Department of Health and Human Resources, 506 So.2d 777 (La.App. 1987).
Swofford v. Cooper, 360 S.E.2d 624 (Ga.App. 1987).
Hinkelman v. Borgess Medical Center, 403 N.W.2d 547 (Mich.App. 1987).
Barnes v. Dale, 530 So.2d 770 (Ala.Sup.Ct. 1988).
Cross v. Lakeview Center, 529 So.2d 307 (Fla.App. 1988).
Evans v. Morehead Clinic, 749 S.W.2d 696 (Ky.App. 1988).
Laird v. Buckley, 539 A.2d 1076 (Sup.Ct.Del. 1988).
Littleton v. Good Samaritan Hospital, 529 N.E.2d 449 (Ohio Sup.Ct. 1988).
Mohan v. Westchester County Medical Center, 535 N.Y.S.2d 431 (A.D. 1988).
Naidu v. Laird, 539 A.2d 1064 (Sup.Ct.Del. 1988).
Weston v. State, 758 P.2d 534 (Wash.App. 1988).
Baldwin v. Hospital Authority of Fulton County, 383 S.E.2d 154 (Ga.App. 1989).
Hokansen v. United States, 868 F.2d 372 (10th Cir. 1989).
Jacobs v. Taylor, 379 S.E.2d 563 (Ga.App. 1989).
Midtown Community Mental Health Center v. Estate of Gahl, 540 N.E.2d 1259 (Ind.App. 1989).
Morton v. Jackson Hospital and Clinic, 548 So.2d 1015 (Ala.Sup.Ct. 1989).
Perreira v. State, 768 P.2d 1198 (Sup.Ct.Colo. 1989).
Sellers v. United States, 870 F.2d 1098 (6th Cir. 1989).
Thomas v. State, 545 So.2d 632 (La.App. 1989).
Goryeb v. Commonwealth, 575 A.2d 545 (Pa.Sup.Ct. 1990).
Hines v. Bick, 566 So.2d 455 (La.App. 1990).
Mahomes-Vinson v. United States, 751 F.Supp. 913 (D.Kan. 1990).
McMillian v. Wallis, 567 So.2d 1199 (Sup.Ct.Ala. 1990).
Morton v. Jackson Hospital and Clinic, Inc., 548 So.2d 1015 (Sup.Ct.Ala. 1990).
Nguyen v. State, 788 P.2d 962 (Sup.Ct.Okl. 1990).
Wofford v. Eastern State Hospital, 795 P.2d 516 (Sup.Ct.Okl. 1990).
Mayer v. United States, 774 F.Supp. 1114 (N.D. Ill. 1991).
Walker v. State, 806 P.2d 249 (Wash.App. 1991).
Annotation: Governmental tort liability for injuries caused by negligently released individual, 6 A.L.R.4th 1155.
Annotation: Liability of governmental officer or entity for failure to warn or notify of release of potentially dangerous individual from custody, 12 A.L.R.4th 722.

3. *Motor Vehicle Injuries*

Kaiser v. Suburban Transportation System, 401 P.2d 350, 398 P.2d 14 (Sup.Ct.Wash. 1965).
Hammontree v. Jenner, 97 Cal.Rptr. 739 (App. 1971).
Freese v. Lemmon, 267 N.W.2d 680 (Sup.Ct.Iowa 1978).
Burroughs v. Board of Trustees, 377 So.2d 801 (Fla.App. 1979).
Watkins v. United States, 589 F.2d 214 (5th Cir. 1979).
Wharton Transport Corporation v. Bridges, 606 S.W.2d 521 (Sup.Ct.Tenn. 1980).
Lopez v. Hudgeons, 171 Cal.Rptr. 527 (App. 1981).
Hasenei v. United States, 541 F.Supp. 999 (D.Md. 1982).
Matter of Estate of Votteler, 327 N.W.2d 759 (Sup.Ct.Iowa 1982).
Davis v. Mangelsdorf, 673 P.2d 951 (Ariz.App. 1983).
Gooden v. Tips, 651 S.W.2d 364 (Tex.App. 1983).
Myers v. Quesenberry, 193 Cal.Rptr. 733 (App. 1983).
Petersen v. State of Washington, 671 P.2d 230 (Sup.Ct.Wash. 1983).
Duvall v. Goldin, 362 N.W.2d 275 (Mich.App. 1984).
Forlaw v. Fitzer, 456 So.2d 432 (Sup.Ct.Fla. 1984).

Anthony v. United States, 616 F.Supp. 156 (S.D.Iowa 1985).
Cartier v. Long Island College Hospital, 490 N.Y.S.2d 602 (A.D. 1985).
Garrison Retirement Home Corp. v. Hancock, 484 So.2d 1257 (Fla.App. 1985).
Welke v. Kuzilla, 375 N.W.2d 403 (Mich.App. 1985).
Cain v. Rijken, 717 P.2d 140 (Sup.Ct.Or. 1986).
Tumelson v. Todhunter, 716 P.2d 890 (Sup.Ct.Wash. 1986).
Joy v. Eastern Maine Medical Center, 529 A.2d 1364 (Sup.Jud.Ct. Me. 1987).
Kirk v. Michael Reese Hospital, 513 N.E.2d 387 (Sup.Ct.Ill. 1987).
Krejci v. Akron Pediatric Neurology, 511 N.E.2d 129 (Ohio App. 1987).
Stebbins v. Concord Wrigley Drugs, 416 N.W.2d 381 (Mich.App. 1987).
Willis v. United States, 666 F.Supp. 892 (W.D.La. 1987).
Johnson Estate v. Condell Memorial Hospital, 520 N.E.2d 37 (Sup.Ct.Ill. 1988).
Laird v. Buckley, 539 A.2d 1076 (Sup.Ct.Del. 1988).
Naidu v. Laird, 539 A.2d 1064 (Sup.Ct.Del. 1988).
Purdy v. Public Administrator of County of Westchester, 526 N.E.2d 4 (Ct.App.N.Y. 1988).
Rebollal v. Payne, 536 N.Y.S.2d 147 (A.D. 1988).
Schuster v. Altenberg, 424 N.W.2d 159 (Sup.Ct.Wis. 1988).
Wilschinsky v. Medina, 775 P.2d 713 (Sup.Ct.N.M. 1989).
Crosby by Crosby v. Sultz, 592 A.2d 1337 (Pa.Super. 1991).
Rollins v. Petersen, 813 P.2d 1156 (Utah S.C. 1991).
Ermutlu v. McCorkle, 416 S.E. 2d 792 (Ga.App. 1992).
Annotation: Liability of physician, for injury to or death of third party, due to failure to disclose driving-related impediment, 43 A.L.R.4th 153.

4. *Managed Care*

O'Neill v. Montefiore Hospital, 202 N.Y.S.2d 436 (A.D. 1960).
Wickline v. State, 228 Cal.Rptr. 661 (App. 1986).
Schleier v. Kaiser Foundation Health Plan, 876 F.2d 174 (D.C.Cir. 1989).
Varol v. Blue Cross and Blue Shield of Michigan, 708 F.Supp. 826 (E.D. Mich. 1989).
Wilson v. Blue Cross of Southern California, 271 Cal.Rptr. 876 (App. 1990).

B. Articles and Books

1. *Duty to Protect and Negligent Release*

Appelbaum, P. S. (1985). *Tarasoff* and the clinician: Problems in fulfilling the duty to protect. *American Journal of Psychiatry, 142,* 425–429.
Appelbaum, P. S. (1988). The new preventive detention: Psychiatry's problematic responsibility for the control of violence. *American Journal of Psychiatry, 145,* 779–785.
Appelbaum, P. S., & Rosenbaum, A. (1989). *Tarasoff* and the researcher: Does the duty to protect apply in the research setting? *American Psychologist, 44,* 885–894.
Appelbaum, P. S., Zonana, H., Bonnie, R., & Roth, L. H. (1989). Statutory approaches to limiting psychiatrists' liability for their patients' violent acts. *American Journal of Psychiatry, 146,* 821–828.
Avins, A. L., & Lo, B. (1989). To tell or not to tell: The ethical dilemmas of HIV test notification in epidemiologic research. *American Journal of Public Health, 79,* 1544–1548.
Beck, J. C. (Ed.). (1985). *The potentially violent patient and the Tarasoff decision in psychiatric practice.* Washington, DC: American Psychiatric Press.
Beck, J. C. (1987). The psychotherapist's duty to protect third parties from harm. *Mental and Physical Disability Law Reporter, 11,* 141–148.
Beck, J. C. (Ed.). (1990). *Confidentiality versus the duty to protect: The risk of foreseeable harm in the practice of psychiatry.* Washington, DC: American Psychiatric Press.
Bobele, M. (1987). Therapeutic interventions in life-threatening situations. *Journal of Marital and Family Therapy, 13,* 225–239.
Brown, J., & Rayne, J. T. (1989). Some ethical considerations in defensive psychiatry: A case study. *American Journal of Orthopsychiatry, 59,* 534–541.
Carlson, G. A., Greeman, M., & McClellan, T. A. (1989). Management of HIV-positive psychiatric patients who fail to reduce high-risk behaviors. *Hospital and Community Psychiatry, 40,* 511–514.
Dickens, B. M. (1986). Legal issues in medical management of violent and threatening patients. *Canadian Journal of Psychiatry, 31,* 772–780.

Feldman, W. S. (1979). Some legal implications of "passes" and "visits." *Journal of Psychiatry and Law, 7,* 93–103.
Felthous, A. R. (1989). *The psychotherapist's duty to warn or protect.* Springfield, IL: Thomas.
Fleming, J. G., & Maximov, B. (1974). The patient or his victim: The therapist's dilemma. *California Law Review, 62,* 1025–1068.
Geske, M. R. (1989). Statutes limiting mental health professionals' liability for the violent acts of their patients. *Indiana Law Journal, 64,* 391–422.
Givelber, D., Bowers, W. J., & Blitch, C. L. (1984). *Tarasoff,* myth and reality: An empirical study of private law in action. *Wisconsin Law Review, 1984,* 443–497.
Goodman, T. A. (1985). From *Tarasoff* to *Hopper*: The evolution of the therapist's duty to protect third parties. *Behavioral Sciences and the Law, 3,* 195–225.
Gostin, L. O. (1990). *AIDS and the health care system.* New Haven: Yale University Press.
Kermani, E. J., & Drob, S. L. (1987). *Tarasoff* decision: A decade later dilemma still faces psychotherapists. *American Journal of Psychotherapy, 41,* 271–285.
Knapp, S., & VandeCreek, L. (1990). Application of the duty to protect to HIV-positive patients. *Professional Psychology: Research and Practice, 21,* 161–166.
Knapp, S., VandeCreek, L., & Shapiro, D. (1990). Statutory remedies to the duty to protect: A reconsideration. *Psychotherapy, 27,* 291–295.
Kroll, J., & Mackenzie, T. B. (1983). When psychiatrists are liable: Risk management and violent patients. *Hospital and Community Psychiatry, 34,* 29–37.
Leonard, J. B. (1977). A therapist's duty to potential victims. *Law and Human Behavior, 1,* 309–317.
Leong, G. B., Eth, S., & Silva, J. A. (1992). The psychotherapist as witness for the prosecution: The criminalization of *Tarasoff. American Journal of Psychiatry, 149,* 1011–1015.
McCarty, C. B. (1989). Patient threats against third parties: The psychotherapist's duty of reasonable care. *Journal of Contemporary Health Law and Policy, 5,* 119–140.
McClarren, G. M. (1987). The psychiatric duty to warn: Walking a tightrope of uncertainty. *Cincinnati Law Review, 56,* 269–293.
Melella, J., Travin, S., & Cullen, K. (1987). The psychotherapist's third-party liability for sexual assaults committed by his patient. *Journal of Psychiatry and Law, 15,* 3–116.
Merton, V. (1982). Confidentiality and the "dangerous" patient: Implications of *Tarasoff* for psychiatrists and lawyers. *Emory Law Journal, 31,* 263–343.
Mills, M. J., Sullivan, G., & Eth, S. (1987). Protecting third parties: A decade after *Tarasoff. American Journal of Psychiatry, 144,* 68–74.
Monahan, J. (in press). Limiting therapist exposure to *Tarasoff* liability: Guidelines for risk containment. *American Psychologist.*
Murphy, J. R., III (1985). In the wake of *Tarasoff:* Mediation and the duty to disclose. *Catholic University Law Review, 35,* 209–243.
Newman, R. S. (1986). The *Tarasoff* progeny: Creating a weaponless policeman with a "deep pocket." *Capital University Law Review, 15,* 699–724.
Perlin, M. L. (1992). *Tarasoff* and the dilemma of the dangerous patient: New directions for the 1990's. *Law and Psychology Review, 16,* 29–63.
Perry, S. (1989). Warning third parties at risk of AIDS: APA's policy is a barrier to treatment. *Hospital and Community Psychiatry, 40,* 158–161.
Poythress, N. G. (1987). Avoiding negligent release: A risk-management strategy. *Hospital and Community Psychiatry, 38,* 1051–1052.
Poythress, N. G. (1990). Avoiding negligent release: Contemporary clinical and risk management strategies. *American Journal of Psychiatry, 147,* 994–997.
Poythress, N. G., & Brodsky, S. L. (1992). In the wake of a negligent release law suit. *Law and Human Behavior, 16,* 155–173.
Price, D. P. T. (1990). Between Scylla and Charybdis: Charting a course to reconcile the duty of confidentiality and the duty to warn in the AIDS context. *Dickinson Law Review, 94,* 435–487.
Roth, L. H., & Meisel, A. (1977). Dangerousness, confidentiality, and the duty to warn. *American Journal of Psychiatry, 134,* 508–511.
Rubin, J. (1987). Mental health professionals and the duty to warn: An economic analysis. *International Journal of Law and Psychiatry, 10,* 311–337.
Schopp, R. F. (1991). The psychotherapist's duty to protect the public: The appropriate standard and the foundation in legal theory and empirical premises. *Nebraska Law Review, 70,* 327–360.
Schwartzbaum, J. A., Wheat, J. R., & Norton, R. W. (1990). Physician breach of patient confidentiality among individuals with human immunodeficiency virus (HIV) infection: Patterns of decision. *American Journal of Public Health, 80,* 829–834.
Slovenko, R. (1988). The therapist's duty to warn or protect third persons. *Journal of Psychiatry and Law, 16,* 139–209.

Sonkin, D. J., & Ellison, J. E. (1986). The therapist's duty to protect victims of domestic violence: Where we have been and where we are going. *Victims and Violence, 1,* 205–214.
Stone, A. A. (1976). The *Tarasoff* decisions: Suing psychotherapists to safeguard society. *Harvard Law Review, 90,* 358–378.
Stone, A. A. (1986). Vermont adopts *Tarasoff:* A real barn-burner. *American Journal of Psychiatry, 143,* 352–355.
Taylor, L., & Adelman, H. S. (1989). Reframing the confidentiality dilemma to work in children's best interests. *Professional Psychology: Research and Practice, 20,* 79–83.
Travin, S., & Bluestone, H. (1987). Discharging the violent psychiatric inpatient. *Journal of Forensic Sciences, 32,* 999–1008.
Treadway, J. (1990). *Tarasoff* in the therapeutic setting. *Hospital and Community Psychiatry, 41,* 88–89.
Turkington, R. C. (1989). Confidentiality policy for HIV-related information: An analytical framework for sorting out hard and easy cases. *Villanova Law Review, 34,* 871–908.
VandeCreek, L., Knapp, S., & Herzog, C. (1987). Malpractice risks in the treatment of dangerous patients. *Psychotherapy, 24,* 145–153.
Weinstock, R. (1988). Confidentiality and the new duty to protect: The therapist's dilemma. *Hospital and Community Psychiatry, 39,* 607–609.
Wettstein, R. M. (1984). The prediction of violent behavior and the duty to protect third parties. *Behavioral Sciences and the Law, 2,* 291–317.
Wexler, D. B. (1979). Patients, therapists, and third parties: The victimological virtues of *Tarasoff. International Journal of Law and Psychiatry, 2,* 1–28.
Winslade, W. J. (1981). Psychotherapeutic discretion and judicial decision: A case of enigmatic justice. In S. F. Spicker, J. M. Healey, & H. T. Engerlhardt (Eds.), *The law-medicine relation: A philosophical exploration.* Dordrecht: D. Reidel.
Wise, T. P. (1978). Where the public peril begins: A survey of psychotherapists to determine the effects of *Tarasoff. Stanford Law Review, 31,* 165–190.
Wulsin, L. R., Bursztajn, H., & Gutheil, T. G. (1983). Unexpected clinical features of the *Tarasoff* decision: The therapeutic alliance and the "duty to warn." *American Journal of Psychiatry, 140,* 601–603.
Zonana, H. (1989). Warning third parties at risk of AIDS: APA's policy is a reasonable approach. *Hospital and Community Psychiatry, 40,* 162–164.

2. *Psychiatric Aspects of Motor Vehicle Accidents*

Carr, D., Jackson, T., & Alquire, P. (1990). Characteristics of an elderly driving population referred to a geriatric assessment center. *Journal of the American Geriatrics Society, 38,* 1145–1150.
Carr, D., Schmader, K., Bergman, C., Simon, T. C., Jackson, T. W., Haviland, S., & O'Brien, J. (1991). A multidisciplinary approach in the evaluation of demented drivers referred to geriatric assessment centers. *Journal of the American Geriatrics Society, 39,* 1132–1136.
Cushman, L. A., Good, R. G., & States, J. D. (1990). Psychiatric disorders and motor vehicle accidents. *Psychological Reports, 67,* 483–489.
Dubinsky, R. M., Gray, C., Husted, D., Busenbark, K., Vetere-Overfield, B., Wiltfong, D., Parrish, D., & Koller, W. C. (1991). Driving in Parkinson's Disease. *Neurology, 41,* 517–520.
Gilley, D. W., Wilson, R. S., Bennett, D. A., Stebbins, G. T., Bernard, B. A., Whalen, M. E., & Fox, J. H. (1991). Cessation of driving and unsafe motor vehicle operation by dementia patients. *Archives of Internal Medicine, 151,* 941–946.
Hansotia, P., & Broste, S. K. (1991). The effect of epilepsy or diabetes mellitus on the risk of automobile accidents. *New England Journal of Medicine, 324,* 22–26.
Krumholz, A., Fisher, R. S., Lesser, R. P., & Hauser, W. A. (1991). Driving and epilepsy: A review and reappraisal. *Journal of the American Medical Association, 265,* 622–626.
Oster, G., Huse, D. M., Adams, S. F., Imbibo, J., & Russell, M. W. (1990). Benzodiazepine tranquilizers and the risk of accidental injury. *American Journal of Public Health, 80,* 1467–1470.
Reuben, D. B., Silliman, R. A., & Traines, M. (1988). The aging driver: Medicine, policy, and ethics. *Journal of the American Geriatrics Society, 36,* 1135–1142.
Simel, D. L., & Feussner, J. R. (1990). Driving-impaired patients leaving the emergency department. *Annals of Internal Medicine, 112,* 365–370.
Tsuang, M. T., Boor, M., & Fleming, J. A. (1985). Psychiatric aspects of traffic accidents. *American Journal of Psychiatry, 142,* 538–546.
Underwood, M. (1992). The older driver: Clinical assessment and injury prevention. *Archives of Internal Medicine, 152,* 735–740.

U.S. Department of Transportation, Federal Highway Administration. (1991). *Conference on psychiatric disorders and commercial drivers* (Pub. No. FHWA-MC-91–006). Washington, DC.

3. *Managed Care*

Chittenden, W. A. (1991). Malpractice liability and managed health care: History and prognosis. *Tort and Insurance Law Journal, 26,* 451–496.
Hinden, R. A., & Elden, D. L. (1990). Liability issues for managed care entities. *Seton Hall Legislative Journal, 14,* 1–63.
Hirshfeld, E. B. (1990). Economic considerations in treatment decisions and the standard of care in medical malpractice litigation. *Journal of the American Medical Association, 264,* 2004–2012.
Morreim, E. H. (1992). Whodunit? Causal responsibility of utilization review for physicians' decisions, patients' outcomes. *Law, Medicine, and Health Care, 20,* 40–56.
Newman, N., & Bricklin, P. M. (1991). Parameters of managed mental health care: Legal, ethical, and professional guidelines. *Professional Psychology: Research and Practice, 22,* 26–35.
Schessler, C. E. (1992). Liability implications of utilization review as a cost containment mechanism. *Journal of Contemporary Health Law and Policy, 8,* 379–406.

4. *Assessment of Dangerousness*

See "Risk Assessments of Violence" in Bibliography of Chapter 3, pp. 77–78.

Table 8.1. Duty to Protect Cases (Legal Citations Provided Above in Reference Section)

Tarasoff v. Regents of University of California ("Tarasoff II")
STATE AND DATE: California, 1976
VICTIM: Acquaintance
CASE: Outpatient at a university counseling center informed his therapist of his intention to kill the victim, without specifically naming her, and was taken into police custody but released. He killed her two months later.
OPINION: A therapist has a duty to use reasonable care to protect an intended victim against his patient, if he determines or should determine that his patient "presents a serious danger of violence."

McIntosh v. Milano
STATE AND DATE: New Jersey, 1979
VICTIM: Ex-girlfriend
CASE: A 17-year-old in outpatient treatment for two years for an adjustment reaction and substance abuse fatally shot his ex-girlfriend, five years older. The patient had never threatened to injure her but had once fired a BB gun at her or her boyfriend's car in jealousy, and carried a knife with him for protection. Plaintiff argued that defendant should have known of the risk to the victim.
OPINION: A therapist has a duty to protect an identified member of the public from a patient who presents a "probability of danger." The physician prevailed at the malpractice trial.

Thompson v. County of Alameda
STATE AND DATE: California, 1980
VICTIM: Five-year-old boy stranger
CASE: Juvenile delinquent inmate killed a child one day after release from custody after threatening to kill an unspecified child in the community.
OPINION: There is no liability by parole officials for failing to warn police or the victim's mother of the release of an inmate without a specified victim.

Lipari v. Sears, Roebuck & Co., and United States
STATE AND DATE: Nebraska, 1980
VICTIM: Strangers
CASE: Former Veterans Administration outpatient, who had withdrawn from treatment one month earlier, opened fire with a shotgun in a nightclub. He had purchased the weapon while still in treatment.

(continued)

Table 8.1. (*Continued*)

OPINION: Therapist is required to do that which is "reasonably necessary to protect potential victims of his patient." The legal duty is limited to foreseeable victims or class of victims. The plaintiff is not required to prove that the defendant knew the identity of the victim.

Cairl v. Minnesota
STATE AND DATE: Minnesota, 1982
VICTIM: Two sisters and apartment complex
CASE: Delinquent, mentally retarded 16 year-old was released on two-week holiday home visit from state facility, and set fire to mother's apartment killing one sister and injuring another.
OPINION: Duty to warn third parties only exists "when specific threats are made against specific victims." The client made no specific threats, and mother was aware of her son's previous firesetting.

In the Matter of Estate of Votteler
STATE AND DATE: Iowa, 1982
VICTIM: Estranged husband's lover
CASE: Outpatient assaulted plaintiff by driving automobile over her causing fatal injuries. Patient had previously threatened plaintiff and twice attempted to run her and the patient's husband down with an automobile.
OPINION: There is no duty to protect third parties when the foreseeable victim already knows of the danger from the patient.

Hedlund v. Superior Court of Orange County
STATE AND DATE: California, 1983
VICTIM: Five-year-old boy, son of girlfriend
CASE: Outpatient shot and injuried girlfriend with a shotgun. She threw herself over her son, seated next to her, to protect him, but he suffered emotional injuries.
OPINION: It was foreseeable that the patient posed a risk of harm to bystanders and those in close relationships with the intended victim such as the son.

Brady v. Hopper
STATE AND DATE: Colorado, 1984
VICTIM: U.S. President's press secretary
CASE: John Hinckley, Jr., in outpatient treatment with Dr. Hopper, shot James Brady.
OPINION: Under Colorado law, a psychiatrist has no duty to protect a third party from his outpatient unless the patient threatens a specific person. The plaintiff's injuries were not foreseeable.

Peck v. Counseling Service of Addison County
STATE AND DATE: Vermont, 1985
VICTIM: Barn
CASE: A 29-year-old client at a counseling center set fire to his parents' barn following an argument with his father. He had a history of impulsive assaultive behavior.
OPINION: Counseling center knew or should have known that the client presented an unreasonable risk of harm to his parents, and thus had the duty to warn parents of his earlier threat to do so. The therapist acted without adequate information about the client or consultation with other staff.

Schuster v. Altenberg
STATE AND DATE: Wisconsin, 1988
VICTIM: Patient's adult daughter
CASE: Outpatient with manic depression was a driver in a fatal automobile collision in which her daughter, a passenger, was injured.
OPINION: Therapist could be held liable for failing to warn the patient of the side effects of medication, including a caution against driving, when an accident with harm to the patient and third parties is foreseeable. A therapist has a duty to warn a potential victim or institute commitment proceedings even in the absence of threats to an identifiable target.

Hamman v. Maricopa
STATE AND DATE: Arizona, 1989
VICTIM: Stepfather

(*continued*)

Table 8.1. (*Continued*)

CASE: A son with schizophrenia assaulted his stepfather two days after an outpatient psychiatric evaluation.
OPINION: The psychiatrist has a duty to exercise reasonable care to protect the foreseeable victim of danger. The foreseeable victim is one who is within the zone of danger, that is, subject to a probable risk of the patient's violent conduct, even in the absence of a specific threat to the victim.

Boynton v. Burglass
STATE AND DATE: Florida, 1991
VICTIM: Acquaintance
CASE: Outpatient shot and killed victim, possibly motivated by jealousy over a mutually known female.
OPINION: Psychiatrist has no duty to control a voluntary outpatient or to warn victim that patient posed a threat to him.

Table 8.2. Negligent Release Cases (Legal Citations Provided Above in Reference Section)

Underwood v. United States
STATE AND DATE: Alabama, 1966
VICTIM: Ex-wife
CASE: Using a military weapon, an Air Force officer shot and killed his ex-wife 20 days after release from hospitalization in a military facility.
OPINION: Air Force was aware of the risk of violence that the patient posed to former wife but did not transmit the information to the discharging physician. He was negligently returned to duty without restrictions on his access to weapons.

Merchants National Bank & Trust v. United States
STATE AND DATE: North Dakota, 1967
VICTIM: Wife
CASE: Husband attempted to run his wife down and then shot and killed her 13 days after release from involuntary hospitalization.
OPINION: VA liable for discharge which lead to wife's death due to failure to diagnose the patient's delusional disorder and recognize his risk of violence.

Semler v. Psychiatric Institute of Washington, D.C.
STATE AND DATE: Virginia, 1976
VICTIM: Girl, stranger
CASE: One month after release from a partial hospitalization program, a man killed the victim. He was on probation for previously abducting a young girl, and had a history of molesting other girls.
OPINION: Hospital and probation officer held liable for not following court order to obtain court approval before discharge from treatment.

Janusko v. State
STATE AND DATE: New York, 1979
VICTIM: Girl, stranger
CASE: The patient fatally stabbed a girl five months after release from a state hospital.
OPINION: The state was not liable for death of the child because the homicide was not foreseeable at the time of discharge. Any negligence by the state was not the proximate cause of the girl's death.

Bradley Center v. Wessner
STATE AND DATE: Georgia, 1982
VICTIM: Wife
CASE: While on an unrestricted weekend pass during a voluntary hospitalization, the patient shot and killed his wife and her lover. He had made several violent threats within the week prior to this.
OPINION: Jury verdict for plaintiffs was upheld because hospital failed to exercise control over the patient they knew, or should have known, was likely to be violent to his wife and her lover.

(*continued*)

Table 8.2. (*Continued*)

Petersen v. State of Washington
STATE AND DATE: Washington, 1983
VICTIM: Stranger
CASE: Five days after release from an involuntary hospitalization for a drug-induced psychosis, the patient drove through a red light at excessive speed and injured plaintiff.
OPINION: Hospital was liable for not taking reasonable precautions to protect foreseeably endangered persons, including seeking recommitment, when they should have known of patient's potential violence while under the influence of drugs.

Novak v. Rathnam
STATE AND DATE: Illinois, 1987
VICTIM: Stranger
CASE: Fourteen months following discharge from an involuntary hospitalization in Illinois, a man with chronic schizophrenia shot and killed the victim in an armed robbery in Florida.
OPINION: The patient's release from the hospital and the subsequent homicide were "too far removed in time to establish the requisite causal connection" between them.

Littleton v. Good Samaritan Hospital
STATE AND DATE: Ohio, 1988
VICTIM: Infant daughter
CASE: A woman in a post-partum depression administered a fatal overdose of aspirin to her two-and-one-half-month-old daughter fourteen days after her discharge from a voluntary hospitalization.
OPINION: The court adopted the "professional judgment" rule to apply in those cases in which there are no professional standards by which to evaluate the defendant's conduct: The psychiatrist "must exercise good faith judgment based on a thorough evaluation of all relevant factors."

Naidu v. Laird
STATE AND DATE: Delaware, 1988
VICTIM: Stranger
CASE: Five months after his release from a voluntary state hospitalization, a man with chronic paranoid schizophrenia deliberately drove his car into the victim, who died.
OPINION: Jury verdict for plaintiff finding gross negligence was proper given evidence that defendant psychiatrist failed to take reasonable precautions to protect potential victims such as extending commitment, referral to an outpatient program, or monitoring medication compliance after release.

Perreira v. State of Colorado
STATE AND DATE: Colorado, 1989
VICTIM: Police officer on duty
CASE: Victim fatally shot four months following the release from involuntary hospitalization of a patient with chronic paranoid schizophrenia who had refused antipsychotic medication during hospitalization.
OPINION: The treating psychiatrist of an involuntarily hospitalized patient has a duty of due care in determining whether to release the patient from commitment. The duty can be discharged by extending the commitment or placing restrictions and conditions on the patient's release, such as petitioning for an order prohibiting the patient to have access to weapons.

9

Competency and Guardianship

I. Types of Competency • II. Impact of Competency in the Treatment Setting • A. Competence to Consent to Health Care • B. Competency Evaluations • C. Competency Standards • D. When the Person Is Decisionally Incapacitated • **III. Court Proceedings for Adjudicating Incompetence** • A. Definition of Incompetence • B. Initiating Proceedings • C. Rights at the Hearing • D. Role of the Mental Health Professional • E. Finding of Incompetency • **IV. Rights Affected by Being Declared Incompetent** • A. Incompetent as to the Estate • B. Incompetent as to the Person • **V. Appointment of a Guardian •** A. Selection of the Guardian • B. The Guardian's Authority • C. Surrogate Decision Making: Principles and Practices • **VI. Dealing with the Guardian in the Treatment Setting • VII. Restoration to Competency • VIII. Other Protective Devices •** A. Representative Payee • B. Adult Protective Services • C. Elder Abuse Reporting • D. Public Guardian • E. Advance Directives • F. Surrogate Consent Law • **IX. Conclusion • X. Commonly Asked Questions • XI. Bibliography**

By itself, the concept of competency is one that we rarely think about. It is only when doubt arises about someone's mental ability to make rational decisions regarding his person or property that decisions about competency become important to us. The law presumes that adults are competent to manage their personal lives and their finances. In contrast, those under 18 years of age are deemed "minors" and for most purposes are considered legally incompetent. Competency forms the basis for being able to exercise our legal rights. These cover a wide range of areas, from personal decision making, such as marriage and refusal of treatment, to commercial transactions, such as purchasing a home. Legal competence serves as the foundation for participating in a variety of activities sanctioned by law, ranging from voting for elected officials to holding a professional license. One form of legal competence is required to participate in the trial process as a defendant and another to participate as a witness in court.

A legal declaration of incompetency restricts or negates an individual's decision-making authority. Many of the rights we take for granted are routinely denied to incompetent persons. A declaration of incompetency means that a court has determined that the person does not have the necessary mental or physical capacity to make decisions regarding his property and/or his person. This finding is designed to protect the mentally or physically disabled person from himself as well as others.

Legal competence and incompetence have a long history. As early as the first century B.C., the Romans had a mechanism for protecting the property of the mentally disabled. During the medieval period, this responsibility fell to the lord of the manor. In colonial America, many colonies enacted laws which provided the means to protect the property of those deemed mentally incapable. These laws were based on the notion that the "insane" or "idiots" should not become burdens on the community, and their assets should be protected for the sake of their heirs. From this concept developed the notion of guardianship. The guardian became the person responsible for making decisions on behalf of the incompetent person (the "ward").

Because a declaration of incompetence has such a substantial impact on the person, a number of legal protections are afforded before a person can be adjudicated incompetent. The appointment of a guardian and a delineation of his duties are the state's means of providing a substitute decision maker. The trend in the law, but not always the practice, is to limit the authority of the guardian to those areas in which the incapacitated person does not have the ability to make rational decisions. Courts retain jurisdiction over the case beyond the adjudication of incompetency so they can intervene when necessary for the protection of the incompetent.

For mental health professionals, legal competence is a more frequent concern. Competence is often a problematic concept when one is dealing with mentally disabled persons. There may be uncertainty about the point at which the patient's mental disorder interferes with his ability to make a rational decision. This is important whenever informed consent to health care is required. By state law, informed consent is required for medical and psychiatric treatment and is also necessary to participate in a research program (see Chapter 5).

This chapter will discuss legal competence, competency evaluations, and guardianship. It will emphasize the impact of these concepts in the treatment setting. The legal mechanisms for declaring someone incompetent and the impact of that declaration are described. The powers and duties of the guardian are also discussed. The chapter concludes with a discussion of how a person is restored to competency, and other protective devices used for those who are incapable of making and implementing decisions.

I. TYPES OF COMPETENCY

For present purposes, we will consider two overall types of competence: legal competence and clinical competence. Legal competence signifies that the person has not been declared incompetent by a court of law. All adults are presumed to be legally competent, and they remain so until formally determined to be incompetent. Children are legally incompetent for most purposes, while adolescents are granted some legal competencies in health care decision making. Legal competence is a binary concept; a person is either legally competent or legally incompetent. Every state has a procedure for declaring a person legally incompetent, which is based on a court's finding that the individual is incapable of managing his assets, unable to make personal decisions regarding his care and welfare, or unable to perform in some other sphere. The underlying reasons for adjudicating incompetence include mental disorder (including substance abuse), mental retardation, physical handicap, or severe medical disorders. Few mentally ill persons have been declared legally incompetent; most mentally ill persons are capable, when their illness is under control, of making decisions related to their welfare. Many severely or profoundly retarded individuals have been declared incompetent upon becoming adults. Upon an adjudication of incompetence, the court-appointed guardian becomes the decision maker for the incapacitated person.

In the past, civil commitment to a mental hospital resulted in, or was equivalent to, a declaration of incompetence and a loss of one's civil rights. Upon release from the hospital, legal competence was automatically restored. Today, almost all state mental health codes specifically provide that an involuntarily hospitalized person remains legally competent to perform all his responsibilities unless determined to be incompetent in a separate hearing. Unfortunately, there appear to be some people in the community who were committed decades ago, who, through oversight or flaws in the law, have not been restored to competence. In those cases, if the person has been functioning in the community for some period of time, he should be presumed competent even if there is no indication that his legal competence was ever in fact restored.

Thus, the law presumes that an adult is competent in all spheres until declared incompetent by a court. Only then is the person legally incompetent, and then only in those areas of functioning specifically adjudicated as such. Except in the case of temporary guardianships, in which the period of incompetence expires after a defined interval, another court proceeding is necessary to restore the legally incompetent ward's decision-making authority.

There are a variety of legal competencies which are specified by the law, both civil and criminal. Specific civil competencies include the competence to consent to medical care, consent to psychiatric care, manage personal affairs, manage financial affairs, contract, vote, drive, marry and divorce, parent a child, function in an occupational or professional capacity, testify in court, sue and be sued, and write a will. Specific criminal competencies include the competence to act as one's own attorney, confess, plead, testify in one's own behalf, stand trial, be sentenced, and be executed. The law defines and distinguishes each specific legal competence from the others; incompetence in one sphere does not necessarily indicate incompetence in another. A court may adjudicate someone to be globally incompetent or incompetent only in certain areas of functioning.

In contrast, clinical competence is not quite so straightforward. Clinical competence, preferably referred to as *decision-making capacity*, simply means that the person is capable of performing a task. The person is expected to understand his current situation, as well as the proposed changes or interventions, and to share this understanding with others. He therefore must have a level of cognitive functioning which renders him able to understand the consequences of his decisions, as well as to communicate them to others. Though there are no degrees of legal competence in that the person is either legally competent or legally incompetent, clinical decision-making capacity is variable in degree. A person can have different levels or degrees of ability to function in a particular area, which are not fixed over time and situation. A person who is considered "competent" may be said to have a sufficient, or threshold amount of, capacity to perform a given task under specified circumstances.

There are many people who are legally competent but who are decisionally incapacitated, at least to various degrees. Adolescents, for example, may be considered clinically competent in some spheres of life but are not legally recognized as competent. A clinician's judgment of functional incapacity may result in petitioning a court for an adjudication of incompetence and the appointment of a legal guardian. Even without a judicial declaration of incompetence, a clinician's judgment of functional incapacity will have a significant impact in the treatment setting, often resulting in a family member's acting as surrogate decision maker for the patient.

II. IMPACT OF COMPETENCY IN THE TREATMENT SETTING

A. Competence to Consent to Health Care

There are a variety of specific legal competencies in the context of health-care decision making. These include competence both to consent to and to refuse recommended care: diagnostic procedures (e.g., biopsy), medical hospitalization, specific interventions such as cancer chemotherapy or surgery, nursing-home care, and medical research. For psychiatric care, these competencies usually include the competence to consent to, or refuse, hospitalization, psychotropic medication, electroconvulsive therapy (ECT), or to participate in research. These various legal competencies may be specifically defined by statute, regulation, or case law.

In medical settings, mental health professionals are usually consulted by the hospital or clinic staff when a patient refuses a recommended diagnostic procedure, form of treatment, placement in a nursing care facility, or is a management problem in some way. Consultations also occur when the staff have doubts about the patient's capacity to consent to medical care or when the patient and family members disagree about the proposed treatment. Thus, requests for mental health consultation in hospitals and clinics are often requests for capacity or competency evaluations, which in turn are requests for permission to force treatment on a refusing patient.

In mental health care settings, clinicians perform capacity assessments on their own patients. These occur on an informal basis during the course of the day-to-day work with the patient. Clinicians also perform formal capacity assessments which occur when a question is raised about the patient's decision-making capacity on the informal assessment. Clinicians may also act as independent consultants charged with performing capacity assessments for patients of other clinicians.

B. Competency Evaluations

Legal competency evaluations are often difficult determinations involving matters which are unfamiliar to treating clinicians. They are time consuming, and require some familiarity with the relevant law. Though similar to consultations performed by consultation–liaison clinicians, there are important differences. Several general recommendations for performing evaluations of legal competence can be offered, whatever the specific legal competence at issue (health care, independent living, finances, parenting, etc.). These procedures are summarized in Table 9.1.

1. Obtain the informed consent of the patient or evaluee prior to beginning the assessment. This is especially important if the evaluee is not in treatment with the evaluator. The evaluee should be informed of the reason for the assessment, the procedures involved, and the use of the information obtained, including its nonconfidentiality if applicable. If the evaluation is court-ordered, then the evaluee should be told this.

Table 9.1. Competency Assessment Procedures

Obtain informed consent to the evaluation.
Evaluate on more than one occasion.
Become familiar with the relevant issues of the competency area.
Know the legal definition and criteria for competency.
Witness information being provided to the evaluee and ensure its adequacy.
Consider the effect of the evaluation setting on the evaluee.
Assess the evaluee's personal values and goals.
Consider the effect of the evaluator on the evaluee.
Invite reassuring third parties into the room.
Pose hypothetical questions to the evaluee.
Perform a functional assessment.
Use structured functional assessment inventories, using information provided by third parties.
Evaluate performance under the conditions relevant to the competency.
Conduct a multidisciplinary evaluation.
Observe functioning and performance rather than infer it.
Assess the reason and the rationale for the patient's decision.
Consider the affective and cognitive dimensions of decision making.
Defer the ultimate competency decision to the court.

2. Evaluate capacity over a period of time. Capacities fluctuate over time. A person may have impaired decision-making capacity one day and little or no impairment another day, whether because of delirium, fatigue, mood alteration, or other problems. Two shorter evaluations are often preferable to one longer one.

3. Become familiar with the specific functional abilities and behaviors that are relevant to the legal competence at issue. If the evaluator is not familiar with the content issues at stake (e.g., the nature of the treatment, its risks, benefits, and alternatives), then he will be unable to properly assess the evaluee's capacities in this regard. Each legal competency is distinguishable from every other. Few clinicians are knowledgeable about the content matters for the entire range of legal competencies, whether they are in health care (e.g., cancer chemotherapy) or financial matters (e.g., contracts, estates, and trusts).

4. Know the law's definition and criteria for the specific legal competence at issue.

5. Make sure that the evaluee has been adequately informed about the proposed intervention or issue. If the treating physician has not informed the patient about the nature, benefits, and risks of a potential treatment, then the competency evaluator will not be able to assess the evaluee's capacity to consent to, or refuse, it. If possible, the evaluator should be present during the presentation of this information to the evaluee.

6. Consider the effect of the setting of the evaluation on the evaluee's performance. An evaluee may perform better in a familiar environment, such as his own home, than in the office or a hospital. In addition, conditions such as noise or crowds in the interview room may be significant in reducing the evaluee's performance and may thus result in an inaccurate conclusion about functional capacity.

7. Obtain a values history from the evaluee, family members, or service providers. Capacity assessments and competency determinations are not value free. Differing professional opinions about an evaluee's capacities and needs sometimes occur because of disagreement or uncertainty about the person's personal values. It is important to consider the evaluee's prior attitudes and beliefs, cultural and moral values, personal goals, and behavior with regard to the specific competency at issue; the present decision making should be consistent with the values history. Evidence of these is the person's past health care compliance, refusal of treatment, tolerance for pain and disability, expressions of individual autonomy and self-determination, and importance of spending versus saving money.

8. Consider the effect of the evaluator on the evaluee. Capacity determinations are a dyadic process; an evaluee may be more or less capable with one clinician than another. Evaluators from different racial, religious, or socioeconomic backgrounds from the evaluee may have difficulty assessing his responses to questions. Patients of certain religious or social-cultural groups have attitudes and values about health care which differ from those of the rest of Western society.

9. Invite a third person into the assessment room. The presence of a family member, friend, or nurse may be comforting to an elderly, distrusting, or disabled evaluee and may enhance his performance, so that a more accurate assessment is obtained.

10. Ask the evaluee counterfactual or hypothetical questions. This approach is especially useful in the medical setting when dealing with a patient who refuses treatment because of denial of illness. Examples include "What would you do if you really did have a gangrenous foot?" and "What should someone else do if they really did have a gangrenous foot?"

11. Perform functional assessments rather than diagnostic ones. Competency evaluations differ in fundamental respects from ordinary psychiatric or psychological assessments, which usually attempt to identify symptoms, establish a diagnosis, clarify the course of a mental disorder, or formulate a treatment plan. The presence of psychiatric symptoms (disorientation, amnesia, thought disorder, delusion, or hallucination) or a psychiatric disorder (psychosis, dementia, or major depression) alone does not mean that the person is thereby clinically or legally incompetent. Certainly, any substantial mental disorder (whether of thought, mood, or behavior) can interfere with decision-making capacity. While evaluations for legal competence include these issues, they are mainly concerned with assessing the functional performance of the individual as a result of any possible mental disorder. Thus, these evaluations are referred to as *functional status* or *behavioral assessments*. Such behavioral assessments include feeding, grooming, self-care, clothing, housekeeping, physical functioning, sensory functioning, telephoning, managing money, and social interaction.

12. Use functional assessment instruments. A patient's functional status can be measured in several ways:

a. By interviewing the patient.
b. By interviewing the caregiver.
c. By observing the patient's performance (at home, office, or hospital).
d. By administering structured measures of performance.

A variety of functional assessment inventories are available to assist in performing legal competency evaluations. These are not competency "tests" *per se*, but they provide a structured means of obtaining the information necessary to a competency evaluation, whether from service providers in the community, caregivers, family members, or physicians. These can be useful to ensure that all the relevant information about the functioning of the person will be obtained. They differ to some extent in their purpose and emphasis.

In evaluating elderly individuals for guardianship, for example, the OARS (Older Americans Resources and Services) Multidimensional Functional Assessment Questionnaire may be a useful instrument. The general dimensions of functioning which are assessed by this instrument include social resources, economic resources, mental health, physical health, and activities of daily living. Similarly, the Guardianship Individual Functional Assessment Tool by Casasanto, Covert, Saunders, and Simon (1987) can help to identify performance limitations which may interfere with a person's decision-making abilities.

13. Consider the relationship between the evaluee's abilities and the situational demands of the legal competence. The evaluator must focus on the evaluee's performance or functioning given a certain anticipated situation. A person's mild memory deficits or other cognitive impairment, for example, might interfere with managing a complex estate but not a simple one.

14. Some legal competency evaluations are best conducted by a multidisciplinary team. It can be useful to involve mental or physical health care professionals from different areas of practice. For example, neurological signs and symptoms can be assessed by a neurologist or gerontologist, psychiatric symptoms and disorders can be assessed by a psychiatrist, psychometric assessments can be performed by a psychologist or neuropsychologist, and assessment of daily functioning can be conducted by a nurse or an occupational therapist. The data can be compiled by a psychiatrist, a psychologist, or other mental health professional trained and experienced in multidisciplinary capacity evaluations.

15. When possible, observe the evaluee's actual functioning under the specific conditions required by the legal competency. While history from the evaluee or others is useful in obtaining background information about the evaluee's functioning, the best capacity assessment is observational rather than inferential. Thus, assessment of independent living skills is best conducted in a real kitchen or apartment, perhaps by an occupational therapist experienced in these evaluations. Similarly, it is more useful to ask the evaluee to write out checks for utilities and other services (or to examine his recent bank statements and cancelled checks) than to rely on his self-report of his ability to do this.

16. Assess the reason (and the reasoning process), psychology, or psychodynamics of the patient's decision. Important life decisions may be based on fact, fantasy, miscommunication, or emotion. Psychopathology often impairs decision-making clarity, especially in a stressful situation such as acute illness or impending loss.

17. Consider the emotional as well as the cognitive dimensions of the evaluee's decision making. Subtle forms of decision-making incapacity can result from depressive cognitions such as hopelessness, pessimism, catastrophization, feelings of guilt, or need for punishment, even though the person otherwise appears to be thinking clearly. Similarly, elevated mood results in denial of illness or impaired ability to weigh risks and benefits of treatment.

18. Only the judge or jury has the legal authority to decide whether the evaluee has sufficient capacity to be considered (legally) competent in a particular area. The

evaluator's responsibility is to provide the court with adequate information about the evaluee's mental and physical abilities to make a decision and then execute that decision. Conclusory psychiatric diagnoses, without the supporting diagnostic and functional data, whether in written reports or in court testimony, provide minimal information about functional status and should be avoided.

C. Competency Standards

While performing the capacity evaluation, the evaluator must focus on the criteria or standards by which the patient's capacity is assessed. Unfortunately, the law will often not specifically define the operational criteria used to determine whether the person meets the law's conception of legal competence. In other words, legal competencies are constructs or abstractions, and the court must decide whether an individual's particular abilities satisfy its view of legal competency. Nevertheless, a number of competency criteria have been used, especially in the context of competence to consent to, or refuse, medical treatment. They generally involve communicating choices, understanding information, and appropriately processing it. These can be presented in a hierarchy, from less strict to more strict criteria, though there is nothing fixed about this procedure. The criteria apply regardless of whether the patient consents to, refuses, or offers no decision about the proposed issue.

1. Is the patient generally aware of his present situation (e.g., in a health care setting with treatment staff, faced with an important decision to make, undergoing a competency assessment, and cooperating with staff and evaluator)?
2. Does the patient verbally accept or reject the proposed intervention (e.g., make and communicate his decision about treatment or residential placement)?
3. Is the patient's decision a reasonable one (i.e., the result or outcome of the decision)?
4. Is there a rational basis for the decision (i.e., the decision-making process that the person used to make his decision; can the patient mentally synthesize or manipulate information in the decision-making process?)?
5. Is the patient able to understand the risks and benefits of, and the alternatives to, the proposed intervention after they have been explained (e.g., medication side effects, risks of surgery or biopsy, living independently in an apartment, or managing his checking account)?
6. Alternatively, does the patient actually understand the risks and benefits of, and the alternatives to, the proposed intervention?
7. Does the patient have a critical and reflective appreciation of his current situation (e.g., does he understand the nature of his current situation [i.e., illness] based upon personal and emotional considerations, rather than in the abstract or as applied to someone else?)?

Given the range of competency criteria, the evaluee will "pass" or satisfy some but "fail" those which are more demanding. In addition, the patient may have more than one problem at issue (e.g., cancer, depression, parenting a child, and living independently), so that his functional and legal competency must be addressed specifically and separately with regard to each. The person, for example, may have adequate capacity to live independently but not to parent a child or refuse ECT.

The level of functional capacity needed to be considered competent to consent to a treatment varies with the complexity of the decision making; competency is "task-specific" and more complex decisions require more ability than those which are simpler. In practice, this "sliding scale" notion of competency is often taken a step further. Commonly, the standard of decision-making competency varies with the risks and benefits to the patient; now, competency is "risk-specific." For example, consent to a research project which has no potential harmful side effects might require a lower level of understanding of the research than consenting to participate in research which is highly risky. Consenting to a treatment which is highly beneficial to the patient might require a lower level of understanding than consenting to a treatment which is less beneficial to the patient. The more potential for harm to the individual as a result of the intervention, the greater the capacity to consent that may be required. Similarly, the less the potential benefit to the individual, the greater the capacity to consent that may be required. Thus, the level of capacity which is needed for one to be considered clinically competent to consent or refuse often varies with the nature of the proposed intervention and its risks and benefits. This risk-specific approach, however, leads to the counter-intuitive and controversial idea that a patient might be considered *competent to consent* to a highly beneficial and minimal risk procedure but *incompetent to refuse* it. This pair of judgments can occur simultaneously because a treatment refusal is often a more complex decision than a treatment consent; the patient needs to understand the consequences of refusal and weigh them against the potential benefits.

D. When the Person Is Decisionally Incapacitated

If the clinician determines that the patient is clinically incapacitated but consent for treatment is needed, or there are financial matters to be managed, the clinician must consider whether a court should determine if the person is legally incompetent. Court involvement in competency determinations is recommended when:

1. The patient's decisional capacity is uncertain and the decision is significant.
2. The patient's incapacity is substantial and likely to be prolonged.
3. The choice of any substitute decision maker is controversial or there is substantial family disagreement about the proposed plan.
4. The decision of any substitute decision maker significantly differs from the views of the patient, or perhaps from medical opinion.

The declaration of incompetency will usually result in the appointment of a legal guardian, who, in most cases, will be able to provide the needed consent. Adjudication of incompetence and appointment of a guardian can be done only by a court, following certain procedures. In many cases, a temporary guardian can be appointed quickly, or the court will simply order the treatment without appointing a guardian. The clinician should begin the process by consulting with the family and by having them initiate the incompetency proceedings. The court will also initially look to a family member to serve as the guardian. If such a person is unavailable or unwilling to serve as guardian, the clinician should contact the facility attorney. Petitioning for guardianship of the disabled person will best protect the patient as well as the clinician by ensuring that the person making necessary medical decisions is mentally and physically capable of doing so.

III. COURT PROCEEDINGS FOR ADJUDICATING INCOMPETENCE

Every state has legal procedures for adjudicating someone as incompetent. This is usually included as part of a probate act. The rights of the individual in incompetency proceedings vary, but certain concepts generally underlie the proceedings. The goal is to ensure that before a declaration of incompetency has been made, the person clearly warrants this finding, and there is no less restrictive alternative finding or disposition. At the same time, the court will want to assure itself that the person appointed as guardian will be capable of acting in the best interests of the incompetent person.

A. Definition of Incompetence

The definition of incompetence varies from state to state. The trend in the law has been to abandon the term *incompetent* and refer to the person as *incapacitated* or *disabled*, since this is less pejorative. Mental illness, mental retardation, alcoholism, drug dependence, and sometimes old age serve as the basis for a finding of incompetency when these disorders result in the individual's inability to make decisions about his person or his property. The Uniform Probate Code, for example, defines an "incapacitated person" as "any person who is impaired by reason of mental illness, mental deficiency, physical illness or disability, advanced age . . . or other cause to the extent that he lacks sufficient understanding or capacity to make or communicate responsible decisions concerning his person." This definition has served as a model for many of the states. Thus, there must be a psychiatric or medical disorder as well as some resulting functional impairment. Other definitions provide that the incompetent be someone who is incapable of managing his property or caring for himself or both. Regrettably for the clinician, most legal definitions of incompetence are not behavioral in type.

B. Initiating Proceedings

In the vast majority of states, the initiation of the incompetency proceedings may be done by "any interested person." This could be any adult who is familiar with the alleged incompetent, who is also called the *respondent*. The petitioner might be a relative, a friend, or an administrator from the treatment facility. A number of states even provide that the person may initiate his own incompetency proceedings. The initiator of the proceedings is required to file a petition which brings the case before the appropriate court. In the petition there will be certain allegations as to why the person is allegedly incompetent and needs a guardian appointed. It is important that the initiator of the proceedings complete the petition properly and file it with the proper court. Assistance of an attorney is beneficial for this process. In addition, most states require a certificate from a health professional describing the person's disability and needs for services.

C. Rights at the Hearing

Every legal proceeding requires legal notice in which the nature and character of the proceedings are described to the person who is a party to it. In guardianship proceedings, the alleged incompetent person must be notified that a petition has been filed seeking to declare him incompetent. He will receive a copy of the petition and will be notified when a hearing is scheduled. Because of the nature of the proceedings, the vast majority of states provide that notice must also be given to a close relative of the disabled person, his representative, or any party potentially affected by it. If neither the respondent nor his representative is present at the hearing because they were not properly served notice, then the entire proceeding will be delayed until service has been completed.

Half the states specifically recognize the right of the allegedly incompetent person to appear at the hearing, though few respondents do in practice. Some states require that the court find a good reason for the respondent's absence from the hearing. In many states, the court can close the hearing to the public or hold the hearing in chambers to protect the disabled person.

Since a legal declaration of incompetency results in a significant loss of rights, it may be argued that the state is constitutionally required to provide indigent persons with the assistance of an attorney. In the majority of states, representation by counsel in guardianship hearings is required by law, and in the others, the court has the discretion to require this. The attorney may perform several different roles depending upon the jurisdiction. Often the attorney acts as a "guardian *ad litem*." The guardian *ad litem* determines what would best meet the needs of the allegedly incompetent person and presents this to the court. The guardian *ad litem* will also present to the court the wishes of the respondent. If there is a disagreement between the guardian *ad litem* and the respondent, the court may also appoint an attorney to represent the position of the alleged incompetent in seeking to avoid a declaration of incompetency. In other jurisdictions, a court investigator or "visitor" screens guardianship petitions and potential guardians to determine if the case necessitates the appointment of a guardian, and if the guardian is an appropriate one. This procedure helps to divert cases which are inappropriate for guardianship into other dispositions. The investigator also informs the proposed ward and guardian of their legal rights and makes recommendations to the judge.

Approximately half the states do not address the issue of whether the allegedly disabled person is entitled to a determination by jury. In the remaining states, a jury is available upon request.

Guardianship court proceedings are usually informal, rather than rigorously adversarial like criminal trials. In some jurisdictions, it is all too common for the respondent to be found legally incompetent even though he was not present at the hearing, he was not represented by an attorney, no expert testified at the hearing, and no court officer or investigator reviewed the allegations of incompetency or the appropriateness of the guardian. Few guardianship petitions are contested or subsequently appealed. Such procedural weaknesses in the laws have prompted calls for reform of guardianship, which is underway in many jurisdictions.

D. Role of the Mental Health Professional

In many states, the statutes provide for the certification or examination of the allegedly incompetent person before there can be an adjudication of incompetency. Such an examination should be conducted as outlined above for competency assessments. It may be requested by an attorney for a party to the litigation, or independently by the court. In most jurisdictions, the law requires a physician's evaluation. In a growing number of jurisdictions, other health care professionals, especially psychologists, are deemed qualified. The clinician responsible for the patient's treatment, or a consulting clinician, may perform this evaluation. Typically, the clinician is not required to be present in court but files a report or an affidavit.

Often, the clinicians who recommend guardianship are confronted by family members who are reluctant or refuse to petition for incompetency or guardianship. Many minimize or deny the extent of the patient's functional incapacity or are aware of the social stigma attached to adjudications of incompetency. Some family members will challenge or threaten to sue the clinicians for filing a guardianship petition. The clinician may need to provide information and reassurance about the benefits of a guardianship court proceeding and the absence of other less restrictive dispositions.

E. Finding of Incompetency

Once the hearing has been completed, the court will render a decision regarding legal competency. In most states, the individual can be determined to be incompetent as to (l) his estate, (2) his person, (3) or both. In a growing number of jurisdictions, limited guardianship is possible. Under this concept, the limits on the disabled person's (and the guardian's) decision-making authority are specifically detailed by the court. Limited guardianship applies to incompetency of the estate as well as incompetency of the person (medical care, residence, etc.).

If an individual is incompetent as to his estate, it means he is unable to make financial decisions and manage his assets. It is possible for someone to be incapable of managing his finances, but capable of making reasonable personal decisions. This is most likely when the assets are large and complex. Unfortunately, it is not unusual to see family become upset with an aging parent who is dissipating his assets either through poor financial judgment or by spending his funds on someone the family disapproves of. In these cases, the family may seek to have the individual declared incompetent as to his estate in order to preserve his assets for themselves. The fact that an individual makes poor financial decisions or spends his money in a way his family disapproves does not by itself indicate that he is incapable of managing his assets. However, if the poor financial decisions are the result of a mental disability, such as manic-depressive illness or dementia, then it is appropriate to have a declaration of incompetency made to preserve the assets and protect the individual as well as his family.

IV. RIGHTS AFFECTED BY BEING DECLARED INCOMPETENT

A declaration of incompetency serves two purposes. First, it is a formal means of protecting and caring for the incompetent person. It ends his right to make decisions which may be harmful to him and establishes a guardian to protect his interests. It is the state's way of exercising its *parens patriae* powers for the protection of the individual. Second, the formal declaration of incompetency provides protection for society. The legal decision becomes part of the public record. It informs the world that this individual no longer has the mental capacity to make one or more important decisions for himself. Since these decisions may affect all those who deal with the incompetent person, the legal declaration provides them with notice that this person no longer has the capacity to make decisions, and that his decisions will not be legally enforceable.

A. Incompetent as to the Estate

A declaration of incompetency as to one's estate affects a wide range of financial decisions. After entry of the court order of estate guardianship, banks, credit card companies, title companies, and financial institutions which request financial information about the incompetent person will be informed that the person has been declared incompetent. These institutions do not want to conduct new business with an incompetent person because contracts with an incompetent person are legally unenforceable.

Upon a declaration of incompetency as to the estate, the incompetent person can no longer enter into contracts. This means that any decisions regarding his assets or any purchases he desires must be performed by someone else, since it has been determined that he has no legal capacity to make such decisions. Since the leasing or purchase of a home is a type of contract, this can no longer be done by the incompetent, but only by a guardian in his name. In those instances where the goal is to sell property of an incompetent, such as his home, stocks or other assets, the sale usually can be accomplished only by the estate guardian through an order of the court. This procedure then gives the new buyer clear title to the property.

Having been adjudicated incompetent to manage one's estate also can affect one's right to make or change one's will. All states require that the person writing a will (the "testator") be of "sound mind" or be "competent" in order for the will to be valid; this is termed *testamentary capacity*. This ensures that, when someone plans for the distribution of his estate upon his death, he is aware of the purpose of a will, his assets, and his natural beneficiaries (his family). If a will was written before the person was declared incompetent, it will be presumed valid. A will speaks only upon the death of its author. At that time, the issue of the testator's competency can be raised, but such an action is backward looking. The will can be set aside only if the testator is determined to be incompetent at the time he wrote the will. In some states, a person under guardianship, whether of estate or person, can still write or change his will; such a will would not automatically be invalid. The level of functional capacity needed to write or change a will is low—lower than that required to manage one's estate or person. Acceptance of a will written when a person was under guardianship may require proof of the person's capacity at the time he wrote or changed his will. As in the case of the person who has not been adjudicated incompetent, there may be a challenge to the person's testamentary capacity after the incompetent person's death.

B. Incompetent as to the Person

Being declared incompetent to manage one's personal affairs means that the individual no longer has the legal right to make any personal decisions nor to participate in many of the activities otherwise taken for granted. The incompetent is similar to a child in the eyes of the law; this is sometimes referred to as *civil death*.

From the health care professional's prospective, this means that the legal guardian, or sometimes a court, must make treatment decisions. Once the patient is declared incompetent, the health care provider should be consulting and seeking approval from the guardian. This will be advantageous where the patient was of questionable competency and had previously made irrational treatment decisions.

The incompetent person can no longer participate in the legal process. He cannot serve as a juror nor appear as a witness. If suit is brought against him for events which occurred during the period of his incompetency, he will not be held liable. In addition, he cannot sue or be sued in his own name. This must be done through the guardian. In many states, the statute of limitations for filing a lawsuit by an incompetent person will be "tolled" or extended to some period beyond the time he is restored to competency. This is similar to how the law treats injuries to minors. For example, assume an incompetent person wanted to sue his physician as a result of complications from surgery; if his state has a two-year statute of limitations for bringing a malpractice suit, the person could bring the suit up to two years beyond the point at which he regained his legal competency.

Legally incompetent persons also lose the privileges of citizenship. They are no longer eligible to vote, hold public office, or obtain civil service employment.

Adjudicated incompetent persons are not permitted to marry, and if married, they will usually not be granted a divorce until a guardian has been appointed to represent their interests. Even then, many courts will not order the divorce, unless the disabled person had already filed for the divorce prior to his adjudication of incompetence. This provision ensures that at the time of a divorce, the incompetent person's interests and assets will be well protected. In divorces under these circumstances, the court will carefully review the ward's finances, trying to provide as much protection as possible to the ward.

A person's motor vehicle license can also be affected by an adjudication of incompetency. A driver's license is a privilege the state grants its citizens, rather than a fundamental civil right. Each state establishes the standards and procedures for granting, suspending, and revoking this privilege. If someone is declared incompetent, he is no longer eligible to hold a driver's license. Even if a person is not declared incompetent, a history of hospitalization for a mental disability will sometimes raise the issue of whether the person should hold or retain his driver's license. When a person has a mental or physical disorder which impairs his ability to drive, the state has the authority to withdraw the license. Suspending or revoking a disabled person's driver's license does not, regrettably, stop some people from driving. It may fall to the family to remove the person's car keys or sell the motor vehicle to stop him from driving.

Finally, an adjudication of incompetency can result in the denial or suspension of a professional license. There are a wide variety of occupations which are licensed by the states. These include barbers, beauticians, nurses, social workers, marriage and family counselors, psychologists, physicians, attorneys, and teachers, among others. By denying or withdrawing the license of one who is incompetent, the state protects the public against someone who does not have the mental ability to make rational decisions or adequately perform his job. Even without a declaration of incompetency, the state can suspend, limit, or revoke the license of an individual who appears to be having psychiatric problems, whether they are due to a mental illness, alcoholism, drug abuse, or some other condition.

V. APPOINTMENT OF A GUARDIAN

A. Selection of the Guardian

The court has the authority to select who will act as the guardian for the incompetent person. One, two, or multiple guardians may be appointed to handle personal decisions and act as guardians of the estate. The goal of the court is to appoint individuals, institutions, corporations, or organizations which will act in the best interests of the incompetent person. In about half the jurisdictions, the law provides that a preference should be given to the nearest relative. In some states, the court will honor the request of the incompetent person as to the identity of the guardian, if it is a reasonable one. Usually the court will seek to find someone to act as guardian of the person who knows the ward, is interested in him, or has had a significant relationship with him. In all states, the guardian must be an adult, viewed as a person of good character, and without decision-making incapacity. Some states specifically exclude convicted felons, disbarred attorneys, or anyone who has a conflict of interest with the incompetent person.

B. The Guardian's Authority

The declaration of incompetency and the appointment of a guardian can be accomplished only through a court order. The court always retains jurisdiction of the case and will have the legal authority to supervise the guardian. Depending upon the applicable law, the court will specify what decisions the guardian has the authority to make, those that the ward retains the authority to make, and those which require court approval. The court could also require a detailed accounting of the expenditures made by the guardian. When the court is concerned about the abilities of the guardian in a certain sphere, the court could assume the responsibility for making those decisions or appoint a limited guardian. The court exercises the state's *parens patriae* powers in ensuring that the needs of the incompetent person will be met.

1. *Guardian of the Estate (Conservator)*

In many instances, the guardian of the estate—known as a conservator in some jurisdictions, since his duties are to conserve the assets—will be different from the guardian of the person. The guardian of the estate may be a bank, a financial institution, or someone with financial experience and training who may be better able to protect the incompetent's assets than the average citizen. Sometimes, a family member will be appointed to act as guardian of the person, and a bank will be guardian of the estate. At other times, the family member and the financial institution will be appointed as co-guardians of the estate, in which case each co-guardian has decision-making authority. This mechanism ensures considerable protection for the ward, particularly when the assets are substantial.

The guardian of the estate has a great deal of authority. He will initially provide an inventory of the estate's property to the court. He will then make all decisions related to the finances of the ward. The estate guardian will decide how best to preserve and, if possible, increase the assets. He will be limited to investing the ward's assets in secure investments. He will be responsible for paying the debts of the ward, as well as the ongoing expenses, such as housing, food, or medical care.

When there is a family business, the estate guardian may become the director of the business or will be responsible for ensuring its successful continuation. The buying and selling of any stocks, bonds, and property will also be part of the responsibilities of the guardian of the estate. If litigation needs to be initiated to protect the ward's estate or enforce his property rights, it is the estate guardian's responsibility to do so. In many instances, the court will require giving its specific approval before certain items can be bought or sold. These may include any major assets or may be limited to certain assets such as the family home or business. The role of the court will depend on who is appointed as the guardian of the estate, the size of the estate, the court's confidence in the guardian, and local law.

When the estate guardianship is initiated, it is common for the court to require the guardian of the estate to post a bond that equals or exceeds the value of the estate. In some states this bond is mandatory. The cost of the bond, which must be periodically renewed, is borne by the ward's estate. This bond ensures that if the guardian breaches his fiduciary duty to the ward, then the estate will be protected from the loss.

In many states, the estate guardian must file an annual accounting of the estate's financial transactions and inventory. This accounting will set forth the assets of the incompetent and what expenditures have been made. Receipts may be needed to document these expenses. A financial institution which acts as guardian of the estate will be entitled to fees for its work, which are paid out of the estate. Court approval may be needed before the fees can be paid. Individual family members or friends who are appointed estate guardians are ordinarily not entitled to fees for their services, but their expenses in managing the estate are compensated. Such individual estate guardians are not expected to use personal funds to pay for their ward's expenses.

While, on paper, state laws attempt to protect the ward's estate, unfortunately the courts are typically unable to monitor the financial activities of an estate of an incompetent person. Most courts which handle guardianships are inadequately funded to properly supervise the hundreds if not thousands of existing guardianships under their purview. Most courts become aware of problems with the estate guardian or the estate only when an interested party brings a suspicion of fraud or misuse to their attention. Some courts, though, routinely audit some of their estate guardianships or screen for abuse. While guardians incur both civil and criminal liability for misuse of their ward's estate, this does not appear to deter misconduct by some guardians. Misconduct is much less of a problem when the guardian is an attorney or professional guardian or affiliated with an institution.

2. *Guardian of the Person*

The guardian of the person is legally responsible for the day-to-day decisions affecting the ward apart from those that are financial. These range from the details of everyday life (e.g., clothing, grooming, bathing, place of residence, socialization, and travel) to major medical and psychiatric decisions. When the guardianship petition is prompted by the need for medical treatment, the court will try to appoint someone who is familiar with the ward's personal values and views before the mental disability arose. There are certain personal decisions which may be beyond the authority of the legal guardian and thus require court approval. In some states, the guardian cannot admit the ward to a mental hospital or nursing home without court approval. Consent for some types of medical procedures, such as ECT, psychosurgery, sterilization, organ transplantation, and, in an increasing number of states, psychotropic medication, must be obtained from the court. In some jurisdictions, guardians may consent to medical treatment, but may not discontinue some treatments, especially those which are life-sustaining. The guardian of the person is obligated to do everything possible to ensure the best quality of life for the ward, given the circumstances.

3. *Plenary Guardian*

A plenary guardian is one who is both a guardian of the person and the estate and who has authority to make all decisions. In most cases, this position is served by one person. In some cases, though, two or more individuals have independent decision-making authority over the ward's personal and financial affairs.

4. *Temporary Guardian*

The need for a temporary guardian arises in three circumstances. The first occurs when there is a need for medical treatment or placement in a nursing home, which cannot be postponed during the time it would take to appoint a permanent guardian through a formal legal proceeding. In these circumstances, the court will dispense with some of the formalities which surround the appointment of a permanent guardian. A judge, may, for example, take telephone testimony from a physician or briefly visit the patient in the hospital or nursing facility. The temporary guardianship will last for only a specified period of time, until a permanent guardian is appointed or until the medical treatment has been provided. Many temporary guardianships never proceed to permanent guardianships. This occurs typically when the person under temporary guardianship receives medical or psychiatric care which restores his functioning.

Concern about financial mismanagement by the disabled person is the second situation which might give rise to the need for a temporary guardian. This could occur when someone is in a manic state and depleting his assets or when there is fear that some other party is improperly using the assets of the alleged disabled person. The court can act quickly to protect the assets by appointing a temporary guardian and, if necessary, freezing financial accounts for a temporary period.

The third situation requiring a temporary guardian arises when the permanent guardian dies. In this case, the court will need to appoint a successor guardian. In some instances where the guardian was a spouse or parent, through a will they can nominate or appoint a testamentary guardian. The courts will generally honor this appointment. When this is not done, and a guardian is needed immediately, the court will attempt to appoint someone who will be able to respond immediately to the needs of the ward.

The length of a temporary guardianship varies with the state. It may be as brief as 30 days or as long as six months. In many places, the appointment of a temporary guardian triggers the procedures necessary to appoint a permanent guardian. A permanent guardianship is effective until the ward's competency is restored in another competency hearing or until the person's death.

5. *Limited Guardian*

The trend in the law of guardianship is to recognize that the mental and physical abilities of a person can be measured along a continuum. Often a person with questionable mental judgment is neither fully capable of making decisions for himself nor fully incapacitated. This may be particularly true of a mentally retarded person who has some abilities but may not be able to make complicated decisions regarding himself. The goal of a limited guardianship is to permit the disabled person to handle those decisions he is competent to handle. This preserves for the person as much autonomy as possible and encourages the development of maximum self-reliance and independence. The guardianship is tailored to reflect the particular needs of the ward.

Although almost all of the states provide for limited guardianship, the courts generally do not use this concept because it requires defining what the individual can and cannot do, which even well-trained mental health professionals often find difficult. Some judges contend that the petitioner or guardian will inevitably return to court to increase the scope of his authority when the ward becomes even more incapacitated and additional substituted decision-making authority is necessary. Thus, these judges argue that ordering limited guardianship wastes the courts' resources.

In limited guardianship, the appointment is specific as to what decision-making authority is retained by the ward, and what authority is provided to the guardian.

6. *Co-guardians*

In some cases, two or more individuals or parties are appointed to act as co-guardians over a single aspect of the ward's functioning. They may be a family member and an institution (e.g., a bank) or, more commonly, two family members. The latter sometimes occurs because both family members are seeking control over the ward's functioning, neither trusts the other to do so, and the court decides to appoint them jointly as guardians. While this may seem like an amicable arrangement, cooperation between guardians who had conflicts prior to the guardianship is likely to be a problem.

C. Surrogate Decision Making: Principles and Practices

Once a person has been appointed legal guardian over one or several aspects of the ward's functioning, the court will charge him with acting on behalf of the ward. However simple this may sound in theory, it is often a problem in practice.

The guardian makes decisions for the ward on the basis of the following considerations.

1. *Best Interests of the Ward*

This perspective on proxy decision making requires that the guardian decide what is in the ward's best interests. This is viewed from a neutral or objective standard (i.e., the guardian determines what is objectively in the ward's best interests and decides accordingly), rather than from the ward's particular viewpoint. Most courts have this in mind when they charge the guardian with proxy decision-making authority over the ward.

2. *Substituted Judgment*

This decision-making perspective requires that the guardian determine what the ward would have wanted to do in the present situation had the ward been able to decide for himself. Thus, the guardian must try to reconstruct the ward's views about solutions to the present situation from whatever written or verbal information the ward provided prior to his incapacity. The ward's prior statements, behavior, and use of any written advance directives (e.g., a living will, a power of attorney, or a letter of instruction) will be useful here. In addition, the ward's religious and personal values will be reviewed. Substituted judgment decision making may be difficult to accomplish, even when the guardian is the spouse of the ward, since many people do not specifically or even generally discuss their views about many medical or other decisions in advance of the problem. The standard cannot be used when the person never had decision-making capacity, as in the case of the profoundly mentally retarded person. The courts are increasingly instructing guardians to use this decision-making perspective, though it is used less frequently than the standard of the best interests of the ward.

3. *Prudent Person or Prudent Administrator*

This is the surrogate decision-making standard employed by financial institutions, that is, those which become bank guardians for the ward. Here, the bank makes financial decisions on the basis of what it thinks is prudent to do with the ward's assets, rather than on the basis of what the ward would have done or what his family members would have done. In this approach, for example, in order to preserve the estate, the bank would refuse to continue the ward's previous pattern of providing substantial gifts to his grandchildren. The ward's assets will be invested in a financially conservative manner.

4. *Best Interests of the Guardian*

Regrettably, some guardians make decisions for the ward on the basis of what is in the guardian's best interests, or what is most convenient for him in the situation. This is not what the court has in mind when it charges the guardian with making substituted decisions for the ward.

5. *Best Interests of a Third Party or the Family*

Again, some guardians are unable or unwilling to decide for the ward on the basis of the ward's best or previously expressed interests and do so on the basis of the interests of another family member or of the family as a whole. There may be a domineering family member who for years strongly influenced all family members in their life decisions; a guardian in this decision-making perspective would defer to this third party. This is also not what the court intends the guardian to do in making decisions for the ward.

Making decisions for others is even more difficult than deciding for ourselves, particularly with regard to important decisions such as medical or psychiatric care. Thus, we should not be surprised to see that guardians make substituted decisions based on any of these perspectives. Sometimes one perspective is employed for a particular decision, and another is used for another decision. The guardian might combine elements of these in reaching a decision.

VI. DEALING WITH THE GUARDIAN IN THE TREATMENT SETTING

Once a person has been adjudicated incompetent to manage his medical or personal affairs, he is no longer legally authorized to consent to or refuse health care services. All health care providers must then obtain legal consent from the appointed legal guardian or guardians. Such substituted consent is required for all types of health care services from the most minor (e.g., X-rays or prescription of sleeping medication) to the major (e.g., surgery or cancer chemotherapy). This does not mean, however, that clinicians should ignore the now legally incompetent patient's wishes and requests. Clinicians should still attempt to maximize the patient's participation in the decision-making process regarding treatment, as well as his participation in the treatment itself. This requires questioning the patient about his views and informing the patient of the treatment plan and its likely impact upon him.

Unfortunately, health care providers are often unaware that the person has been found legally incompetent and a guardian appointed. This typically occurs when the patient is new to the clinician, and the guardian either does not accompany the patient to the appointment or does not adequately explain the nature of their legal relationship to the clinician. The clinician cannot expect the patient to volunteer this information, as most wards will not themselves be aware of it or able to communicate it. When family members or others indicate that the patient has been found incompetent, the clinician must attempt to clarify the nature of the decision-making authority. This is often difficult to do and may require that the responsible guardian bring the court papers and court order to the clinician for verification. Recent research has demonstrated that many guardians are unfamiliar with the extent of their decision-making authority; some estate guardians, for example, will claim that they have personal or plenary authority. Others who are representative payees will claim that they are legal guardians for the patient.

Another dilemma in dealing with obtaining substituted consent is that the responsible guardian may abdicate his decision-making authority or delegate it to others, whether family or friends. Here, whether by design or default, the legal guardian involves others in decisions about the ward. In such situations, which may be more typical than is commonly realized, the clinician may have to deal with a large number of family members, even though only the guardian is empowered to consent to health care. For many important decisions (e.g., about ECT), there is often a division of opinion in the family, and this complicates the clinician's task of informing the decision makers and obtaining a consent or refusal. This situation is distinguished from one in which the guardian retains decision-making authority but family members challenge his judgment and decisions, demand that the clinician accept their substituted decision, and even threaten to sue the clinician or the guardian. Here again it is useful for the clinician to be certain of the legal authority of the family members. When there is a dispute among family members, the clinician can advise the family to seek legal counsel or a court order.

In short, it is not always as easy as it seems to deal with substitute decision makers. Most legal guardians receive little or no orientation or training to be guardians, and few receive any written information about their responsibilities. Many parties may have an interest in the incapacitated person, and they may or may not have legal decision making authority. Co-guardianships of the person, where two or more parties have legal decisional authority, are uncommon but also complicate decision making. Estate guardians, while not formally empowered to make health care decisions, often impact upon personal or medical guardians because of the importance of financing health care services.

A final consideration for the clinician in a substituted judgment situation is that of the guardian who himself appears incapacitated. A spouse of an elderly ward may have significant cognitive, sensory, or physical limitations which prevent him from processing information and making complex medical decisions. Thus, the clinician may conclude that the guardian has reached a poor decision, or even none at all, from the perspective of the ward. In these cases, it may be necessary for the clinician to work intensively with the guardian in trying to educate him about the problem at hand or by involving other family members in the decision. Alternatively, it may be necessary for the clinician to request that the family petition the court for another guardian, whether family or others, or simply to notify the court of the dilemma. As noted earlier, guardians may make what the clinician considers to be a wrong decision because of the guardian's self-interest, rather than the ward's best interest or substituted judgment.

VII. RESTORATION TO COMPETENCY

When an adjudicated incompetent person is no longer functionally incapacitated, he, or any interested person on his behalf, can petition the court to restore him to legal competency. This requires an additional judicial hearing, since once adjudicated incompetent, the person is presumed incompetent, no matter what his actual or functional capacity. If the restoration hearing is successful, the incompetency is terminated, the guardian is discharged, and the person's rights are restored. The court would then no longer have legal jurisdiction over the individual. In practice, restoration to competency is an infrequent event.

VIII. OTHER PROTECTIVE DEVICES

A number of other protective devices help protect those mentally disabled persons with decisional incapacities. These include the representative payee, adult protective services, elder abuse reporting, public guardians, advance directives, and surrogate consent statutes.

A. Representative Payee

Perhaps the most widely used protection for the funds of mentally disabled persons is the representative payee (this topic is discussed extensively in Chapter 4). This system, which is common for the payment of Social Security and veterans benefits and pensions to the mentally disabled, appoints a person to receive the funds the disabled person is entitled to. The appointed person, known as a *represen-*

tative payee, will often be a relative with whom the disabled person is living. In the case where the disabled person is institutionalized, the representative payee may be an official of the institution. The funds are then expended to benefit the disabled person. This system has the benefit of not requiring a formal competency court hearing with the resulting expenses, when these funds are the only asset. However, there are many documented cases where the payee fails to utilize funds in the best way to meet the needs of the disabled person.

B. Adult Protective Services

Adult protective services are a legislative mechanism that allows the state, through its caseworkers, to provide a coordinated system of health and social services without appointing a guardian or relying on civil commitment. This system is utilized for people who live in a community, including the developmentally disabled, the mentally ill, and the elderly. The goal is to keep the people in the community and make sure their needs for care and safety are met. Available services include investigation by a protective services worker, homemaker support services, home health services, exploration of alternative living arrangements, referral, petition for guardianship, and transfer to a nursing home or hospital. Services may be recommended for the elderly person in need as well as for any caretakers. Under some adult protective services statutes, these services can be provided involuntarily to the disabled person after some procedural protection has been provided to the person. In others, emergency court orders can be obtained. Generally, services are provided in accordance with the least restrictive alternative principle. Some protective service agencies provide direct services, while others only refer to, or contract with, outside agencies.

Since adult protective services are relatively new, it is unclear how successful they have been in meeting the needs of the disabled in a way which permits them to remain in the community. Adequate implementation depends upon the financial resources available to the program, the availability of alternative social service programs for the elderly, and interagency cooperation. Some jurisdictions have had their protective services periodically eliminated for budgetary or political reasons.

C. Elder Abuse Reporting

In response to a variety of issues, almost every state has enacted elder abuse or dependent adult reporting statutes. Analogous to child abuse reporting, elder abuse reporting seeks to identify and prevent elder abuse, which is typically at the hands of family members. The ideal elder abuse reporting law contains provisions for reporting, investigation, and service delivery.

Some elder abuse reporting statutes apply to all adults age 18 and older who are considered mentally or physically disabled but were intended to apply primarily to the elderly. Others only apply to the elderly. The definitions of elder abuse vary widely from state to state and may cover physical neglect, psychological neglect, self-neglect, verbal abuse, physical abuse, psychological abuse, sexual abuse, financial exploitation, and theft, but the presence of suspected substantial physical harm or injury is a common denominator. In some areas, reporting is optional or elective as opposed to mandatory, in that there is no civil or criminal penalty for failure to report the suspected abuse. Those parties who are subject to mandatory elder abuse reporting typically include health care professionals, while a few states mandate reporting by any citizen who has reasonable cause to believe its occurrence. Ordinarily, however, citizens are subject only to voluntary reporting. As in child abuse reporting, there is immunity from civil or criminal liability for all reports made in good faith. In addition, some states which mandate reporting by employees of long-term care facilities provide protection from retaliation or discipline by the facility.

Reports of suspected elder abuse include the name and address of the victim and the alleged offender, the nature and extent of the injury, and any other relevant information. Reports of suspected elder abuse are filed with the police, social services agencies, or departments of aging operated by the city, county, or state. Some jurisdictions have "elder abuse hotlines" which provide information or secure reports by telephone. Telephoned reports typically require subsequent written reports on the appropriate form.

Investigation and substantiation of elder abuse reports are usually the responsibility of a social services agency, which, in severe cases, may refer the matter for prosecution. Agencies may petition the court for authorization to conduct the investigation, but sometimes the statutory authority to do so is unclear. Emergency services, protective placement, protection ("no contact") orders, or guardianship may be available to the abused elderly person, but intervention and service delivery are often secondary priorities in elderly abuse reporting law and practice.

As in the case of child abuse reporting laws, there is much controversy about the success of elder abuse reporting provisions in detecting new cases of abuse, providing needed services, and protecting the abused person against further abuse. There is also disagreement about the extent of state intrusion into the lives and civil liberties of its legally competent elderly citizens. At present, elder abuse appears to be significantly underreported. Since elder abuse reporting is relatively new, many professionals and citizens are unfamiliar with its availability and provisions. In addition, both the elderly abused and their family abusers are reluctant to report or acknowledge neglect and abuse. Service delivery systems are often underfunded and poorly coordinated. Nevertheless, clinicians who work with the elderly need to retain a high index of suspicion of elder abuse, to be familiar with the available social service agencies, and to become knowledgeable about their legal responsibilities in this area.

D. Public Guardian

In approximately three-fourths of the states, there is a public guardian. This publicly funded official guardian serves as the "guardian of last resort" for a disabled person when there is no one else to fill this role. This is usually the case when the disabled person has a small estate or has been institutionalized for a lengthy period of time. In many jurisdictions, the public guardian serves as the coordinator of services for the disabled person. These offices are funded by a state, county, or local governmental agency. If the disabled person has available funds, the public guardian may collect a fee for the services the agency provides. Public guardians serve as guardians of the person, of the estate, or both, depending upon the jurisdiction.

In some state psychiatric hospitals, patients are routinely screened for financial decision-making incapacity. Should the patients be judged by the clinical staff to be incapable of handling their personal finances, then hospital administrators act as estate guardians for the patient, as long as the patient is hospitalized there. The administrator would typically have no authority as guardian once the patient leaves the facility. Sometimes, such administrators also assume responsibility for personal or medical decisions as well as financial ones.

Public guardianship is not without its critics, for several reasons: (1) there may be conflicts of interest between the public guardian and the ward; (2) bureaucratic government agencies make it difficult to establish personal relationships with the ward; and (3) inadequate funding and staffing reduce the likelihood that the public guardian will be able to perform his responsibilities. On the other hand, public guardians are available to serve people with small estates and serve as an agency of last resort for people who have no one else to take responsibility for their care.

E. Advance Directives

Guardianship, as it is currently practiced throughout the United States, does not involve the incapacitated person in either the preadjudication or postadjudication phase. As noted earlier, the person may not be present at his guardianship hearing, may have little or no input into the selection of a guardian, and typically has little or no input into the guardian's decisions made on his behalf. Further, it is a process which is not initiated until the person becomes incapacitated.

In contrast, a variety of personal or financial decision-making mechanisms are available which are prospective, or forward-looking, in design. These "advance directives" are initiated by a person who currently retains decision-making functioning but anticipates a future decline in functional capacity. These mechanisms, promoted by recent federal law, include living wills, power of attorney, durable power of attorney, and health care power of attorney.

1. Patient Self-Determination Act

Effective in 1991, the Patient Self-Determination Act (PSDA) (42 U.S.C. 1395, 1396) requires that Medicare- and Medicaid-funded programs (including hospitals, nursing homes, home health care programs, health maintenance organizations, and hospices) provide patients written information on the state laws and facility policies regarding the right to accept or refuse treatment including the execution of an advance directive. The goal of this federal law is to encourage the use of advance directives with the hope that people will make known their views on life-sustaining medical care before becoming disabled.

The PSDA appeared in response to the 1990 U.S. Supreme Court decision in *Cruzan v. Director, Missouri Department of Health*. In this case, Missouri challenged the decision of Nancy Cruzan's family to discontinue her artificial feeding and hydration after she had been in a persistent vegetative state since 1983. The Court affirmed the right of competent patients to refuse life-sustaining treatment, including artificial nutrition and hydration. In denying the family's petition, it also ruled that had Nancy Cruzan clearly and convincingly expressed a wish to discontinue life-sustaining medical care before she became disabled in an automobile accident, those views would have been followed.

Both the *Cruzan* case and the passage of the PSDA have spurred more states to enact provisions for advance directives for health care and surrogate consent laws. Legislators have recognized that an individual's rights to self-determination should be preserved by decision making by the person himself if competent or others designated by him if not, rather than by a court or governmental agency. As part of the PSDA, many hospitals and nursing homes are not only informing patients of the applicable law and policy in this area, as is required, but are also providing copies of living wills or powers of attorney for health care for patients to complete. Unanswered by the regulations are the special needs and the accompanying sensitivities of informing psychiatric and post-trauma rehabilitation patients about advance directives at the time of their admission to a psychiatric unit or rehabilitation facility.

2. *Living Wills*

Living wills were initiated in 1976 in California in the form of a Natural Death Act. A living will is typically a brief written document, signed by a legally competent person (the "declarant"), which directs the person's physician to withhold, withdraw, or consent to life-sustaining medical treatment should the person ever become terminally ill. A terminally ill person's wishes regarding treatment should always be ascertained when such treatment is proposed, of course, but many terminally ill people are unable to make or communicate treatment decisions as their illness progresses. A living will thus provides evidence of the patient's wishes while the person is able to decide. It will also relieve the family of much of the burden of the uncertainty about treatment decisions for their terminally ill relative. Living wills can always be modified or withdrawn by a competent declarant. Nevertheless, conflicts sometimes arise between the patient's refusal of treatment in the living will and the family's or physician's wishes to continue treatment; for example, some living wills authorize the withholding or withdrawal of artificial feeding, but family members or the attending physician might be opposed to this.

Living wills are limited to terminating treatment only for a person who is terminally ill, or hopelessly ill, or one whose death is imminent, and it is not always clear what is terminal, hopeless, or imminent. Severely demented patients, or ones in persistent vegetative states or coma, for example, are usually not considered terminally ill, and living wills would not be invoked, although some state courts have defined persistent vegetative states as terminal illness. Finally, since living wills cannot anticipate all relevant terminal medical dilemmas, it will sometimes be unclear what the person would have wanted the physicians to do in a particular case. More recently enacted living-will statutes thus provide the opportunity for the patient to appoint a proxy who can make treatment decisions for the patient if the patient is incapacitated. Finally, most living will statutes provide for immunity from civil or criminal prosecution for health care professionals who carry out the patient's wishes expressed in a living will. A physician who is unable or unwilling to execute the patient's wishes in a living will is obligated to transfer that patient to a physician who will.

In most jurisdictions, signing of the living will must be witnessed by one or more persons, often unrelated to the patient. A person who executes a living will should let his family or friends know where the original is kept. Copies should also be provided to the family and the treating physician.

3. *Powers of Attorney*

Power of attorney is another decision-making mechanism signed by a competent person who wishes to delegate decision-making authority. This mechanism permits a competent person, the principal, to delegate personal or financial decision-making authority to another person, sometimes, but not necessarily, an attorney. The designated decision maker, referred to as the *attorney in fact*, continues to make decisions for the principal as long as instructed to do so. At any time, the principal can terminate the power of attorney. The power of attorney need not be filed with a local court, but this option is sometimes used to publicly record it. A power of attorney cannot be created by a person who is either legally incompetent or too functionally incapacitated to realize what he is doing. The states vary as to the extent of authority which may be conveyed by a power of attorney. A recent development is that powers of attorney are used for health care decision making of various kinds rather than only for financial decisions. A power of attorney for health care is generally broader and more useful than the living will and can address medical decision making when the person is not terminally ill. Health care powers of attorney avoid the need for guardianship and court supervision of medical decision making.

A significant limitation of the traditional power of attorney is that it ceases to be effective once the principal becomes incapacitated. Thus, a traditional power of attorney is less useful for granting decision-making authority to the attorney in fact during progressive or terminal medical illnesses. In contrast, a durable power of attorney survives the principal's incapacity; that is, once appointed, the attorney in fact with durable power continues to make treatment or financial decisions for the principal even after the principal becomes unable to make treatment decisions for himself. Some durable powers of attorney become effective immediately upon signing, while others become effective only after the principal has become incompetent, or they designate the event which will give rise to their effectiveness. Generally, they cease in authority at the death of the principal.

All 50 states and the District of Columbia currently have durable power of attorney statutes. Some explicitly provide for withholding and withdrawing life support, while others authorize consent to treatment. There may be particular requirements in signing durable powers, such as witnesses or filing documents in court. Some permit the principal to nominate a person who will serve as personal or financial legal guardian in the event that a guardian is ever appointed. Like living wills, the power of attorney will not be useful unless its existence is known. Copies of the power of attorney should be provided to family members. When the power of attorney is written for health care decision making, a copy should be provided to the treating physician.

Written instruction directives such as living wills and powers of attorney for health care are useful in that they provide a mechanism for a person to express his views and decisions about his future health care needs should he become unable to make or communicate them at a later date. Yet they, especially living wills, have their limitations: Written documents are typically made too far in advance of the need for the treatment decision, and people have often changed their views by then; medical practice may have been significantly changed since the written document was signed; it is unlikely that one can anticipate every detailed medical dilemma; and some laws limit their application and either do not provide for or explicitly exclude decisions such as the withdrawal of feeding tubes and nutrition or participation in medical research. It is thus important to nominate a proxy through a living will or a durable power of attorney for health care, a trustworthy person who is familiar with the person's values and history, and who will be authorized to make treatment decisions which may not be specified by a living will.

F. Surrogate Consent Law

Without a guardianship, specific court order, or durable power of attorney for health care, the legal authority for family or interested others to make decisions for a decisionally impaired person is generally uncertain. Nevertheless, family members have historically acted as informal guardians, especially in the medical area. Some states, however, have enacted surrogate consent statutes which legally recognize the substituted decision of family members even in the absence of a prior designation of decision making authority by the patient. There may also be case law which provides for this. These surrogate decision-making provisions may be contained in the living-will statutes, in the informed consent to treatment laws, or elsewhere. These laws often enumerate a priority list of family members who could provide substituted consent or refusal for the patient. Such a sequence might include spouse, adult child, either parent, sibling, other relative, or interested nonfamily member. The family surrogate decision maker must be available, willing to serve as surrogate, and not decisionally incapacitated himself. These laws sometimes restrict the surrogate's authority to certain interventions or at certain times (e.g., the use of life-sustaining care in the presence of a terminal illness). To invoke the surrogate's decision-making authority and avoid petition to the court, the treating clinician (and sometimes a required second medical opinion) must certify the patient's decision-making incapacity. The use of a priority list of surrogates is particularly helpful when there is dissent in the family about treatment, since only the decision of the family member with the highest priority is to be effected. Petition to court is still sometimes available to resolve family disputes regarding consent. These surrogate consent acts often have a variety of technical requirements which make it necessary for clinicians to be intimately familiar with their provisions.

IX. CONCLUSION

Competency is perhaps the most central concept in mental health law. Nearly every legal issue faced by mental health clinicians relates to the patient's functional capacity or legal competency in one way or another. In fact, the law treats patients with mental disorders differently from those with physical disorders because of an underlying suspicion that the mental disorder renders them incompetent in some, often undefined way.

Despite the importance of competency in the law, there is little consensus about the minimum standard of capacity which renders a person competent or incompetent in the eyes of the law. Legal competencies are usually not operationally defined but are largely abstract concepts.

Nevertheless, mental health clinicians are called on to perform capacity or competency assessments on a regular basis, both informally and formally. Clinicians are often pressured by family or treating therapists to find the patient incapacitated so that a guardian can be appointed, the estate secured, or treatment provided. Such assessments involve difficult clinical, legal, and ethical judgments. Familiarity with standard assessment procedures and competency criteria will lighten the therapist's burden in this area. The clinician needs to remember that the ultimate judgment about a patient's legal competency is the responsibility of a court, not the clinician.

In practice, any one of the many types of legal guardianships can usually be obtained without much difficulty. Guardianship hearings are rarely truly adversarial, though respondents have some legal rights in this area. Legal reforms in guardianship in the future may result in increasing legal protections for allegedly disabled persons, more courtroom challenges to allegations of incompetency, and more accountability of guardians. Once a guardianship has been obtained, clinicians are responsible for working with the guardian as well as the patient. Since guardianship is costly and deprives a person of his civil rights in one or more areas, alternatives to guardianship should be used as much as possible.

X. COMMONLY ASKED QUESTIONS

1. Can a legal guardian of a person admit his ward to a psychiatric hospital?

States vary as to the legal authority of a guardian to consent to psychiatric treatment for the ward. Some states permit a guardian to consent to involuntary hospitalization, involuntary medication, or ECT. Others require a specific court order for these forms of psychiatric treatment. Others permit some combination of these or even none at all. Civil commitment may be needed to hospitalize an adjudicated incompetent person when the guardian lacks the legal authority to do so.

2. A suicidal patient who is voluntarily admitted to the hospital consents to undergo a course of ECT treatments. Upon questioning about the nature of the treatment, however, he states that he welcomes the ECT because he knows that it will kill him. Should the staff accept his assent?

No. While staff typically welcome a patient's consent to treatment and dread a treatment refusal, not all apparent consents should be accepted as valid. Staff should first attempt to educate the patient about ECT and treat his apparent suicidality or depression as much as possible without ECT. Should continued treatment fail to alter the irrationality of his assent, temporary medical guardianship should be considered, perhaps with the family's involvement.

3. The staff and family of the patient in Question 2 above decide to proceed with guardianship. After the guardian has been appointed, must the patient's legal admission status be changed to civil commitment since he no longer is deemed legally competent to consent to voluntary hospitalization?

Some states are likely to view an initial consent to voluntary hospitalization as surviving any adjudication of incompetency. Others will interpret their admission and commitment laws so that, in effect, each consent is valid only so long as the patient is capable of providing it. In the latter case, the patient would now need to be civilly committed.

4. *How does one evaluate testamentary capacity?*

Testamentary capacity, the ability to write a will, in the absence of undue influence from others, can be assessed when the person ("testator") is alive or deceased. Evaluating testamentary capacity postmortem requires a retrospective determination of the testator's mental capacity when he executed his will at some time in the past. An evaluator who never previously met the testator must use the available medical, psychiatric, and financial records, in conjunction with interviews with family, friends, attorneys, and others, to determine whether the testator knew the nature and purpose of a will, the extent of his estate, and his natural beneficiaries at that time. Evaluating testamentary capacity is more accurately accomplished with a living testator who can be personally interviewed about these matters. His capacity can be documented by means of audiotape and videotape recordings in the presence of witnesses at the time he makes a will.

5. *Should a therapist become a legal guardian for a patient if no one else is available?*

No. The unavailability of potential legal guardians of the person for elderly or disabled individuals is an increasingly prevalent problem. Acting in a dual capacity as the patient's therapist and legal guardian inherently creates a conflict of interest and must be avoided. Those who deliver health care services should not also be responsible for supervising or paying for those services. It is preferable to identify another health care professional, an administrator of the facility, an attorney, or a community volunteer familiar with the relevant issues to act as personal guardian for the patient. When there is doubt about a potential conflict of interest for the proposed guardian, the court should be consulted.

6. *If a therapist for a patient with a legal guardian of the estate believes that the guardian is mishandling the patient's funds, what should he do?*

The therapist might consider several approaches to this situation depending upon the nature and extent of the mismanagement, the patient's capacity to understand it, and the therapist's relationship with the patient, the guardian, and the family. The therapist might initially confront the guardian or inform family members of the problem. Should this be unsatisfactory, the therapist could bring the situation to the attention of the court charged with supervising the guardianship.

7. *A patient refuses a recommended medical procedure or treatment, asserting religious reasons. Must the clinician respect this refusal?*

The clinician must determine (a) the presence, nature, and extent of any mental disorder; (b) the organization and history of the patient's religious beliefs to learn whether this is an organized religion or the patient's idiosyncratic and bizarre beliefs; and (c) whether the religious beliefs are in fact the basis for the refusal or only a pretext for them, when the genuine reason is mental disorder or denial of illness. If the clinician determines the patient is making a competent decision to refuse treatment, the decision must be honored.

8. An adult patient's family member tells the therapist that he would like to discontinue a patient's treatment. Must the therapist comply with the family's request when the patient continues to consent to treatment?

The clinician must evaluate the patient's capacity to consent to treatment. If the patient consents to treatment, and the consent is assessed as being a capable one, then a legally competent patient can continue to receive the treatment as he requests, despite the family's disapproval. It would be advisable under the circumstances to discuss the issue further with the family to resolve the apparent conflict.

9. Can a person who appears mentally incapacitated grant a durable power of attorney?

No. Under state law, in order to grant a power of attorney or a durable power of attorney, the principal must be capable of understanding its nature, purpose, and effect. A durable power of attorney is useful because it survives the person's incapacity, but it must be granted prior to the onset of that incapacity.

10. Can anyone be forced to accept a power of attorney or to act as a legal guardian?

No. Except in the case of an institution or public agency whose professional responsibility is to serve as a substitute decision maker, individuals must agree to accept the power of attorney or to be the guardian.

11. Can a person still legally act on his own after giving a power of attorney to someone?

Yes. After the power of attorney has been granted, the principal can still act, so long as he has not become incapacitated.

12. When a person is appointed to be the guardian of the person or of the estate, must he use his personal funds to provide for the care of his ward?

No. A guardian is required to use only the funds of the ward. If, as a matter of convenience, the guardian finds it necessary to temporarily use his personal funds for the ward, then the guardian should provide proper documentation of these expenses to the court to obtain reimbursement from the ward's estate.

13. Is there a form for a power of attorney for health care?

As more states are recognizing the limitations of living wills, they are enacting specific provisions for health care powers of attorney. A stationery store which carries legal forms will often have copies of the forms to use, if there is such a law in a particular state. They can also be obtained from attorneys who specialize in estate planning. Legal counsel may be useful in tailoring the power of attorney to an individual patient.

14. What are the advantages of a power of attorney for health care?

A power of attorney for health care (a) obviates the need for a legal guardianship, thus saving time and fees; (b) can be broader than a living will, thus addressing medical decisions even when the person is not terminally ill; (c) designates in advance who shall act as the substitute decision maker for the person; (d) provides documentation of the person's views on health care while the person remains able to express his views; and (e) may avoid the need for a personal guardian.

15. Can advance directives be used for psychiatric treatment?

Only one state, Minnesota, has a law specifically permitting a mentally ill person to write an advance directive (a written instruction directive or appointing a proxy decisionmaker) for the future use of antipsychotic medication or ECT. Other states with health care power of attorney provisions do not specifically address whether they apply or do not apply to psychiatric treatments, leaving this matter uncertain. There are likely to be many problems with implementing advance directives for psychiatric treatment, including their conflict with existing standards and procedures for civil commitment, involuntary medication, and ECT. Their use also raises questions about the person's decision-making capacity at the time of their writing.

XI. BIBLIOGRAPHY

I. Competency

A. Cases

Application of President and Directors of Georgetown College, 331 F.2d 1000 (D.C.Cir. 1964). [refusal of blood transfusion due to religious beliefs as a Jehovah's Witness]
In re Guardianship of Mikulanec, 356 N.W.2d 683 (Minn.Sup.Ct. 1984). [competency to marry]
Taylor v. Garinger, 507 N.E.2d 406 (Ohio App. 1986). [testamentary capacity after legal incompetence]
Blattner v. Blattner, 411 N.W.2d 24 (Minn.App. 1987). [competency to divorce]
In the Matter of Beth Israel Medical Center, 519 N.Y.S.2d 511 (Sup. 1987). [competency to consent to surgery]
Julius Cohen Jeweler v. Succession of Jumonville, 506 So.2d 535 (La.App. 1987). [competency to contract to buy jewelry]
In re Milton, 505 N.E.2d 255 (Ohio Sup.Ct. 1987). [treatment refusal due to religious belief in faith healing]
Succession of Sauls, 510 So.2d 715 (La.App. 1987). [testamentary capacity after legal incompetence]
Heights Realty v. Phillips, 749 P.2d 77 (N.M.Sup.Ct. 1988). [competency to sign real-estate-listing contract]
Feiden v. Feiden, 542 N.Y.S.2d 860 (A.D. 1989). [competency to execute deed]
Harper v. Rogers, 387 S.E.2d 547 (Sup.Ct.W.Va. 1989). [competency to execute deed]
Lloyd v. Jordan, 544 So.2d 957 (Ala.Sup.Ct. 1989). [competency to sign annuity contract]
Weir by Gasper v. Estate of CIAO, 556 A.2d 819 (Sup.Ct.Pa. 1989). [competency to transfer real estate]
Craig v. Perry, 565 So.2d 171 (Ala.Sup.Ct. 1990). [testamentary capacity]
Payne v. Marion General Hospital, 549 N.E.2d 1043 (Ind.App. 1990). [competency to request do not resuscitate order]
In the matter of Romero, 790 P.2d 819 (Sup.Ct.Colo. 1990). [competency to consent to sterilization]
Wilcox v. Willard Shopping Center, 579 A.2d 130 (Conn.App. 1990). [competency to bid on property]
In re Marriage of Davis, 576 N.E.2d 972 (Ill.App. 1991). [competency to marry]
Pape v. Byrd, 582 N.E.2d 164 (Sup.Ct.Ill. 1991). [competency to marry]
Shoals Ford v. Clardy, 588 So.2d 879 (Ala.Sup.Ct. 1991). [competency of person in manic episode to buy truck]
Syno v. Syno, 594 A.2d 307 (Pa.Super. 1991). [competency to divorce]
Annotation: Power of court or other public agencies, in the absence of statutory authority, to order compulsory medical care for adult, 9 A.L.R.3d 1391.
Annotation: Mental competency of patient to consent to surgical operation or medical treatment, 25 A.L.R.3d 1439.

B. Articles and Books

Appelbaum, P. S. (1984). Informed consent. In D. N. Weisstub (Ed.), *Law and mental health, Vol. 1*, pp. 45–83, New York: Pergamon Press.
Appelbaum, P. S., & Grisso, T. (1988). Assessing patients' capacities to consent to treatment. *New England Journal of Medicine, 319*, 1635–1638.
Appelbaum, P. S., & Roth, L. H. (1981) Clinical issues in the assessment of competency. *American Journal of Psychiatry, 138*, 1462–1467.

Appelbaum, P. S., & Roth, L. H. (1982). Competency to consent to research: A psychiatric overview. *Archives of General Psychiatry, 39*, 951–958.
Appelbaum, P. S., Lidz, C. W., & Meisel, A. (1987). *Informed consent*. New York: Oxford University Press.
Berlin, R. M., & Canaan, A. (1991). A family systems approach to competency evaluations in the elderly. *Psychosomatics, 32*, 349–354.
Collier, M. M. (1990). The mentally deficient witness: The death of incompetency. *Law and Psychology Review, 14*, 107–137.
Culver, C. M., & Gert, B. (1982). *Philosophy in medicine: Conceptual and ethical issues in medicine and psychiatry*. New York: Oxford University Press.
Culver, C. M., & Gert, B. (1990). The inadequacy of incompetence. *Milbank Quarterly, 68*, 619–643.
Cutter, M. A. G., & Shelp, E. E. (Eds.). (1991). *Competency: A study of informal competency determinations in primary care*. Dordrecht: Kluwer Academic.
Drane, J. F. (1985). The many faces of competency. *Hastings Center Report, 15*, 17–21.
Draper, R.J., & Dawson, D. (1990). Competence to consent to treatment: A guide for the psychiatrist. *Canadian Journal of Psychiatry, 35*, 285–289.
Faden, R. F., & Beauchamp, T. L. (1986). *A history and theory of informed consent*. New York: Oxford University Press.
Gabinet, L. (1986). A protocol for assessing competence to parent a newborn. *General Hospital Psychiatry, 8*, 263–272.
Gurian, B. S., Baker, E. H., Jacobson, S., Lagerbom, B., & Watts, P. (1990). Informed consent for neuroleptics with elderly patients in two settings. *Journal of the American Geriatrics Society, 38*, 37–44.
Gutheil, T. G., & Bursztajn, H. (1986). Clinicians' guidelines for assessing and presenting subtle forms of patient incompetence in legal settings. *American Journal of Psychiatry, 143*, 1020–1023.
Gutheil, T. G., Bursztajn, H., Kaplan, A. N., & Brodsky, A. (1987). Participation in competency assessment and treatment decisions: The role of a psychiatrist–attorney team. *Mental and Physical Disability Law Reporter, 11*, 446–449.
Hoffman, B. F., & Srinivasan, J. (1992). A study of competence to consent to treatment in a psychiatric hospital. *Canadian Journal of Psychiatry, 37*, 179–182.
Kaplan, K. H., & Price, M. (1989). The clinician's role in competency evaluations. *General Hospital Psychiatry, 11*, 397–403.
Kapp, M. B. (1985). *Geriatrics and the law: Patient rights and professional responsibilities*. New York: Springer.
Lidz, C. W., Meisel, A., Zerubavel, E., Carter, M., Sestak, R. M., & Roth, L. H. (1984). *Informed consent: A study of decisionmaking in psychiatry*. New York: Guilford Press.
McCrary, S. V., & Walman, A. T. (1990). Procedural paternalism in competency determination. *Law, Medicine, and Health Care, 18*, 108–113.
McKinnon, K., Cournos, F., & Stanley, B. (1989). *Rivers* in practice: Clinicians' assessments of patients' decision-making capacity. *Hospital and Community Psychiatry, 40*, 1159–1162.
Melnick, V. L., & Dubler, N. M. (Eds.). (1985). *Alzheimer's dementia: Dilemmas in clinical research*. Clifton, NJ: Humana Press.
Pavlo, A. M., Bursztajn, H., & Gutheil, T. G. (1987). Christian Science and competence to make treatment choices: Clinical challenges in assessing values. *International Journal of Law and Psychiatry, 10*, 395–401.
Pavlo, A. M., Bursztajn, H., Gutheil, T. G., & Levi, L. M. (1987). Weighing religious beliefs in determining competence. *Hospital and Community Psychiatry, 38*, 350–352.
Rosner, R., & Schwartz, H. I. (Eds.). (1987). *Geriatric psychiatry and the law*. New York: Plenum Press.
Roth, L. H., Meisel, A., & Lidz, C. W. (1977). Tests of competency to consent to treatment. *American Journal of Psychiatry 134*, 279–284.
Rozovsky, F. A. (1990). *Consent to treatment: A practical guide* (2nd ed.). Boston: Little, Brown.
Saks, E. R. (1991). Competency to refuse treatment. *North Carolina Law Review, 69*, 945–999.
Schwartz, H. I., & Blank, K. (1986). Shifting competency during hospitalization: A model for informed consent decisions. *Hospital and Community Psychiatry, 37*, 1256–1260.
Spar, J. E., & Garb, A. S. (1992). Assessing competency to make a will. *American Journal of Psychiatry, 149*, 169–174.
Spaulding, W. J. (1985). Testamentary competency. *Law and Human Behavior, 9*, 113–139.
Stanley, B., Stanley, M., Guido, J., & Garvin, L. (1988). The functional competency of elderly at risk. *Gerontologist, 28* (Suppl), 53–58.
Stone, A. (1979). Informed consent: Special problems for psychiatry. *Hospital and Community Psychiatry, 30*, 321–327.

II. Guardianship and Substituted Decision Making

A. *Cases*

Vecchione v. Wohlgemuth, 426 F.Supp. 1297 (E.D.Pa. 1977); 558 F.2d 150 (3rd Cir. 1977).
Estate of Early, 673 P.2d 209 (Sup.Ct. Cal. 1983).
In re Gardner, 459 N.E.2d 17 (Ill.App. 1984).
In the Matter of the Guardianship of Opal Ingram, 689 P.2d 1363 (Wash.Sup.Ct. 1984). [court approval needed for amputation]
Pace v. Pace, 513 N.E.2d 1357 (Ohio App. 1986).
Detzel v. Detzel, 521 N.Y.S.2d 6 (A.D. 1987).
In the Matter of the Guardianship of K.N.K., 407 N.W.2d 281 (Wis.App. 1987).
In re Guardianship of Osterman, 515 So.2d 1066 (Fla.App. 1987).
Werner v. Wright, 737 S.W.2d 761 (Mo.App. 1987).
In re Conservatorship of Goodman, 766 P.2d 1010 (Okla.App. 1988).
In re Conservatorship of Estate of Martin, 421 N.W.2d 463 (Neb.Sup.Ct. 1988). ["prudent man" proxy decision-making standard]
In re Interdiction of Thomas, 535 So.2d 1315 (La.App. 1988).
Wahlenmaier, v. Wahlenmaier, 762 S.W.2d 575 (Tex.Sup.Ct. 1988). [guardian's right to obtain divorce for ward]
In re Bailey, 771 S.W.2d 779 (Ark.Sup.Ct. 1989).
Commonwealth of Pennsylvania v. Bean, 558 A.2d 170 (Pa.Cmwlth. 1989).
Goldman v. Krane, 786 P.2d 437 (Colo.App. 1989).
Hill v. Jones, 773 S.W.2d 55 (Tex.Ct.App. 1989).
Pate v. Bobo, 540 So.2d 660 (Sup.Ct.Ala. 1989).
In re Lundgaard, 453 N.W.2d 58 (Minn.App. 1990).
Bryan v. Holzer, 589 So.2d 648 (Sup.Ct.Miss. 1991). [fraud by conservator]
In the Matter of Grinker, 573 N.E.2d 536 (N.Y.Ct.App. 1991). [conservator may not commit ward to nursing home]
In the Matter of Estate of Logan, 815 P.2d 35 (Idaho App. 1991). [guardian's failure to keep records]
Guardianship of Doe, 583 N.E.2d 1263 (Mass.Sup.Jud.Ct. 1992). [terminate feeding and hydration from never competent person]
Annotation: Effect of guardianship of adult on testamentary capacity, 89 ALR 2d 1120.
Annotation: Validity of guardianship proceeding based on brainwashing of subject by religious, political, or social organization, 44 ALR 4th 1207.

B. *Articles and Books*

American College of Physicians. (1989). Cognitively impaired subjects. *Annals of Internal Medicine, 111*, 843–848.
Anderer, S. J. (1990). *Determining competency in guardianship proceedings.* Washington, DC: American Bar Association.
Apolloni, T., & Cooke, T. P. (1984). *A new look at guardianship.* Baltimore: Brookes.
Applegate, W. B. (1987). Use of assessment instruments in clinical settings. *Journal of the American Geriatric Society, 35*, 45–50.
Areen, J. (1987). The legal status of consent obtained from families of adult patients to withhold or withdraw treatment. *Journal of the American Medical Association, 258*, 229–235.
Axilbund, M. T. (1979). *Substituted judgment for the disabled: Report of an inquiry into limited guardianship, public guardianship and adult protective services in six states.* Washington, DC: Commission on the Mentally Disabled, American Bar Association.
Barnes, A. P. (1988). Florida guardianship and the elderly: The paradoxical right to unwanted assistance. *University of Florida Law Review, 40*, 949–988.
Brown, R. N. (1989). *The rights of older persons.* Carbondale: Southern Illinois University Press.
Buchanan, A. E., & Brock, D. W. (1989). *Deciding for others: The ethics of surrogate decision making.* Cambridge: Cambridge University Press.
Cairl, R. E., Pfeiffer, E., Keller, D. M., Burke, H., & Samis, H. V. (1983). An evaluation of the reliability and validity of the Functional Assessment Inventory. *Journal of the American Geriatric Society, 31*, 607–612.
Casasanto, M. D., Covert, S. B., Saunders, A. G., & Simon, M. M. (1987). Individual functional assessment: An instruction manual. *Mental and Physical Disability Law Reporter, 11*, 60–90.

Commission on Legal Problems of the Elderly American Bar Association. (1986). *Statement of recommended judicial practices*. Washington, DC: American Bar Association.
Commission on the Mentally Disabled, Commission on Legal Problems of the Elderly, American Bar Association. (1989). *Guardianship: An agenda for reform*. Washington, DC: American Bar Association.
Denton, P. (1988). Assessing the patient's functional performance. *Hospital and Community Psychiatry, 39*, 935–936.
Emanuel, E. J., & Emanuel, L. L. (1992). Proxy decision making for incompetent patients. *Journal of the American Medical Association, 267*, 2067–2071.
Friedman, L., & Savage, M. (1988). Taking care: The law of conservatorship in California. *Southern California Law Review, 61*, 273–290.
Frolik, L. A. (1981). Plenary guardianship: An analysis, a critique, and a proposal for reform. *Arizona Law Review, 23*, 599–660.
George, L. K., & Fillenbaum, G. G. (1985). OARS methodology: A decade of experience in geriatric assessment. *Journal of the American Geriatric Society, 33*, 607–615.
Grisso, T. (1986). *Evaluating competencies: Forensic assessments and instruments*. New York: Plenum Press.
Gutheil, T. G., & Appelbaum, P. S. (1985). The substituted judgment approach: Its difficulties and paradoxes in mental health settings. *Law, Medicine, and Health Care, 13*, 61–64.
Hafemeister, T. L., & Sales, B. D. (1982). Responsibilities of psychologists under guardianship and conservatorship laws. *Professional Psychology, 13*, 354–371.
Hafemeister, T. L., & Sales, B. D. (1984). Interdisciplinary evaluations for guardianships and conservatorships. *Law and Human Behavior, 8*, 335–354.
High, D. M., & Turner, H. B. (1987). Surrogate decision making: The elderly's familial expectations. *Theoretical Medicine, 8*, 303–320.
Iris, M. A. (1988). Guardianship and the elderly: A multi-perspective view of the decisionmaking process. *Gerontologist, 28*(Suppl), 39–45.
Jecker, N. S. (1990). The role of intimate others in medical decision making. *Gerontologist, 30*, 65–71.
Lamb, H. R., & Weinberger, L. E. (1992). Conservatorship for gravely disabled psychiatric patients: A four-year follow-up study. *American Journal of Psychiatry, 149*, 909–913.
Lichtenberg, P. A., & Strzepek, D. M. (1990). Assessments of institutionalized dementia patients' competencies to participate in intimate relationships. *Gerontologist, 30*, 117–120.
Massad, P., & Sales, B. (1981). Guardianship: An acceptable alternative to institutionalization? *American Behavioral Scientist, 24*, 755–767.
New York State Task Force on Life and the Law. (1992). *When others must choose: Deciding for patients without capacity.* New York: Author.
Nolan, B. S. (1984). Functional evaluation of the elderly in guardianship proceedings. *Law, Medicine, and Health Care, 12*, 210–218.
Parry, J. (1987). A unified theory of substitute consent: Incompetent patients' right to individualized health care decision making. *Mental and Physical Disability Law Reporter, 11*, 378–441.
Parsons, R. J., & Cox, E. O. (1989). Family medication in elder caregiving decisions: An empowerment intervention. *Social Work, 34*, 122–126.
Peters, R., Schmidt, W. C., & Miller, K. S. (1985). Guardianship of the elderly in Tallahassee, Florida. *Gerontologist, 25*, 532–538.
Pfeiffer, E., Johnson, T. M., & Chiofolo, R. C. (1981). Functional assessment of elderly subjects in four service settings. *Journal of the American Geriatric Society, 29*, 433–437.
Pleak, R. R., & Appelbaum, P. S. (1985). The clinician's role in protecting patient's rights in guardianship proceedings. *Hospital and Community Psychiatry, 36*, 77–79.
Rhoden, N. K. (1988). Litigating life and death. *Harvard Law Review, 102*, 375–446.
Robinson, B. E., Lund, C. A, Keller, D., & Cuervo, C. A. (1986). Validation of the Functional Assessment Inventory against a multidisciplinary home care team. *Journal of the American Geriatric Society, 34*, 851–854.
Schmidt, W. C., & Peters, R. (1987). Legal incompetents' need for guardians in Florida. *Bulletin of the American Academy of Psychiatry and the Law, 15*, 69–83.
Schmidt, W. C., Miller, K. S., Bell, W. G., & New, B. G. (1981). *Public guardianship and the elderly*. Cambridge, MA: Ballinger.
Seckler, A. B., Meier, D. E., Mulvihill, M. & Paris, B. E. C. (1991). Substituted judgment: How accurate are proxy predictions? *Annals of Internal Medicine, 115*, 92–98.
Solomon, D. (1988). National Institutes of Health Consensus Development Conference Statement: Geriatric assessment methods for clinical decision making. *Journal of the American Geriatric Society, 36*, 342–347.

Steinberg, R. M. (1985). *Alternative approaches to conservatorship and protection of older adults referred to public guardian*. Los Angeles: Andrus Gerontology Center, University of Southern California.
Tomlinson, T., Howe, K., Notman, M., & Rossmiller, D. (1990). An empirical study of proxy consent for elderly persons. *Gerontologist, 30*, 54–64.
Warren, J. W., Sobal, J., Tenney, J. H., Hoopes, J. M., Damron, D., Levenson, S., DeForge, B. R., & Muncie, H. L. (1986). Informed consent by proxy: An issue in research with elderly persons. *New England Journal of Medicine, 315*, 1124–1128.
Wettstein, R. M., & Roth, L. H. (1988). The psychiatrist as legal guardian. *American Journal of Psychiatry, 145*, 600–604.

III. Elder Abuse and Protective Services

Council on Scientific Affairs, American Medical Association. (1987). Elder abuse and neglect. *Journal of the American Medical Association, 257*, 966–971.
Daniels, R. S., Baumhover, L. A., & Clark-Daniels, C. L. (1989). Physicians' mandatory reporting of elder abuse. *Gerontologist, 29*, 321–327.
Filinson, R., & Ingman, S. R. (Eds.). (1989). *Elder abuse: Practice and policy*. New York: Human Sciences Press.
Kapp, M. B. (1983). Adult protective services: Convincing the patient to consent. *Law, Medicine, and Health Care, 11*, 163–188.
Kosberg, J. I. (Ed.). (1983). *Abuse and maltreatment of the elderly: Causes and interventions*. Boston: John Wright.
Pillemer, K., & Finkelhor, D. (1988). The prevalence of elder abuse: A random sample survey. *Gerontologist, 28*, 51–57.
Quinn, M. J., & Tomita, S. K. (1986). *Elder abuse and neglect: Causes, diagnosis, and intervention strategies*. New York: Springer.
Salend, E., Kane, R. A., Satz, M., & Pynoos, J. (1984). Elder abuse reporting: Limitations of statutes. *Gerontologist, 24*, 61–69.

IV. Advance Directives

A. Cases

Barber v. Superior Court, 195 Cal.Rptr. 484 (1983).
Bartling v. Superior Court, 209 Cal.Rptr. 220 (App. 1984).
John F. Kennedy Memorial Hospital v. Bludworth, 452 So.2d 921 (Fla. 1984).
In Re Conroy, 486 A.2d 1209 (N.J.Sup.Ct. 1985).
Saunders v. State, 492 N.Y.S.2d 510 (Sup.Ct. 1985).
Cruzan v. Missouri Department of Health, 110 S.Ct. 2841 (1990).

B. Articles and Books

Alexander, G. J. (1988). *Writing a living will using a durable power of attorney*. New York: Praeger.
Choice in Dying. (1992). *Refusal of treatment legislation: A compilation of state statutes*. New York: Author.
Clifford, A. D. (1987). *Simple will book: How to prepare a legally valid will*. Berkeley: Nolo Press.
Davidson, K. W., Hackler, C., Caradine, D. R., & McCord, R. S. (1989). Physicians' attitudes on advance directives. *Journal of the American Medical Association, 262*, 2415–2419.
Emanuel, L. L., & Emanuel, E. J. (1989). The medical directive: A new comprehensive advance care document. *Journal of the American Medical Association, 261*, 3288–3293.
High, D. M. (1987). Planning for decisional incapacity: A neglected area in ethics and aging. *Journal of the American Geriatrics Society, 35*, 814–820.
King, N. (1991). *Making sense of advance directives*. Dordrecht: Kluwer Academic Publishers.
Legal Counsel for the Elderly. (1987). *Decision making, incapacity, and the elderly: A protective services manual*. Washington, DC: American Association of Retired Persons.
Meisel, A. (1989 & Suppl.). *The right to die*. New York: Wiley.
Moore, D. L. (1986). The durable power of attorney as an alternative to the improper use of conservatorship for health-care decisionmaking. *St. Johns's Law Review, 60*, 631–673.

Ouslander, J. G., Tymchuk, A. J., & Rahbar. B. (1989). Health care decisions among elderly long-term care residents and their potential proxies. *Archives of Internal Medicine, 149*, 1367–1372.
Overman, W., & Stoudemire, A. (1988). Guidelines for legal and financial counseling of Alzheimer's disease patients and their families. *American Journal of Psychiatry, 145*, 1495–1500.
President's Commission for the Study of Ethical Problems in Medicine and Biomedical and Behavioral Research. (1983). *Deciding to forego life-sustaining treatment*. Washington, DC: U.S. Goverment Printing Office.
Roe, J. M., Goldstein, M. K., Massey, K., & Pascoe, D. (1992). Durable power of attorney for health care. *Archives of Internal Medicine, 152*, 292–296.
Schneiderman, L. J. (1985). Counseling patients to counsel physicians on future care in the event of patient incompetence. *Annals of Internal Medicine, 102*, 693–698.
Soled, A. J. (1988). *The essential guide to wills, estates, trusts, and death taxes*. Glenview, IL: Scott Foresman.
U.S. Congress, Office of Technology Assessment. (1987). *Life-sustaining technologies and the elderly*. Washington, DC: U.S. Government Printing Office.

10

Legal Rights of Children

KATHLEEN M. QUINN, M.D.* AND BARBARA A. WEINER, J.D.

I. Competency • A. Emancipated Minor • B. Mature Minor • **II. The Child Witness** • **III. Access to Medical Care** • A. Emergency Care • B. Parents' Refusal of Treatment • C. Handicapped Infants • D. Parental Consent • E. Child's Role in Treatment Decisions • F. Consent by Nonparents • **IV. Reproductive Rights** • A. Access to Contraceptives • B. Venereal Disease Counseling • C. Abortion • D. Sterilization • **V. Access to Outpatient Counseling** • A. Substance Abuse • B. Mental Health Services • **VI. Psychiatric Hospitalization of Minors** • **VII. Confidentiality of Records** • **VIII. Participation in Research** • **IX. Child Abuse and Neglect** • A. Reporting Abuse and Neglect • B. Investigation of Abuse and Neglect • C. Actions to Protect the Child • D. Liability of the Caseworker • **X. Divorce and Child Custody** • A. Legal Definitions • B. Evaluating the Child's Best Interests • C. Recommending Joint Custody • D. Mediating Custody Disputes • E. Acting as Therapist to One of the Parties • F. Confidentiality Issues • **XI. Access of Disabled Children to an Education** • **XII. Juvenile Justice System** • A. Role of the Mental Health Professional • B. Charging the Child as an Adult • C. The Future • **XIII. Commonly Asked Questions** • **XIV. Bibliography**

Under the legal system in the United States, a child is a person who is under 18 years of age. Age is the determining factor in deciding who can consent to treatment. The treatment provider must be concerned with wishes and rights of the parents as well as the rights of the child. It is usually the parents or guardians who refer the minor for care and define the problem for which they are seeking help. Rarely does the child alone initiate a request for services.

Mental health professionals often describe children by stages of development: infancy, preschool, latency, and adolescence. These terms do not have meaning within the legal system. In general, the closer an individual comes to the age of

*Dr. Quinn is a child psychiatrist who also specializes in forensic psychiatry. She is an Associate Professor and Associate Director, Division of Forensic Psychiatry, at Case Western Reserve School of Medicine. Dr. Quinn is currently a consultant to the criminal, juvenile, and domestic relations courts in Cuyahoga County, Ohio.

majority, the more likely it is that the individual will be treated as an adult. Legally, the rights of children should be viewed as a continuum, with the infant having the least rights and the older adolescent having the greatest rights, but usually fewer than an adult. The health care provider must be concerned about the wishes of the parent/guardian, the wishes of the child, and sometimes the wishes of the state. The state has the authority and responsibility under its *parens patriae* powers to protect children from serious harm when their parents cannot or will not do so. *Parens patriae* refers to the state's traditional obligations to both protect and provide for any persons under a legal disability (such as age) and therefore unable to provide for themselves. Issues regarding minors often include a balancing of the rights of children and the rights and duties of their parents and the state. In day-to-day clinical practice it must be determined who has the authority to speak for the child: the parents, the state, or the child himself.

This chapter will provide a brief overview of the areas the mental health professional is likely to encounter when dealing with children. Rules applying to consent for the medical treatment of minors and the delivery of mental health services to minors will be discussed. The differences in civil commitment laws as well as the laws concerning confidentiality are reviewed. The role of the mental health professional in child abuse and neglect situations as well as child custody determinations is described. The rights of the disabled to an education are briefly summarized. Finally, the chapter concludes with a description of some of the major features of the juvenile justice system. Selected clinical examples are given to illustrate major issues.

I. COMPETENCY

Competency means that an individual has sufficient ability or authority to make personal decisions regarding his life and his assets. Competency is specific to the task required of the individual. Adults are presumed to be legally competent, unless declared otherwise, but children are presumed to be incompetent. Thus, there are a wide variety of decisions they cannot make and activities in which they cannot participate. Legally incompetent persons are unable to decide where they will live, what type of medical care they will receive, and how their finances will be handled. The legally incompetent person is unable to vote, enter into contracts, or write a will. A substitute decision maker will make the decisions necessary for the incompetent person. (See Chapter 9, "Competency and Guardianship.") In the case of a child this will be the parents, unless their parental rights have been terminated.

The age when a child is legally recognized as having the rights and responsibilities of a competent adult has been arbitrarily defined by various statutes. Until the passage of the Twenty-Sixth Amendment to the United States Constitution in 1971, which allows 18-year-olds to vote, the age of majority was 21. The passage of the Twenty-Sixth Amendment resulted in all states' changing a variety of laws concerning the attainment of majority. However, in some states one must be 21 in order to make a will or purchase alcoholic beverages. In contrast, the *Juvenile Justice Standards Relating to Rights of Minors* proposes the adoption of the age of 18 as the age of majority for all cases. However, there is continuing doubt over the age to grant certain rights and privileges and a resulting lack of uniformity of law from state to state concerning issues such as when children may work, drive, marry, or consent to treatment. Laws limiting the rights and activities of children have been upheld as being within the states' discretion in protecting children.

A. Emancipated Minor

Although children are considered legally incompetent for health care decision making, there are exceptions to this rule. In many states a child can petition the court to be declared an "emancipated minor." The child must show that he has the ability and capacity to manage his own affairs. In general, an emancipated minor is one who is married, is living separately from his parents, or is economically self-supporting. Because emancipation requires a court order, it is unusual to find a child who has been declared an emancipated minor.

If one is declared an emancipated minor, he is to be treated as an adult. If a child is emancipated, this new status has a bearing on (1) the child's right to wages and damages; (2) the child's right to sue and be sued; (3) the child's right to parental support; (4) the child's choice of where to live; and (5) the child's power to make contracts. At issue may be the question, for example, of who is liable for a hospital bill, the adolescent or his parent. While the courts have not been unanimous in their resolution of claims, most decisions have ruled that a parent cannot be compelled to pay for services consented to by an emancipated minor unless the parent has specifically accepted financial responsibility. College students, even if financially dependent on their parents, are considered emancipated in most medical contexts. The fact of having borne children does not necessarily mean one is emancipated. Although an adolescent mother may make treatment decisions concerning her own child and herself, the states vary as to whether or not the adolescent mother is considered emancipated for other purposes. The lowering of the age of majority from 21 to 18 has diminished the overall significance of the emancipation issue because many of the previously litigated cases involved persons in the 18-to-21 age group.

When a practitioner is approached by an adolescent who alleges that he is emancipated, the claim of the minor may be taken at face value if he appears reasonable and sincere and as long as the provider has no reason to doubt him and acts accordingly in good faith. Definitive documentation of the emancipation (e.g., the court order) is not required, but the practitioner must use his professional judgment about the claim.

For example, a 14-year-old might come alone to a doctor's office requesting a physical exam before starting a job. Clinically immature, she represents herself as no longer living at home. A practitioner who has any knowledge to the contrary, such as through a recent social contact with family friends who have mentioned this girl's ongoing conflict with her parents while still living at home, would be well advised not to proceed. This minor's situation should be more fully investigated prior to proceeding to treat her as an emancipated minor.

B. Mature Minor

The "mature minor" doctrine is another evolving exception to the presumption of the legal incompetence of children and the general requirement of parental consent to the treatment of minors. This doctrine holds that if a minor is of sufficient intelligence and maturity to understand and appreciate the risks and benefits of a proposed treatment, then the minor may consent to that treatment without parental consent. A mature minor is an adolescent who has demonstrated the ability to participate in the decision-making process. As adolescents come closer to reaching the age of majority, greater weight should be given to their decisions. In many ways the law has recognized the needs of these children by providing various ages at which they can consent to services or treatment without parental consent. These laws are called *minor treatment statutes*. Mature minors differ from emancipated minors in that they are living at home, are not supporting themselves, and are neither married nor parents. The basis of their authority to consent is their level of development and maturity.

II. THE CHILD WITNESS

Another area of competence of children concerns their ability to be witnesses. The legal standards for establishing the competence of a child witness vary substantially from jurisdiction to jurisdiction. The majority of the states by statute or case law prescribe an age at or above which a child is presumed competent to testify. This age has varied from 14 in common law to 10 currently in approximately half the states and 12 in others. In some states, and in federal as well as military law, an age criterion has been abandoned. Below the specified age, the court must determine testimonial capacity on a case-by-case basis. The child needs to have had mental capacity at the time of the occurrence of the event about which he is to testify to form an accurate impression of it. The child's memory must be sufficient to retain an independent recollection of the event. The child must also be able to understand simple questions put to him, and to express himself. In addition, the child must understand the obligation to speak the truth. An understanding of the obligation to speak the truth may be elicited by determining that the child understands the nature of an oath or that the child understands the consequences of telling the truth or telling a lie.

The competency evaluation should take place shortly before the anticipated testimony and should be conducted by a professional with forensic experience. The written report on competency is a direct report to the court that will rule on the child witness's competency to testify after an in-chambers interview of the proposed child witness. For example, a seven-year-old was allegedly physically and sexually abused by a neighbor. When seen for an evaluation of his competency to be a witness, he became afraid, saying, "The bad man will be there [in the courtroom]." He then became disorganized and barricaded himself in the bathroom. Over the course of three appointments, these behaviors were consistently observed and then summarized in a report. The judge observed similar behaviors at the time of the in-chambers interview and found him to be incompetent to be a witness. This case illustrates the way posttraumatic symptoms can interfere with competency to be a witness.

When a child is a witness, issues are often raised concerning age-related differences in memory, the suggestibility of young children, or their capacity to lie. Free recall, the spontaneous account of an event, has repeatedly been shown to be an ability less well developed in preschoolers than in older children and adults. The increased retrieval strategies and selective attention which improve recall develop most fully between the ages of 5 and 10. Because of these age-related differences, children make more errors of omission in giving an account of an event than errors of commission (false elaboration about the event). These age-related differences in memory may be diminished by the use of structured interview protocols to maximize free recall, the use of two or three investigatory interviews, and the use of props such as anatomically detailed dolls or drawings.

Research has demonstrated that preschoolers are more suggestible than older children and adults. Witnesses of any age provide more accurate data on free recall than in response to direct questions. Children's memory of the action of an event is better than their memory of details about its surroundings. These issues suggest that interviewers of preschool witnesses should be particularly careful to avoid leading questioning and also to ask some open-ended questions, such as "Why are you here today?"

Children under four are generally unable to lie successfully. Clues to lying in children are similar to those in adults, including looking for discrepancies in emotional expression in the voice rather than in facial expressions.

Children between the ages of two and seven who are in the preoperational cognitive stage often present their experiences in concrete and fragmentary communications. Time and sequence are difficult issues for a child in this age range. Interviewers should attempt to establish time sequences by use of major events ("Was it before your brother was born?") or persons ("Who was your teacher that year?"). Evaluators will need to inform legal personnel of the expectable developmental limitations which child witnesses may have.

Recent laws have attempted to address the vulnerabilities of the child witness. Some states give statutory authority for videotaping a child's statements and outline conditions for the tape's admissibility. Many other states permit videotaping of the child's testimony. Videotaping has been viewed as having the advantages of (1) preserving details, especially when the trial occurs long after the event; (2) being taken in a relatively informal setting; and (3) possibly inducing a guilty plea. Disadvantages include (1) a child's discomfort with the recording equipment; (2) a single tape giving an incomplete or fragmented description of the crime; and (3) a technically poor interview becoming a focus for the defense.

All special legal procedures accorded child witnesses are likely to result in appellate review because of the accused's right to confrontation guaranteed by the Sixth Amendment of the United States Constitution. The United States Supreme Court, in *Coy v. Iowa* (1988), disallowed the placement of a screen between the child witness and the defendant as a general procedure. However, the Court recognized that there *may* be a compelling state interest in protecting individual child witnesses from face-to-face confrontation with the defendant. In *Maryland v. Craig*, a 1990 case, the United States Supreme Court acknowledged that face-to-face confrontation is not an absolute constitutional requirement. The Court stated that the defendant's right could be superseded by a legal finding that it is necessary to protect an individual child witness from the trauma that would be caused by testifying in the physical presence of the defendant. Legislation has been introduced in Congress which would provide uniform federal rules to govern the testimony of children.

Nearly every state has ruled on the constitutionality of closed-circuit and videotaped prior testimony statements. The courts have upheld those techniques that permit effective cross-examination of the child and have permitted the waiver of the defendant's being able to confront the child face to face, only upon a showing of individualized need. There are still many questions regarding the constitutionality of laws which find alternative ways for children to testify. In 1990, the United States

Supreme Court held that a child's out-of-court statement can be admitted only if the witness is not available to testify and if the statement is likely to be reliable. Few interviews of child witnesses are videotaped because of the expense and the elaborate procedures required. Yet videotaping remains the optimal method of documenting the child's testimony.

III. ACCESS TO MEDICAL CARE

When a child needs medical care, it is the responsibility of his parent or guardian to provide informed consent prior to treatment. Although an informed consent from an older adolescent is clinically helpful to establish rapport with the patient and maximizes compliance with treatment procedures, it is the parent or guardian who has the ultimate decision-making authority regarding consent to treatment. The failure of clinicians to obtain parental consent in a nonemergency medical situation may give rise to a legal action by the parents for assault and battery. Such an action would be based upon the common law principle of the child as property of his parents, who have an almost absolute right to make decisions concerning their children. Yet there are a number of exceptions to this rule.

A. Emergency Care

In an emergency, the first priority is providing the care necessary to save the life of the child or stabilize his condition. Consent under such circumstances is implied from the facts; that is, given the urgency of the health care need, any reasonable parents would wish their child to be treated promptly. An emergency exists where delay, for purposes of obtaining consent, may reasonably be anticipated to endanger the life or adversely and substantially affect the health of the patient. An emergency may consist of a medical condition requiring urgent attention or a condition causing the child severe pain or fear. Courts have recognized bone fractures, lacerations, and more serious injuries as emergencies. The clinical imperative of an emergency situation is the necessity to act reasonably and promptly in order to stabilize and maintain the health of the patient.

Most states now have statutes specifically addressing emergency care of minors. The vast majority of these laws define an emergency in an extremely broad way and give physicians wide latitude in judging when an emergency exists and parental consent need not be obtained. The laws in Arizona, Idaho, and Montana are more narrow. For example, Arizona defines emergency care as procedures necessary for "treatment of a serious disease, injury, or drug abuse, or to save the life of the patient" (Arizona Revised Statutes Annotated, Section 36–2271(c)). Not all health service providers are allowed by statute to determine if an emergency exists. Only physicians are authorized in some states, while in others psychologists are authorized as well. Reference should be made to the specific state law to determine who is permitted to determine if an emergency exists. With few exceptions there is no legal requirement for a physician to obtain a concurring medical opinion that an emergency exists. Only South Carolina, North Carolina, and Oklahoma have second-physician rules and then only if surgery is contemplated. Even these states waive this requirement if a second opinion is not readily available.

Individual states differ as to what efforts, if any, must be made to contact the parents prior to proceeding with emergency care of a minor. Many states authorize the physician to proceed immediately if an attempt to notify the parents would place the minor at increased risk of death or further deterioration of health. Other states describe their notification requirements. For example, the law in Tennessee states that emergency treatment can proceed only after a "reasonable effort" to notify the minor's parents or guardians, if they are known (Tennessee Code Annotated, Section 63–6-222). All efforts should be made to notify the parents after the patient has been stabilized. The hospital chart should document any efforts which were made to notify the parents. In general, the younger the child, the more narrow should be the definition of an emergency. This is based on the principle that the courts would prefer that informed consent be provided whenever possible. If a procedure to be done is irreversible, such as an amputation or other surgery, treatment should proceed only when there is no other medical alternative or efforts to obtain parental consent have been unsuccessful. Parents should be consulted whenever possible about all aspects of their children's care, including an extension of treatment such as during surgery.

B. Parents' Refusal of Treatment

When the health care professional determines that a child requires medical care, and the parents refuse, the attorney for the hospital should be contacted immediately. Traditionally there have been several options, the first being to seek a court order to override the parents' refusal to consent to treatment. Increasingly, however, a second option, reporting to the local child-protective agency, has been exercised. In all states, the withholding of necessary medical care from a child constitutes abuse and/or neglect. It becomes the role of the protective service agency to investigate the report and take protective action if necessary, which may include a court proceeding. In most states, if a parent is refusing treatment for religious reasons, the law will specifically allow the state's child-protective agency to intervene, to obtain temporary custody, and to provide consent for the needed treatment. Most common are cases where the child needs a blood transfusion and parents object because of their religious principles. It is for the court, not the health care professional, to decide when a child can be treated against parental will.

With the pace of new medical technology, the medical/ethical/legal issues in this area have become increasingly complicated. Health care professionals must understand that whatever advances they have made in terms of technology, it is the child and his family who must live with the decisions made regarding the care, and that only the parents can accurately assess the impact of a potential decision on the child and the family unit. It is when the parents and medical care providers come into conflict that the state asserts its *parens patriae* interest in protecting the child. The courts are careful to give deference to the parents, when it appears that they are acting in a reasonable and rational manner.

C. Handicapped Infants

Under the Child Abuse Amendments of 1984 (42 U.S.C., Sections 5101–5103), all states that accept federal child abuse funds must implement procedures for responding to and investigating medical neglect of handicapped infants "as may be necessary to prevent the withholding of medically indicated treatment from disabled infants with life threatening conditions." The only recognized exceptions recommended in model procedures for implementing the law are (1) the infant who is chronically and irreversibly comatose; (2) cases in which treatment merely prolongs dying; and (3) situations in which treatment is "virtually futile." These amendments were enacted after the publicity given in 1983 to two "Baby Doe" cases. The first case involved an Indiana infant known as "Baby Doe," who was born with Down's syndrome and a surgically correctable blockage of the esophagus, who died after his parents and physician elected not to perform surgey and to withhold food from him. The second case involved a New York child known as "Baby Jane Doe" who was born with multiple neural tube defects, including spina bifida, microencephaly (an abnormally small head), and hydrocephalus (an accumulation of fluid on the brain). After consulting with many parties, including their priest, the parents elected conservative medical treatment that would have decreased the chance of infection, but refused surgery intended to correct the baby's defects. Both cases received a great deal of publicity. The New York case was tried in court, and the trial judge ordered that the infant be treated; however, on appeal, the parents' decision to refuse surgery was respected (*Weber v. Stony Brook Hospital*, 1983).

Model procedures for implementing the Child Abuse Amendments also state that proper nutrition, hydration, and palliative medications must be provided. The extent to which physicians and parents will be allowed to try to make decisions in the best interests of many severely impaired infants depends on the sensitivity and skill of the local investigating departments of protective services, the applicable state regulations, and the responsiveness of hospital review committees, which may do case reviews of disabled infants with life-threatening conditions. Health care providers confronted with questions concerning a severely handicapped infant should consult with their own hospital ethics committee or appropriate hospital administrative personnel to ascertain what legal obligations, if any, must be met.

D. Parental Consent

The consent of only one parent for a child's health care is sufficient unless the health professional knows or has good reason to believe that the other parent would object to that care. When parents are separated or divorced, the parent with possession (physical control) of the child at the time the health need arises generally may authorize the treatment, even if he or she is not the legal custodian. The treating professional need not obtain proof of the accompanying parent's custodial status but may proceed in good-faith reliance upon the information given by the accompanying parent. However, if the care to be given is either more than routine or purely elective (e.g., psychotherapy), the professional should inquire concerning the legal status of the custody of the child and seek the consent of the custodial parent. If the care provider is concerned either that an absent parent will object to treatment or that the accompanying parent does not have the legal authority to consent to treatment (e.g., if the child has been kidnapped from a custodial parent), treatment should not proceed without both parents' consent or judicial authorization unless the presenting complaint is a medical emergency.

In cases in which there is a parental dispute concerning the manner in which a child is to be treated, the health professional should attempt to mediate the dispute in a manner which addresses the best interests of the child. If no resolution occurs and the child's health and welfare are threatened by a delay in needed treatment, the care provider should either report the case as one of child neglect, seek a court order authorizing treatment, or advise the parent favoring the needed treatment to seek such an order.

In at least two clinical situations the consent of one or even both parents may not be effective: (1) in most states parents may not consent to the sterilization of a minor child without court order; and (2) some states limit the right of a father of an illegitimate child to consent to his child's health treatments.

E. Child's Role in Treatment Decisions

Developmental theory predicts that adolescents, especially those 14 and older, would be competent to consent to treatment. The prerequisite of having the necessary cognitive skills—namely, formal operations—reaches a point of equilibrium at about age 14. Children begin to develop formal operations at approximately age 11. Research has demonstrated that 14-year-olds do not differ significantly from adults in making decisions about hypothetical treatment situations. Nine-year-olds appear less competent than adults in their ability to reason about and understand information about medical problems. However, the nine-year-olds studied often did not differ in their choice of reasonable preferences about treatment. Based upon this work, children as young as nine appear able to participate meaningfully in personal medical decision making. Although the law does not permit youngsters of this age to make these decisions, they should be included in regular discussions of the proposed treatments.

Health care providers may face a situation where the parent seeks a particular treatment for a child but the child objects. As the child approaches the age of 18, more weight should be given to his decisions and the reasoning behind them. If the child is close to 18 years of age, and treatment can be delayed until he is 18, it would be wise to wait or, if possible, choose a mutually agreed upon treatment modality. If this is not possible, and the child is an older adolescent who is expressing rational reasons why he is opposed to treatment, the health care professional should seek the advice of the hospital's attorney before proceeding with treatment or may wish to refer the patient for a second opinion concerning appropriate treatment. Although the parents are the ultimate decision makers regarding their child's medical care, the courts afford a great deal of weight to the reasoning of a "mature minor."

Most states have statutes which specify an age at which minors may consent to medical treatment. Practitioners need to be informed concerning their state's statute as well as any specific prohibitions concerning certain procedures such as abortions (see the section on reproductive rights). There have been no reported legal decisions within the last 25 years in which a parent recovered damages, even in the absence of a statute concerning the treatment of minors, for care given a child over 15 without parental consent. This care includes both medical and psychiatric treatment. In consultation with the hospital or clinic attorney, the clinician should determine and then document that the proposed treatment is for the benefit of the minor and is necessary but less than major or serious, that the child is 15 years or older and understands both the risk and benefits of the procedure, and that there is good reason, including refusal of the minor to request it, why parental consent cannot be obtained. Clinicians need to be aware that, except in emergency cases, if no effort has been made to contact the parents, the parents will not be held financially liable for any services rendered.

F. Consent by Nonparents

Can any other persons besides the parents and, in the exceptions described above, the minor consent to care for a minor child? Historically, the answer has been no. Under the doctrine of parental sovereignty, parental decisions regarding a minor and his health needs were considered final and beyond review of the state or other individuals. Increasingly in the past 150 years, however, state involvement in family affairs has increased. Many children reside in foster care, where they have been placed by the auspices of the local protective services. Who may consent to the treatment of children in such official placements? Statutes which specifically address this issue generally permit custodial institutions or foster parents to consent to care of the child which is ordinary, routine, or necessary. However, if a treatment is major, high-risk, or elective, the natural parents, not the foster-care authority, probably retain the legal right to consent. This residual legal right to consent to treatment would not remain if a parent's rights have been terminated or if the child has been surrendered for adoption or placed involuntarily. Few states have statutes specifically addressing issues of medical consent for children in placement. The clinician may need to consult the state agency responsible for foster care concerning the applicable administrative guidelines and regulations. If such information is not available, the clinician should inquire of the individual caretaker accompanying the child who may give consent or should call the supervising social service agency. The state has no greater rights over the minor than a natural parent. Therefore, a child in foster care may become emancipated, may be considered a mature minor, may receive contraceptives, and may have the same rights as other minors.

Children who are presented for treatment by relatives other than parents or concerned adults, or who are in informal placements, are covered by the law pertaining to minors accompanied by nonparental adults. There is little legal authority to permit an adult other than a parent to consent to treatment for a minor unless a specific state statute recognizes such consent or the parent has given the caretaker in writing authority to make such decisions. Such written consents are common in school and classroom settings. In addition, parents will often be aware that if someone else is to care for the child for a long period, such as another relative, written consent should be given to them.

IV. REPRODUCTIVE RIGHTS

Most state legislatures have enacted statutes permitting minors afflicted or affected by certain conditions to obtain treatment without parental consent. These include sexually transmitted diseases and pregnancy-related care. The principle behind these statutes has been to encourage prompt care and preventive measures in young people who would not be likely to seek care if parental consent were required. Abortion and contraceptive-care consent issues are the only situations in which a minor's right to self-consent is constitutionally derived based on a minor's presumed right of privacy. The rules which require parental consent for treatment do not generally apply in the reproductive area.

A. Access to Contraceptives

The United States Supreme Court in *Carey v. Population Services International* (1977) held that contraceptives must be made available to minors. Therefore, a majority of states specifically affirm by statute, court decision, or attorney general's opinion the rights of persons under 18 to consent to contraceptive services and to seek these services without their parents' permission or notification. In a few states, substantial barriers are placed to permitting teenagers to have access to contraceptives. The most notable is the requirement that the parent be notified when the child seeks contraceptive services. The constitutionally of such statutes is questionable. With increasing pressure to overturn *Roe v. Wade* (1973), which recognized a woman's private interest in deciding to have an abortion, it is important for health care providers who work in this area to be aware of the current state of the law.

Title XIX (Medical Assistance) and Title XX (Aid to Families with Dependent Children) of the Social Security Act and Title X of the Family Planning Services and Population Research Act of 1970 require that participating states provide family-planning assistance to all eligible minors regardless of marital status, age, or parenthood. Parental consent and/or notification is neither required nor allowed.

B. Venereal Disease Counseling

Most states have laws which permit minors to seek counseling and treatment for venereal disease without notification of their parents or guardians. States differ on questions of the minimum eligible age, posttreatment notification of parents or partners, and public health reporting requirements. For example, Illinois requires the treating professional to make "reasonable efforts" to involve the family. Any public health reporting requirements applicable to adults regarding sexually transmitted disease (STD) also apply to minors. Such public health reporting applies only to the clinician who makes the diagnosis of STD.

C. Abortion

In 1976, in *Planned Parenthood of Central Missouri v. Danforth*, the U.S. Supreme Court held that a Missouri law requiring minors to have their parents' consent to obtain an abortion was unconstitutional. The Court held that minors, like adults, have a constitutional interest in reproductive privacy. While acknowledging the state's obligation to protect the welfare of the minor and the traditional importance of parental authority, the Court found these interests to be outweighed by the minor's constitutional interest in making an independent, private abortion decision. The Court, in subsequent decisions, has nevertheless not granted the minor the same rights as the adult in the abortion area. Most notable is the Court's 1981 decision in *H.L. v. Matheson*, which upheld a Utah law requiring the physician to give notice to the parents when performing an abortion on a minor. The case emphasized the importance of parental consultation in a "decision that has potentially traumatic and permanent consequences, particularly if the patient is immature."

In 1990, the United States Supreme Court asserted that it is constitutional for a state to require a physician to notify one of a minor's parents at the time she seeks an abortion. However, in *Ohio v. Akron Center for Reproductive Health* (1990), the Court did not directly address whether a judicial bypass procedure is required in parental notice statutes. In a related case, *Hodgson v. Minnesota* (1990), a statute requiring the notice of both parents was held unconstitutional. The issue of whether or not notice can be required if the minor is "mature" remains unanswered.

In many states, abortion remains a controversial topic. In some states, the issues of banning abortion or requiring parental consent or notice are raised on a yearly basis in the state legislature. Until the United States Supreme Court more clearly defines the rights of young women in this area, the health care provider should be aware of the law related to abortion in the state of his practice.

D. Sterilization

A minor cannot be sterilized without a court order in the vast majority of states. This is true even if the parent consents or the minor is mature. Sterilizations which are funded out of federal funds, such as Medicaid, have stringent requirements before the sterilization can occur. Incompetent persons and those under the age of 21 cannot be sterilized with federal funds. When one is seeking a federally funded sterilization, there are notice requirements, a 30-day waiting period, and a requirement to provide advice about alternative birth control methods.

The issue of sterilization, because of its irreversibility, is particularly sensitive when it is proposed for a mentally retarded child. In analyzing such cases, the court determines if the minor is permanently mentally incapacitated to make an informed decision. The judge tries to determine if there is proof to a clear and convincing degree that sterilization is in the best interest of the retarded person and will preserve that person's physical and mental health. The court will consider the individual's potential to care for a child, the impracticality of other contraceptive approaches, the need for contraception (i.e., the probability of sexual activity), and the person's physical capacity for reproduction. The court may also consider the medical necessity of sterilization and the psychological impact of both sterilization and childbirth. Before the court proceeding will occur, the disabled person must be given notice and usually an attorney will be appointed to represent her. Often the judge will interview the minor to discuss her wishes. Even if the guardian or parent of a retarded person requests sterilization, a physician should not undertake to perform this procedure without a court order granted after a full hearing. In addition, the physician should have the advice of his own lawyer as to the authority of the court to issue such an order under the law of the state in question.

V. ACCESS TO OUTPATIENT COUNSELING

A. Substance Abuse

More than half of the states have laws which provide that minors have a right of access to information and treatment regarding substance abuse without parental consent. The laws are often not specific regarding the use of alcohol. Since alcohol is recognized as a drug or substance, it is likely that children can obtain alcohol counseling without parental consent. Even in the absence of a state statute, it is likely an adolescent would be found competent to give consent to treatment since the social and personal consequences of continued substance abuse are so devastating. Some states have a minimum age below which parental consent is required. The minimum age is usually in the range of 12 to 14 years.

The states vary on parental notification once treatment is sought or provided to the minor. Some prohibit disclosure (e.g., Connecticut and Iowa), some leave this decision to the professional's discretion (e.g., California, Maine, and Kentucky), some require notification if a minor is hospitalized or remains in treatment a specified time (e.g., Illinois), and some require notification if substance abuse is confirmed but prohibit notification if substance abuse is ruled out (e.g., Montana). If there is no state statute concerning notification, notification should not be done without the minor's permission unless a life-threatening situation (e.g., serious overdose) exists.

Clinically, one cannot successfully treat an abusing adolescent living at home without involving the entire family in treatment. Although confidential access to a treatment facility is essential for initiating the assessment and treatment, it is often possible to negotiate how and when the parents will be told once treatment is under way.

B. Mental Health Services

A minority of states have enacted statutes specifically addressing the ability of minors to consent to outpatient mental health treatment. Typical is the California law, which permits minors 12 or over to consent to outpatient psychotherapy treatment without a parent's consent if the parent's involvement would be "inappropriate." Electroconvulsive therapy (ECT), psychosurgery, and psychotropic medications are excluded. Documentation is required concerning attempts to involve the parents or why it was not appropriate to do so. Other statutes merely state an age at which a person may consent to outpatient treatment. The age of consent ranges from 12 to 18.

In the absence of a specific statute, the state's rules governing medical consent, including emancipated and mature minors, would most likely apply. All licensed psychotherapists could provide services; however, unlicensed personnel may or may not be covered by a state's statutes concerning the treatment of minors. It is hard to imagine a law permitting a minor to consent to surgery but denying the same minor the right to consent to outpatient mental health counseling. Similarly, since nearly all states waive the parental consent in other sensitive health areas such as substance abuse or reproductive health services, by analogy it is likely that a court would view the benefit of confidentiality to a minor in need of mental health care as being of a higher priority than either parental consent or notification. Finally, the constitutional right to privacy may also extend to the communications between a minor and a therapist, lending additional weight to the right of a minor to consent to outpatient treatment.

Community mental health centers would be expected to be covered by the usual rules pertaining to minor consent that apply to other medical treatments. Although treatment could be properly provided such a minor, the therapist could not hold the parents liable for payment. Clinically, the therapist will pursue the issues surrounding parental involvement as a therapeutic issue but clearly must follow the appropriate state statutes regarding consent or notice.

VI. PSYCHIATRIC HOSPITALIZATION OF MINORS

Prior to the 1970s, the majority of states permitted parents and guardians to unilaterally admit their minor children for psychiatric inpatient treatment without review by anyone except the admitting and treatment personnel. Currently, many states continue to allow "voluntary commitment" of a child by his parents. Most states also provide that a preadolescent minor may not leave a mental hospital without approval of his parents. Such policies afford a child significantly fewer protections than an involuntarily hospitalized adult, who may petition for a formal hearing before a court with legal counsel present and due process protections.

During the 1970s, with increased interest concerning children's rights, several state courts began to recognize certain minimal rights of due process for minors prior to their being hospitalized. The most legally stringent approach was applied in North Carolina, where a hearing with counsel appointed for the minor occurred within 10 days of admission. The 1975 case which articulated these standards (*In re Long*) resulted from the direct application of the principles set forth in *In re Gault*, the 1967 landmark U.S. Supreme Court case which had resulted in a substantial increase in legal safeguards for minors in juvenile court. Shortly after the *Long* case, a number of other states enacted similar statutes providing that young children (under 13 or 14) could be admitted voluntarily, but that older minors had a right to a hearing, counsel, and other due process rights automatically or at their own request.

In 1979, the U.S. Supreme Court decided the case of *Parham v. J.L. and J.R.*, in which the essential issue was whether parents may secure psychiatric hospitalization for a minor child on the recommendation of mental health personnel without independent judicial or administrative review. The Court ruled to uphold parental authority for psychiatric admission when accompanied by concurring clinical opinion and periodic review. The *Parham* decision states the constitutional minimum procedural standards which must be applied when admitting minors and upheld the admissions procedures of nearly 30 states. It does not prohibit the states from enacting additional procedural requirements, which 19 other states have done. In some states, this is accomplished by permitting the child to protest the admission, and thus to gain the same hearing an adult would have, with all the due process protections the law provides, such as representation by an attorney. In other states, the minor has a right to sign himself out, and this could initiate the civil commitment process if the staff believes he is committable. Approximately one-third of the states grant the minor or someone on his behalf the right to request to be discharged. If the discharge is not granted by the staff, then a hearing must be held.

The clinical indications for committing minors should follow the state commitment law. In general, children and adolescents who are suicidal, homicidal, or severely mentally ill are committable. Children whose functioning is deteriorating in the face of vigorous outpatient intervention should also be considered committable in those states which have a standard of "being in need of treatment" as a criterion for commitment. Following the guidelines articulated in *Parham*, a psychiatrist must independently conduct an evaluation to determine if a minor requires inpatient hospitalization or, if not, the appropriate services for the child. The evaluation must include an interview of the child alone and a careful review of the child's background utilizing all available sources of information, including parents, the school, and social agencies. After hospitalization, the child's continuing need for inpatient treatment should be periodically reviewed by a similar independent method. Although the U.S. Supreme Court in *Parham* did not specify the required frequency of such a review, some states have done so. For example, Arizona states a review must be done every ten days. In other states, it is as infrequent as every 60 days. A few states have additional rules for minors who are wards of the state.

Some children brought by parents for psychiatric hospitalization are more appropriately handled by the social service agencies, which can arrange alternate placements. One example will illustrate this:

> A 15-year-old chronically conduct disordered adolescent took six aspirins after one of numerous arguments with his alcoholic mother. When seen in the emergency room the adolescent had no active medical problems which required intervention. Psychiatric assessment revealed no signs of psychosis, major depression, or current suicidal ideas or plan. The adolescent was well supported in a residential day school for the severely behaviorally handicapped. The immediate precipitant was the increased family conflict exacerbated by the mother's recent separation from her second husband. There was no indication for an acute psychiatric hospitalization so shelter care was arranged when the mother refused to take the boy home. Outpatient mental health and substance abuse services were also arranged for the boy and his mother.

Most states also permit minors beyond a certain age to voluntarily admit themselves into the hospital for mental health services. This age ranges from 12 in Georgia to 17 in Florida. Other states require either a combination of *both* adult and minor consent after a child reaches a certain age or an application for admission from either a parent or an eligible minor.

When a minor refuses admission for inpatient mental health care, many states simply permit the minor to be hospitalized based on parental consent. If the state does not permit such a "voluntary commitment," procedures must be followed for emergency psychiatric hospitalization.

Another issue which may arise is the involuntarily hospitalized minor who refuses treatment, most frequently medication. Unless there is a specific statute or regulation to the contrary, the facility should obtain the consent of the parent to provide treatment over the minor's refusal. However, where the treatment is one which is viewed as unusual or hazardous, such as ECT or unusually high dosages of a drug, then the consent of the parent may not be sufficient in light of the minor's refusal. Protection against potential liability is best obtained with a court order requiring the treatment. Before seeking such a court order, the health care professional should be prepared to demonstrate that there is no less burdensome treatment, that the benefits outweigh the risks, and that because of his mental incapacity, the minor is not able to participate appropriately in the decision-making process.

In summary, the rules governing a minor's admission to a mental hospital are complex and vary widely. The clinician is urged to become informed about local statutes concerning hospitalization in order to commit properly when necessary. Following the proper procedures is critical to avoid charges of malicious commitment or false imprisonment.

VII. CONFIDENTIALITY OF RECORDS

The legal responsibility for release of information concerning the care of an unemancipated child or adolescent rests with the parents or legal guardian. Many of the states permitting a minor to consent to health care treatment will not allow record release without the consent of the minor. In general, however, the laws concerning confidentiality have not kept apace of the laws concerning minors' rights to treatment. A few states prohibit the disclosure to parents of records concerning sexually transmitted diseases and/or abortions without the minor's consent. The clinician should release only data relevant to the particular purpose for which consent has been obtained.

Clinicians should emphasize protecting children so they will not be stigmatized as adults for their childhood behavior. This can most clearly be seen in the juvenile justice system, where the criminal record is not disclosed, except under limited circumstances. Methods for expunging the record are also often provided. Efforts must be made to ensure that the records of children are used only for the purposes for which they are being kept. In juvenile court, for example, examining clinicians should determine that the contents of their reports are used only to determine the need of immediate medical or psychiatric care or to answer the question of the ultimate disposition of the case. The content of interviews should not be used for the guilt-finding phase of the proceeding. School personnel and health care providers have been sensitized to keeping accurate records which truly reflect the facts, rather than making unsupported inferences.

Parents (both custodial and noncustodial) now have a statutory right to review their child's educational record based on the Family Educational and Privacy Act of 1974 (Buckley Act). Most states with statutes conferring nearly unlimited access to physicians' office records or hospital records have exceptions for psychiatric records. However, some states do permit access to therapeutic records by parents and the minor patient. It is important to recognize that the child's right to privacy may conflict with his parents' right to access to his records. Sensitive therapeutic issues (e.g., sex or gender) are best detailed in a separate file of working notes held by the mental health practitioner. Health providers usually may keep any personal working notes from patient access, but such notes are generally not immune from subpoena. An alternate method is to record only necessary data in the formal chart, data which are specific only to the degree that is necessary for documentation and therapeutic purposes. For example, the notation "increasingly close relationship with boyfriend" would describe an adolescent in need of reproductive counseling. The use of separate files may also clarify what material given by family members about themselves or others is confidential in the context of family-oriented treatment.

The legal standing of minors to review their records is uncertain. Minors appear to have the right to review records of health care that they consented to and received on their own. On the other hand, it is less clear whether minors have access to records concerning treatment rendered upon the consent of their parents. Clinically, it appears wise to review the chart entries with the patient as a way to foster trust. Obviously, as with adults, a patient's right of review may be denied if the clinician reasonably believes the risk for harm to the patient by disclosure outweighs the benefits. Such denial, and the reasons for such denial, must be charted.

Several issues arise for the mental health professional who provides treatment to a child or engages in family therapy. The professional should anticipate that the minor may gain access to records upon reaching adulthood. Data such as the previously unknown adoption or paternity of the minor should not be included in the records unless the issue is a major focus of the intervention. Such clinical issues argue for the separate files described above.

Questions often arise about the extent of the parents' knowledge of their child's mental health contacts. Since young children are virtually never treated without a family-centered therapeutic focus, this conflict arises infrequently in practice with them. However, fantasy material, dreams, and strong negative emotional responses to family members may not need to be explicitly discussed or may be summarized in a general way if the clinician believes it is in the best interest of the child's treatment for the parent to be informed. In treatment with an adolescent, no information should be revealed without the child's consent except in emergencies, such as when a minor is suicidal or homicidal. Parental guidance advice can often be given without revealing specific details of the teen's communication. Often, the adolescent can be assisted in communicating sensitive material directly to the parent in conjoint sessions if the therapist assesses that such communication is in the adolescent's best interest.

When the parents are divorced or there has been a change in the guardianship of the child, the therapist is often faced with the dilemma of which parent has a right to access to the records. The clinician should request a copy of the court order granting custody and then, if questions remain, consult with his attorney. Ideally, both parents should be apprised of the child's status, but in some cases this may only add to the conflict.

VIII. PARTICIPATION IN RESEARCH

At times, children are eligible to participate in a medical research protocol. The research may be aimed at treating an illness that affects only children or is prevalent among them. The protections promulgated through federal regulations are based upon the estimate of risk to the minor participant and whether or not a direct therapeutic benefit to the individual is anticipated.

In 1983, the United States Department of Health and Human Services published federal regulations specifying protections for children involved as research subjects (45 C.F.R. 46). One notion incorporated here is that children can have the ability to assent to being part of a research protocol, and that such assent should be required since research participation must be voluntary. *Assent* is defined as a child's affirmative agreement to participate in research, not just the failure to object to it, and is to be distinguished from *consent*, which can be given only by those permitted by law to consent to treatment. These regulations authorize the individual Institutional Review Board (IRB) to determine the child's role in the decision making about participation in research. In determining the child's role, the IRB must consider the child's age, his maturity, his psychological state, and the nature of the research.

A minor's assent may be waived in circumstances where (1) the risk to the minor is minimal, *and* (2) the waiver does not violate the rights and welfare of the minor, *and* (3) the research cannot be practically carried out without waiver of the minor's assent, *and* (4) the minor will be provided with any relevant information after participation in the research, if appropriate (45 C.F.R., Section 46.116(d)). A minor's assent may also be waived if the methods involved in the research hold the prospect of direct therapeutic benefit for the minor which is available only in this manner (45 C.F.R., Section 46.408(a)).

In most circumstances involving research procedures, the written informed consent of a parent or guardian is required. If a proposed procedure involves more than minimal risk without any direct therapeutic benefit, the consent of both parents should be obtained when reasonably possible, unless only one parent has legal custody. The requirement of parental consent can be waived when such a requirement is deemed not reasonable to protect the child. Clearly, most adolescents should be able to provide an informed assent. There is no requirement for parental consent if the adolescent has reached the age of consent to the treatment procedures involved in the research. For example, minors who have sexually transmitted diseases, are substance abusers, are pregnant, or need contraception can consent to procedures involving these conditions. The need for parental consent may also be waived if it is not "a reasonable requirement to protect the subjects . . . provided an appropriate mechanism for protecting the children . . . is substituted" (45 C.F.R., Section 46.408(c)). For example, research in child abuse is an example of an area of research in which parental consent may not be reasonable.

Research must conform to the state or local laws concerning informed consent as well as to any determination of the IRB. The IRB at the facility where research is proposed must generally approve the research protocol when minors are involved.

IX. CHILD ABUSE AND NEGLECT

A. Reporting Abuse and Neglect

The mental health professional may become the first or only one aware that a child is being abused. Abuse may become known through the child, another family member, or a third party. The law in all states is that when child abuse is suspected there is an obligation to report the abuse. Most but not all reporting statutes require the reporting of suspected abuse, no matter what the source of information. (See Chapter 6 for a discussion of the civil and criminal liability faced by the mental health professional for not reporting child abuse.) Reports are filed immediately by telephone, and subsequently in writing, to either the designated social service agency or the police.

The legal definition of child abuse and child neglect varies from state to state. The most frequently used clinical definition of child abuse is "the nonaccidental physical injury (or injuries) that is the result of the acts (or omissions) on the part of parents or guardians that violate the community standards concerning the treatment of children." It is estimated that 125,000 cases of physical abuse to children occur annually in the United States. Nonaccidental trauma is the most easily identified type of maltreatment. Characteristically, the injuries are more severe than could have resulted from, or are incompatible with, the alleged cause.

Child neglect, a far more common clinical entity than abuse, can be defined as the failure of a parent or other person legally responsible for a child's welfare to provide an adequate level of care for the child's basic needs. Neglect tends to be chronic and involves inattention to the child's minimal needs for nurturance, food, clothing, shelter, medical care, safety, and education.

Child sexual abuse is the exploitation of a child by an adult or another child for sexual gratification or profit. Sexual abuse is often long-standing and perpetrated by someone known to the child. It can range from exhibitionism and fondling to penetration or the use of a child in the production of pornographic materials. Child sexual abuse often includes a progression of acts over time and emotional coercion of the child to enforce secrecy. Frequently, sexual intercourse or physical force is not involved.

In 1985, the American Medical Association issued diagnostic and treatment guidelines concerning child abuse and neglect. These guidelines emphasize the need for multidisciplinary teams to address the problems of managing cases of child abuse and neglect. Mental health professionals are well advised to obtain a copy of their jurisdiction's reporting laws on child abuse and neglect and to familiarize themselves with the available community services for these families. Clinicians may then better assume the role of advocates for their child and family patients.

In most jurisdictions, if the mental health professional reasonably suspects that abuse or neglect exists, the case must be reported. It is unnecessary to attempt to substantiate the complaint prior to reporting. All state statutes provide that a professional required to make a report is immune from any suit for negligence or defamation if the abuse allegation report was made in good faith. The clinician must not attempt to second-guess the adequacy of the social service agency which must investigate and intervene in reported cases. It is always better for the mental health professional to err on the side of protecting the child. Only when someone becomes aware of the abuse and reports it is there any hope that the child can be protected.

Therapists who determine that they are obligated to report suspected abuse or neglect should attempt to actively engage the family in the reporting process. This may include informing the parents of the therapist's obligation to report and enlisting their assistance in reporting while they are in the office. If the parents refuse to cooperate, the therapist must proceed to report whether the parent is present during the reporting (the preferable procedure) or not. The therapist should inform the parents as well as the child victim of the therapist's legal obligation to report, the basis for the report, and the need for a protective service investigation. If there is any doubt concerning the child's safety, the child should be detained until seen by protective service personnel. The therapist should offer no promise to the family concerning the outcome of the investigation or possible interventions.

The major purpose of child abuse reporting statutes is the protection of children who have been abused and the prevention of future abuse. Therapists may experience issues of conflict between therapist–patient confidentiality and the duty to report the abuse of children. Therapists should be familiar with the details of their reporting law to determine, for example, if present and also past abuse must be reported. Mandated reports may require only the identification of the suspected victim, although in some states the alleged perpetrator must also be named.

B. Investigation of Abuse and Neglect

Clinicians involved in investigations of abuse complaints should establish a structured, nonleading format in their investigatory interviews. Therapists already treating the child should not conduct these interviews. Treating mental health professionals should maintain a clear separation of roles from those professionals mandated to conduct the investigation. Investigatory personnel should maintain meticulous documentation of their evaluation, including, where possible, verbatim responses from the victim to maximize their future admissibility in court. Careful documentation of the process of the interview (both questions and answers) will also allow investigators to answer any concerns over possible leading or coercive techniques used in their interviews. Several structured interview protocols are available, though no protocol has been found to be superior to any other. The key clinical issue is that investigators use one general format for all their interviews to maximize consistency, gain experience in children's response to the interview format, and maximize the validity of their investigations. Anatomical dolls are helpful props with the preschool age group; research has shown them to be of particular assistance with three-year-olds. Anatomical drawings may be used as aids during interviews of school age and early adolescent children.

Documentation may range from notes taken within the interview to videotaping. Videotaping, when available, is the preferred method because of its accuracy. More than a dozen states give statutory authority for videotaping a child's statement and outline conditions for the tape's admissibility in court. Many other states permit the taping of a child's testimony. Clinicians using videotape should consult the relevant state statutes. Expense and lack of equipment often preclude either audiotape or videotaping. Investigators should then attempt to preserve as much of the interview as possible by using either a trained observer taking notes behind a one-way mirror or personal taking of notes during the interview. A minimum of two and a maximum of three interviews with the child are recommended in order to assess the consistency of the report and also to minimize contamination of the child's statements.

C. Actions to Protect the Child

The immediate intervention of child welfare investigators consists of removing the child from the home or removing the parent from the home, if there is an immediate risk of reinjury or molestation. The reporting mental health professional may be asked for any clinical data relevant to this decision. Situations suggesting the need for taking the child into protective custody include (1) a child who is seriously injured; (2) a child who has been sadistically tortured; (3) a parent who has displayed a reckless disregard for the child's safety; (4) a home in which the physical conditions are so dangerous they pose an immediate threat of serious injury; (5) a child who has been sexually abused by a perpetrator within the home and a nonoffending parent who will not require the perpetrator to leave or who will not leave with the children; (6) parents who have systematically withheld food from the child; (7) parents who refuse to obtain or consent to medical or psychiatric care for the child which is needed to prevent or treat a serious injury or disease; (8) parents who cannot provide for the child's minimal basic needs because of severe mental illness, mental retardation, or substance abuse; (9) parents who have abandoned the child; and (10) the parents who may flee with a child who appears to be neglected or abused. Finally, the siblings of an abused child may be removed for their own protection.

Once the initial action has been taken, a longer-term strategy will be developed with the goals of preventing further abuse to the child and, if the family has been separated, family reunification. These strategies usually take one of three forms or a combination: (1) therapeutic and/or education efforts designed to change the parents; (2) efforts which focus on the situational factors which gave rise to the abuse, with the intent of reducing environmental stress; and (3) interventions designed to ameliorate the effects of the abuse and neglect on the child.

D. Liability of the Caseworker

The enormous expansion of programs to prevent child abuse and neglect has saved many children from injury and death. Of concern to child-welfare workers is the growing number of legal cases concerning criminal and civil liability for their official conduct, which has been the subject of a United States Supreme Court decision (*DeShaney v. Winnebago County Department of Social Services*, 1989).

Four major areas of liability exist for caseworkers: (1) failure to protect a child adequately, including inadequate investigation and monitoring of cases; (2) violation of parental rights; (3) inadequate foster-care services; and (4) liability for children who remain in foster care indefinitely. This liability is variously actionable as a deprivation of the constitutional or statutory rights of the children or may be brought as a violation of tort law (negligence). To protect themselves against liability, caseworkers are advised to (1) obtain adequate training; (2) carefully document observations, assessments, and rationale for interventions; (3) seek consultation from supervisors and other professionals, including multidisciplinary teams; and (4) obtain malpractice insurance. The ongoing tension in protective service work is avoiding either too little or too much intervention. Approximately 1,000 child fatalities occur annually because of abuse, often in cases already known to the child-protective agency. On the other hand, parents and children may be subjected to unnecessarily intrusive investigation, malicious prosecution, or wrongful removal of their children because of poorly conducted investigations and case management. Nationwide, fewer than 50% of allegations of abuse (both physical and sexual) are substantiated. These figures reflect the relatively low standard of reporting ("reasonable suspicion"), the clinical problems of verifying abuse, and the infrequent cases of false allegation.

To safeguard family privacy, all states have laws making child-protective records confidential. In most states, unauthorized disclosure is a crime. In addition, violation of such a criminal statute would go toward establishing civil liability for breach of confidentiality. The information may be shared with those individuals who make crucial case-handling decisions. These include police, physicians, foster-care agencies, treatment programs for the family, the courts, specified state officials, and researchers.

X. DIVORCE AND CHILD CUSTODY

The divorce rate in the United States for new marriages is 50%, with a newborn child predicted to have a 40% chance of living in a single-parent home by the time he graduates from high school. Of all children, 35% will experience remarriage, and 20% a second divorce. Although the vast majority of divorces result in parental agreement regarding the visitation and custody of the children, it is estimated that approximately 20% of divorcing families dispute custody.

A father fighting for custody of his children was almost unheard of 20 years ago.

Today, this is an accepted proposition. The laws have changed to make it easier for fathers to succeed in a custody dispute. These changes began in the 1960s with the increased emphasis on the equality of the sexes. Perhaps the most notable reason for the increase in custody litigation both during and after divorce proceedings is the changing role of women in our society, which at the same time has changed the role of men. More than half of mothers with preschool children now work outside of the home. For working mothers to be able to manage a job and a household, fathers have generally had to become more involved in the care of the children and in household management. The increased involvement of fathers in the home makes it easy to understand why they wish to continue their daily involvement with their children even after the marriage has ended, and why the courts are no longer as willing to conclude that mothers are necessarily better or uniquely qualified compared to fathers to meet the children's needs.

The states have rejected the concept that the custody of a child of "tender years" (usually under 10 years of age) should automatically be awarded to his mother. All states have adopted the custody standard of the "best interests of the child." This standard is sex-neutral and does not give automatic preference to either mothers or fathers; it reaches a decision based on the child's needs. The recognition of the importance of involving both parents and continuing the involvement of the noncustodial parent has led more courts to encourage joint custody arrangements and frequent visitation for noncustodial parents.

The mental health professional may take on a variety of roles during a custody or visitation dispute. The professional may be the therapist to either of the parents, the children, or the family. In providing counseling through a school or work situation, the professional may need to provide advice to a family member in a custody dispute. Often a mental health professional is asked for a referral to a colleague with expertise in the area of custody and visitation. In addition, the courts will turn to mental health professionals for evaluations to determine which parent should be given the legal custody of the child, and what the visitation with the noncustodial parent should be.

Much has been written about performing child custody determinations, and we will only briefly highlight the major legal and clinical issues, beginning with some legal terminology. Prior to evaluating a family concerning custody and visitation, a mental health professional should review the prevailing legal standards and procedures, study a curriculum of didactic material, and have supervised experience in order to develop clinical competence in this area. Because of their lack of expertise, most clinicians do not and should not do these evaluations. In order to make appropriate referrals, such clinicians should acquaint themselves with the names of colleagues in the community who perform these evaluations competently and routinely. The following discussion is offered to permit the mental health professional to know the prevailing clinical standards concerning custody and visitation cases.

A. Legal Definitions

The standard of the *best interests of the child* has been adopted by every state to determine which parent can best meet the needs of the child at the time of the dispute. The factors to be considered in reaching a conclusion regarding the child's best interests are the wishes of the parents; the wishes of the child; the interaction and interrelationship of the child with his parents, siblings, and any other involved persons; the child's adjustment to his home, school, and community; and the mental and physical health of all involved individuals. This standard recognizes that a child's psychological parent may not necessarily be the child's biological parent, although an award of custody is given to a nonparent only after the finding that the parent is unfit. The standard also states that the court shall not consider the conduct of a proposed custodian that does not affect his relationship to the child (such as cohabitation or a homosexual lifestyle).

Legal custody refers to the parent who has the right to make the major decisions regarding the child, including those related to education, religious training, and medical needs. In an intact family, each parent has legal custody. In a divorced family, the courts determine which parent has legal custody and thus the authority to make these decisions.

Physical custody or possession refers to the person who has the physical possession of the child. For example, during visitation, the noncustodial parent will have the physical custody of a child.

Joint custody is based on the concept that, in certain circumstances, both parents should retain the right to make decisions in major areas affecting their child, and to share the child's physical custody. A joint custody decision has two parts: decision-making authority and physical custody. The trend in the law is to encourage joint custody arrangements though not to require it.

When joint legal custody is awarded, both parents have the right to be involved in the major decisions related to the child. Joint physical custody then describes how each parent will share the physical custody of the child. Any arrangement which will work for the child and the family is acceptable, and there is no requirement of equal time.

It is possible to establish joint legal custody while giving the physical custody primarily to one parent. This has the advantage of recognizing who has been the primary caretaker while keeping the other parent actively involved in decision making concerning the child.

Modification of custody is the court-ordered change of custody after the initial custody order at the time of divorce. All courts empowered to award custody retain their jurisdiction over the child until he is no longer a minor. The states' criteria vary for modification of custody. Some states retain the general best interest standard; others maintain a stricter standard of a need to show a change in circumstances since the divorce decree which endangers the child's welfare. Professionals performing custody evaluations must familiarize themselves with the standards in their state. Most states provide that no changes can occur within a specified time (usually two years) unless the child's physical or emotional health is in immediate danger. This provision is meant to allow the child a period of stabilization.

Visitation or access to the child by the noncustodial parent is a child's right. Longitudinal research has demonstrated the best psychological outcomes for children who have regular and consistent access to the noncustodial parent. Almost every state specifically recognizes the rights of children to grandparent visitation. Legally, visitation by any person must be shown to be in the child's "best interests."

B. Evaluating the Child's Best Interests

The decision of a judge in a child custody case is based in part on the recommendations of mental health professionals who have evaluated the family to determine how to meet each child's best interests. It is recommended that professionals performing custody evaluations perform court-ordered examinations of both parents and all the children. These evaluations are viewed as impartial and carry greater weight with the court than those evaluations done at the request of the attorney for one of the parents. Some clinicians may assess only one parent in a divorce dispute at that parent's attorney's request. Such an evaluation can address only that parent's strengths and limitations in parenting and overall mental health and does not possess the data to speak to the issue of custody or visitation without data from the other parent. The value of the report under these circumstances is usually so limited as to be worthless.

When the quality of each parent's relationship with the child is closely matched, a critical factor is which parent will encourage visitation with the noncustodial parent and be supportive of the noncustodial parent's continued involvement with the child. In addition, if there have been important extended family relationships, it is important to consider which parent will continue to promote these relationships.

A growing number of state laws recognize the preference of the child in custody decisions. Depending on the state, children from the ages of 14 to 18 can choose the parent with whom they wish to live. The courts will honor their choices if it is in the child's best interest to do so. The preferences of younger children are assessed by the evaluator, who takes into account the age of the child and the reasons for the preference.

The splitting of siblings is rare in custody decisions. The sibship is believed to offer considerable support and buffering against parental conflict. However, when it can be demonstrated to the court that dividing the children between the parents is in the children's best interest, such an award will be ordered.

C. Recommending Joint Custody

The concept of joint custody is controversial among both mental health professionals and attorneys. Those who support joint custody argue that it provides the child the advantages of having two involved parents who continue to participate actively in the child's life. The child does not have to divide loyalties. It has also been suggested that under joint custody neither the child nor the parent experiences the sadness, sense of loss, or loneliness that often occurs when one parent is awarded custody. Joint custody seems to assure the child greater access to both parents. Research has offered conflicting data as to whether there is less postdecree litigation when joint custody is awarded.

In contrast, those who question the viability of joint custody suggest that shared decision making may do nothing but expose the child to unnecessary conflict and confusion. Their concern is that the child will be shuttled between two homes with differences in lifestyle, approach to discipline, socioeconomic status, and religious upbringing. They believe that these inconsistencies will subject the child to more instability than in a sole custody arrangement.

Although there is still much research to be done on the effects of divorce on children, it is generally believed that, for joint custody to work successfully, both parents must be committed to making it work. This entails being able to set aside the differences that led to the divorce and being able to communicate well on issues related to the child. In addition, the parents need to have similar views on child rearing. Ideally, they should live in the same neighborhood so that the child's life will not be drastically disrupted during moves from one residence to the other. Recent work suggests that it is the quality of the continuing relationships with each parent, not the nature of the custody arrangement, which is key to a child's positive post-divorce adaptation.

Even when parents are ideally suited for a joint custody arrangement, they must be flexible enough to recognize that the arrangement may not be workable for a particular child. Younger children may find the changes inherent in joint physical custody more difficult than school aged children and adolescents. Initial joint custody plans will require negotiated modifications as the needs of the children change. A forum should exist for the parents to discuss any required changes either alone or with a designated third party.

D. Mediating Custody Disputes

Another trend is for the courts to encourage mediation of custody and visitation disputes as opposed to going to trial. In some jurisdictions, the court sponsors mandatory mediation sessions on these issues. Mediation involves a neutral third party who attempts to foster open and honest discussion of the issues between the parents so that they can reach a voluntary agreement about child issues. This is an agreement reached by the parties, not one suggested by the mediator. In cases in which the parents have some ability to communicate and there is a skillful mediator, this process has the advantage of resolving many of the issues in a way which is satisfactory to both parties. When the issues involve children, the mediator should ensure that the arrangement will be developmentally appropriate for the child. Mediation is a good approach for those couples who are capable of participating equally in such a process. For others, where one parent is more dominant than the other or there is no real ability to communicate, mediation is unlikely to work.

Although ethical standards in the mediation of custody disputes are just beginning to be developed, the mental health professional who is called upon to play such a role must be neutral. Having been a therapist to one of the parties would disqualify one from being either a mediator or a family evaluator. If, however, the professional has served as a family therapist and both parents agree to the professional's serving as the mediator, this would be appropriate. The professional should keep in mind that the arrangements worked out may have legal and tax consequences for both parties. Therefore, before any arrangement is finalized, consultation with an experienced divorce attorney by each parent is essential.

E. Acting as Therapist to One of the Parties

One of the most frequent reasons a person seeks mental health services is trouble in his marriage. Unless the couple is engaged in marital therapy, it is important for the therapist to remember that he is hearing only one side of the problem. This is important should the marital problems lead to a dispute over custody or visitation. In that circumstance, the treating therapist may be called upon to reveal information about what has occurred in therapy or the therapist's assessment of the client's parenting skills. Records or information should not be released without discussion with the client and obtaining his permission. Unless the treating therapist has seen both parents and the child, he will be unable to render an opinion concerning the ultimate issue of custody or visitation and should state this limitation in his report and/or testimony.

F. Confidentiality Issues

A clinician who has been a therapist to either parent or child is commonly asked, subpoenaed, or ordered to testify in custody cases. The courts have generally held that the therapist–patient testimonial privilege does not apply in custody cases. The right of the parent/client to confidentiality in mental health treatment is considered less important than establishing the evidence to determine the best interest of the child. Therefore, a trial judge may have the authority to order a therapist's testimony about a client in any custody case in which the judge has determined that the therapist has information relevant to the determination of what is in the child's best interest. This finding is made after an in-chambers review by the judge of the therapist's knowledge and records pertaining to his client. However, a therapist may not testify about a client or reveal any information without the client's consent unless a court order has been obtained. A therapist who testifies without the client's consent before being ordered to do so by a court may be subject to a malpractice suit for breach of confidentiality.

In a case in which a clinician has been appointed by the court as an independent evaluator, his testimony is not covered by a therapist–patient confidential testimonial privilege. The lack of confidentiality should be explained at the beginning of each interview conducted for court purposes.

XI. ACCESS OF DISABLED CHILDREN TO AN EDUCATION

Until 1975, many jurisdictions offered little or no education for disabled children. At that time, over two million school-age children were out of school. These children were handicapped, poor, nonwhite, or non-English speaking. In 1975, Congress passed the Education for All Handicapped Children Act (EAHCA), Public Law 94–142. The act requires the states to provide a "free appropriate public education" to all handicapped children between the ages of 3 and 21. Handicapped children are defined as including the mentally retarded, learning disabled, physically handicapped, and emotionally disturbed. Congress has authorized large annual appropriations to aid the states that are in compliance with the mandated services of P.L. 94–142.

P.L. 94–142 requires that all handicapped children, regardless of the severity of the handicapping condition, be provided a free, appropriate public education in the least restrictive environment appropriate to the needs of the child. The act avoids prescribing specific educational programs and instead outlines the procedure by which a program can be determined for any individual child. This process includes (1) development of the child's Individualized Educational Program (IEP); (2) procedural safeguards; and (3) parental involvement.

An IEP is a "written statement for each handicapped child" that is developed at a meeting among the child's parents, teacher, and a qualified school representative.

Either the school or the child's parents can initiate the individual planning and placement process. Under P.L. 94–142, parents have the right to be notified of any proposed school actions and of their rights under the law. They must be included in the development of the child's IEP through conferences with responsible school personnel.

The first step in developing an IEP is a multidisciplinary and racially nondiscriminatory educational evaluation conducted by school personnel to determine the extent of the child's special-education needs. After this evaluation, a meeting is held in which parents and school personnel meet as equal partners to write a formal educational plan for the child. This plan must outline short-term and long-term goals and the services to be provided to achieve these goals. If agreed upon and signed by both the parents and the school district, the IEP becomes a binding contract that can be enforced through either administrative hearings or civil litigation. If the parties do not agree, the parents are entitled to an "impartial due process hearing" before a hearing officer who is not an employee of the agency involved in the education of the child. The issue may be appealed up from the local level to the state agency for review and then for civil action in a state or federal court.

The IEP is the key to obtaining needed services. Even if a school district does not have the program specified in an IEP, it must arrange for such a program from other public or private agencies. These services are provided at no cost to the parent and must be in the least restrictive setting appropriate to the child's needs. P.L. 94–142's goal of "full educational opportunity" for all handicapped children and the provision of "a free appropriate public education" include the provision of both special educational instruction and "related services." These related services, which are all specified in the IEP, may include transportation, speech therapy, psychological services, physical and occupational therapy, recreation, and diagnostic medical services.

P.L. 94–142 has had a profound effect on all its participants: children, parents, and educators. The limits of P.L. 94–142 continue to be defined by the developing educational case law. In 1982, the United States Supreme Court in *Board of Education v. Rowley* held that "a free appropriate public education" is satisfied when the state provides personalized instruction with sufficient support services to permit the handicapped child to benefit educationally from that instruction. Such instruction and services must be provided at public expense, must meet the state's educational standards, must approximate the grade levels used in the state's regular education program, and must comport with the child's IEP. The Court specifically held that this was not a guarantee of the best possible education for the child, but one that was adequate and tailored to the child's individual needs.

Financial issues around placement have been repeatedly litigated in the courts. Numerous cases have stated that the child must remain in the current placement during the pendency of administrative and judicial proceedings unless the parents and the school officials agree to a change. Unilateral special placements by parents will not be reimbursed.

Finally, one of the most difficult and controversial areas concerning P.L. 94–142 has been the procedures necessary to expel students who argue that their behavior is a result of a handicap. The majority of recent cases state that expulsion constitutes a change in educational placement that requires the procedural protection of P.L. 94–142, and that expulsion never justifies a complete cessation of educational services.

XII. JUVENILE JUSTICE SYSTEM

In the early 1900s in the United States, the juvenile justice system developed in response to children's being housed with adult criminals and being given long prison sentences. The goal of the new juvenile court system was to evaluate and treat the child. The emphasis was on rehabilitation, not punishment. Each case was viewed individually with no systematic notions of what punishment should fit the offense. The court was given wide discretion in what actions could be taken.

As part of the emphasis on treating children differently from adults, a language has been developed to emphasize the differences in philosophy between juvenile and adult criminal court. Juvenile offenders are *delinquents,* not *defendants;* the legal proceedings are *adjudicatory and dispositional hearings,* not *trials.* Children are not sent to *prison,* but to *training* or *reform schools.*

By the mid-1960s, it was recognized that the juvenile justice system had many failings. Clinical research demonstrated that children who committed "status offenses" such as truancy and running away were housed with delinquents who had committed violent crimes. In such circumstances, the status offenders quickly modeled themselves after the delinquents. Other children were incarcerated longer in the reform school for their behavior than they would have been had they been tried as adults. Children neither had the benefit of an approach which was effective in helping them become responsible adult citizens nor had the due process protections afforded to adults charged with crimes.

At the same time, major changes in the rights of juveniles came in a series of United States Supreme Court decisions. In *Kent v. United States* (1966), the first Supreme Court case considering the juvenile court system, Justice Fortas noted, "[t]here may be grounds for concerns that the child receives the worst of both worlds, he gets neither the protections accorded to adults nor the solicitous care and regenerative treatment postulated for children." In *In re Gault* (1967), the Court extended to juveniles many of the same rights afforded to adults, including being given notice of the charges against them, representation by an attorney, and the right to examine and cross-examine witnesses. The Court said that "Neither the Fourteenth Amendment nor the Bill of Rights is for adults alone." In 1970, in *In re Winship,* the Court found that, to convict a child of an offense, proof of the offense must be established beyond a reasonable doubt, the same standard applied to adult criminals.

Although these cases substantially ensured that juveniles would have the same rights at criminal hearing as adults, they still are not entitled to trial by jury, nor to the right to appeal. There is also no set sentencing procedure for juveniles in many states. When a juvenile is detained, his name will not be released; juvenile court proceedings are not open to the public, and juvenile records are not available. Each of these procedures is designed to ensure that a child will not be stigmatized at the time of the proceeding or in the future.

Approximately one million children are arrested each year in the United States. Nearly half the thefts and one-third of violent crimes committed in this country are committed by children between the ages of 10 and 17. However, longitudinal studies have shown that one-half of children diagnosed with conduct disorder do not continue in this behavior as adults. Addressing the problems created by juvenile offenders is a major political as well as mental health issue.

The definition of delinquent behavior varies from state to state. Generally, any act considered a crime when committed by an adult is considered delinquent behavior when committed by a juvenile. The juvenile courts have jurisdiction over delinquents and children committing status offenses, as well as over abuse and neglect cases. When a child is detained, the response to the behavior at issue will also vary greatly from state to state, depending on the resources available within that state and the jurisdiction's view of juvenile offenders. Although there is still concern about rehabilitation, in many circumstances there is a greater concern about safety and procedural safeguards. The trend is toward making the proceedings more like adult criminal trials. The current emphasis is on setting a sentence which is proportionate to the crime committed, rather than giving the court wide discretion in its response to a particular juvenile offender. The emphasis is also on offering separate services to delinquent youth and to status offenders.

A. Role of the Mental Health Professional

The professional who works in the juvenile justice system is most likely to be called upon to make dispositional recommendations or to offer a recommendation concerning whether a child should be tried as an adult. Thus far there are few good empirical studies to give the professional information on which to base these clinical decisions. The range of options is often limited by the volume of cases and the limited funds spent on juvenile services. The professional must review each case to determine what treatment approach is appropriate for the child. Each youth referred for a diagnostic assessment should be carefully assessed for treatable disorders, such as attention-deficit hyperactivity disorder. The strengths and limitations of the youth and his family situation should be communicated to the court in concise, well-written reports free of jargon or theoretical bias. Most useful to court personnel are specific behavioral observations and historical data which support any recommended interventions. Care must be taken not to overlook adolescents with psychotic disorders, intellectual deficits, and specific learning disabilities as well as neurological conditions which contribute to acting-out behavior. All clinical assessments done pursuant to a court order will require a warning concerning lack of confidentiality and how the information may be used.

The mental health professional in the community may receive a court-ordered referral to evaluate a juvenile as either an inpatient or an outpatient. The mental health professional should clarify what is the status of the juvenile court proceeding as well as what are the referral questions. If the juvenile delinquency charge has not yet been tried, particular care must be taken to minimize detailed discussions of the alleged offenses unless clinically indicated (e.g., a juvenile's need to discuss guilt over involvement in a homicide). Clear statements must be made to the juvenile concerning the limitations on confidentiality, the length of treatment contracts, and the power of the court to determine a disposition.

B. Charging the Child as an Adult

In the vast majority of jurisdictions, when a minor has committed a serious crime, such as rape, murder, or attempted murder, the prosecution will consider trying him as an adult. This process is called *waiver* or *bind over* of the juvenile to adult court. In each state, the statute sets forth the standards that determine when a child should be tried as an adult. In many states, this can occur to an adolescent as young as 13 years of age. Typically, the law will require that the act be aggressive and premeditated. The court will consider the minor's previous history of delinquent behavior and past attempts at rehabilitation in the juvenile justice system. If there is a history of other violent acts, then it is more likely the child will be tried as an adult. Another factor will be whether the interests of the child and the public will be served in having him held for a period beyond his minority. Under the juvenile justice system, when a child is committed to juvenile facility he will remain there only until he reaches majority, or until he reaches 21. Over half the states permit the death penalty for those who commit homicides as adolescents.

The professional performing a waiver evaluation should restrict the focus of the report to mental health issues. The mental health assessment should inform the court of the pattern and chronicity of antisocial acting out, the presence of violence toward others, and the role of treatable conditions, such as substance abuse or attention-deficit disorder, which may further impair the youth's impulse control. A waiver report should detail any past attempts at treatment and the child's response. The report should describe any recommended treatment approaches. The opinion section should directly address the positive and negative prognostic indications for the child, leaving the court to address the ultimate bind over issue.

In addition to determining when a child might be tried as an adult, the mental health professional may be called upon to make recommendations regarding the death penalty. In these circumstances the professional may find factors which would argue against sentencing the juvenile to death, such as retardation, psychosis, depression, or psychosocial stressors such as the victim's having abused the defendant.

C. The Future

It is likely that the next decade will see major changes in the juvenile justice system. The focus will continue to be on attempts to classify youth at high risk for repeated offenses, the development of specialized mental health services for juvenile offenders, and safeguards of their legal rights.

XIII. COMMONLY ASKED QUESTIONS

1. *Does a teenager who has had a child have the right to make medical decisions for her child and herself?*

The only medical decisions the teenage mother can make without the permission of her parent or guardian relate to reproductive health issues. In most states, but not all, she would also be capable of consenting to medical treatment for herself which does not involve reproductive issues. She also has the right to consent to care for her child, if her parental rights have not been terminated.

2. *When nonemergency psychiatric treatment such as medication is prescribed for a teenager but the teenager refuses it, what options are available to the therapist?*

Under most state laws, the parent has the ultimate authority to determine what medical and psychological care the child receives. This, however, will vary with the age of the teenager, since the closer the teenager is to 18 years of age, the more likely his treatment refusal will be managed in the same manner as an adult's refusal. In some states, adolescents who refuse medication for their psychiatric illness will be given the same rights as an adult who refuses medication. This may involve an informal administrative hearing or a court hearing, depending upon the state. In an emergency, the adolescent does not have a right to a hearing. However, an emergency can not last for days, only for a brief period.

3. *Does a civilly committed adolescent have the same rights as a civilly committed adult?*
The adolescent's ability to challenge the commitment varies widely from state to state. A significant number of states provide the same procedural safeguards for adolescents as for adults. If a minor is competent to consent to treatment, it is probable that he also has the right to refuse treatment. Medication refusal on the basis of psychotic beliefs or grossly disorganized behavior suggests an inability to make a competent decision. The parents or guardian could authorize treatment over the adolescent's refusal.

4. *What happens when the treatment team determines that a child should be released from the hospital, and the parents refuse to take the child home?*
In many states, the parents may have a right to request a hearing to determine if discharge is appropriate. If the hearing determines that the discharge should occur but the parents refuse to take the child back into their home, then the child should be viewed as neglected, and the child-protective agency should be notified so that some other living arrangement can be provided.

5. *In a custody dispute in which both parents seem to have significant parenting deficits, what options are open to the forensic evaluator?*
The issue for the evaluator then becomes which parent is more appropriate given the circumstances. If there is no indication of suspected child abuse or neglect, the clinician should decide the least detrimental alternative. It is possible to inquire whether there are other relatives willing to assume the role of custodian. In cases where finances permit, a boarding school may be a better alternative than having the child live with one parent on a full-time basis.

6. *Can a mature minor decide on the parent with whom he wishes to live?*
In almost all states, a child over a certain age, usually 14 to 16, can make a decision as to which parent he wishes to live with. The court will honor that decision if it is shown to be in the child's best interest.

7. *Can an adolescent who runs away from home consent to medical treatment without parental consent?*
A recent survey has estimated that over 730,000 young people leave home annually without parental consent. Therefore, a health professional is commonly asked to provide services to adolescents who do not meet the formal definition of emancipation since they have only recently left their parents' home and have not established a separate residence. If an emergency exists, normal emergency considerations will apply. If there is no present emergency, then the treating facility should attempt to notify and obtain the consent of the parents. If the minor refuses to

cooperate, the facility should document that the minor did not agree to parental notification and refused to provide information which would have permitted parental notification to occur. It is also recommended that health professionals document the attempts to convince the minor to involve his parents. Support for providing health care to runaways can also be found in the mature minor doctrine. A review of case law concerning the treatment of minors without parental consent suggests that physicians are rarely held liable for providing needed medical care to runaways without parental consent even in nonemergencies.

8. Can a minor legally consent to contraceptive services and, if necessary, prenatal care?

Many states have specific statutes which address the right of a minor to consent to the prevention or treatment of pregnancy. It is likely that this care would include pregnancy testing, pelvic examinations, and prenatal care. Even in the absence of a specific state statute, however, minors probably have a constitutionally protected privacy right to consent to sex related health care, including pregnancy-related health care, assuming, of course, that the minor can give informed consent.

Statutes in some states state that the provider may notify the minor's parents only if failure to do so would jeopardize the minor's health. Although it is usually beneficial to involve the parents with the minor's consent, notification is not a requirement. Issues such as possible abuse (physical and sexual) or parental rejection must be considered.

9. As a result of the Baby Jane Doe case, which limited when care could be terminated for a seriously ill infant, at what age is a child considered an "infant" under the Child Abuse Amendments of 1984?

An infant is defined in these amendments as a child less than one year of age or, in certain circumstances, a child older than one year with a long-term disability. Any treatment needed by a child initially qualifying under the amendments could not be discontinued when the child passed his first birthday.

10. What clinical issues should be addressed in the evaluation of a juvenile sex offender?

The first issue to be assessed is whether inappropriate sexual behavior has occurred. Generally, a sexual offense is recognized to have occurred if there is a five-year or greater age difference between the offender and victim and/or if any form of coercion (by overt violence or threat of violence) occurred.

Other important issues to be examined include the type of sexual activity exhibited, the persistence of the sexual activity, any evidence of progression in the nature or frequency of the sexual activity, and whether there are any distinguishing characteristics about the victims. A key issue to be explored is the nature of the fantasies that preceded or accompanied the adolescent's abusive behavior. In addition, the history should address whether the adolescent was acting out problems (such as a personal victimization) in a sexual way and whether there are other serious mental disorders, such as psychosis, mental retardation, or substance abuse further impairing the adolescent's impulse control. The clinician must also review the family attitudes or behaviors which precipitated or perpetuated the sex offenses.

11. When an adult client tells of having been abused as a child, must the therapist report this as a case of child abuse?

No. The point of child abuse reporting statutes is to protect a child who may be in danger of being harmed. Although the adult may continue to suffer psychologically as a result of the past child abuse, the child-protective agency will no longer have jurisdiction. In addition, given the time that has passed, criminal prosecution will probably be barred.

12. *In a divorce situation in which one parent has custody, may the other parent bring the child for a psychological evaluation?*

Therapists are well advised not to get caught in a dispute between parents involved in postdivorce proceedings related to custody. Absent an emergency, consent for the child's psychological care should be obtained from the custodial parent. Otherwise, the noncustodial parent should obtain a court order to perform an evaluation on a child when the noncustodial parent does not wish the custodial parent to be aware of the evaluation. There are also circumstances when the court order setting forth the rights of the parents specifically addresses what type of consent is necessary before mental health services can be rendered. When in doubt, the clinician should request a copy of the court order or marital settlement agreement which addresses the child custody issues.

13. *Can the custodial parent deny the noncustodial parent access to the child's mental health record?*

In most states, the divorce statute will provide that both parents shall have access to all the child's records including school, health, and mental health records. In some states adolescents can determine who may see a copy of their record. Additionally, the court order in the divorce action may address this issue. Requiring a court order before releasing records may be necessary if the applicable law and the court decree are not clear. Child therapists and evaluators should remember that, when providing services to children, there is a probability that those records may become part of a divorce or postdivorce proceeding. The mental health professional must be careful when these issues arise and legal consultation is often advisable.

XIV. BIBLIOGRAPHY

I. General

Besharov, D. J. (1985). *The vulnerable social worker: Liability for serving children and families*. Silver Spring, MD: National Association of Social Workers.

Besharov, D. J. (1986). The misuse of foster care: When the desire to help children outruns the ability to improve parental functioning. *Family Law Quarterly, 20*, 213–231.

Davis, S. M., & Schwartz, M. D. (1987). *Children's rights and the law*. Lexington, MA: Lexington Books.

Henning, J. S. (1982). *The rights of children: Legal and psychological perspectives*. Springfield, IL: Thomas.

Holder, A. R. (1982). *Legal issues in pediatrics and adolescent medicine* (2nd ed.). New Haven: Yale University Press.

Melton, G. B., Petrila, J., Poythress, N. G., & Slobogin, C. (1987). *Psychological evaluations for the courts*. New York: Guilford Press.

Reppucci, N. D., Weithorn, L. H., Mulvey, E. P., & Monahan, J. (Eds.). (1984). *Children, mental health and the law*. Beverly Hills, CA: Sage Publications.

Schetky, D., & Benedek, E. (Eds.). (1992). *Clinical handbook of child psychiatry and the law*. Baltimore: Williams & Wilkins.

II. The Child as a Witness

A. Cases

Coy v. Iowa, 108 S.Ct. 2798 (1988).
Idaho v. Wright, 110 S.Ct. 3139 (1990).
Maryland v. Craig, 110 S.Ct. 3157 (1990).
White v. Illinois, 112 S. Ct. 736 (1992).

B. Articles and Books

Benedek, E. P., & Schetky, D. H. (1986). The child as witness. *Hospital and Community Psychiatry, 37,* 1225–1229.
Ceci, S. J., Toglia, M. P., & Ross, D. F. (1987). *Children's eyewitness memory.* New York: Springer-Verlag.
Goodman, G. S. (Ed.). (1984). The child witness. *Journal of Social Issues, 40*(2), 1–175.
Marin, D. V., Holmes, D. L., Guth, M., & Kovac, P. (1979). The potential of children as eyewitnesses. *Law and Human Behavior, 3,* 295–305.
Melton, G. B. (1981). Children's competency to testify. *Law and Human Behavior, 5,* 73–85.
Myers, J. E. B. (1992). *Evidence in child abuse and neglect cases.* New York: Wiley Law Publications.
Nurcombe, B. (1986). The child as witness: Competency and credibility. *Journal of the American Academy of Child Psychiatry, 25,* 473–480.
Quinn, K. M. (1986). Competency to be a witness: A major child forensic issue. *Bulletin of the American Academy of Psychiatry and the Law, 14,* 311–321.

III. Consent to Treatment

A. Abortion and Contraception Cases

Griswold v. Connecticut, 381 U.S. 479 (1965).
Roe v. Wade, 410 U.S. 113 (1973).
Planned Parenthood of Central Missouri v. Danforth, 428 U.S. 52 (1976).
Carey v. Population Services International, 431 U.S. 678 (1977).
Bellotti v. Baird (II), 443 U.S. 622 (1979).
H.L. v. Matheson, 450 U.S. 498 (1981).
Hodgson v. Minnesota, 110 S.Ct. 2926 (1990).
Ohio v. Akron Center for Reproductive Health, 110 S.Ct. 2972 (1990).

B. Articles and Books

Ambuel, B., & Rappaport, J. (1992). Developmental trends in adolescents' psychological and legal competence to consent to abortion. *Law and Human Behavior, 16,* 129–154.
Beeman, D. G., & Scott, N. A. (1991). Therapists' attitudes toward psychotherapy informed consent with adolescents. *Professional Psychology: Research and Practice, 22,* 230–234.
Croxton, T. A., Churchill, S. R., & Fellin, P. (1988). Counseling minors without parental consent. *Child Welfare, 67,* 3–14.
Demetriou, E., & Kaplan, D. W. (1989). Adolescent contraceptive use and parental notification. *American Journal Diseases of Children, 143,* 1166–1172.
Gaylin, W. (1982). The competence of children: No longer all or none. *Journal of the American Academy of Child Psychiatry, 21,* 153–162.
Holder, A. R. (1987). Minors' rights to consent to medical care. *Journal of the American Medical Association, 257,* 3400–3402.
Kopelman, L. M., & Moskop, J. C. (Eds.). (1989). *Children and health care: Moral and social issues.* Dordrecht: Kluwer Academic.
Lewis, C. L. (1987). Minor's competence to consent to abortion. *American Psychologist, 42,* 84–88.
Melton, G. B., Koocher, G. P., & Saks, M. J. (1983). *Children's competency to consent.* New York: Plenum Press.
Morrissey, J. M., Hoffman, A. D., & Thorpe, C. (1986). *Consent and confidentiality in the health care of children and adolescents: A legal guide.* New York: Free Press.

Reilly, P. R. (1991). *The surgical solution: A history of involuntary sterilization in the United States*. Baltimore: Johns Hopkins.
Rozovsky, F. A. (1990). *Consent to treatment: A practical guide* (2nd ed). Boston: Little, Brown.
Scherer, D. G. (1991). The capacities of minors to exercise voluntariness in medical treatment decisions. *Law and Human Behavior, 15*, 431–449.
Weithorm, L. A., & Campbell, S. B. (1982). The competency of children and adolescents to make informed treatment decisions. *Child Development, 53*, 1589–1598.

IV. Psychiatric Hospitalization of Minors

A. *Cases*

In Re Long, 25 N.C. App. 702 (1975).
Kremens v. Bartley, 431 U.S. 119 (1977).
Parham v. J.R., 442 U.S. 584 (1979).
Sec. of Public Welfare v. Institutionalized Individuals, 442 U.S. 640 (1979).

B. *Articles*

Amaya, M., & Burlingame, W. V. (1981). Judicial review of psychiatric admissions: The clinical impact on child and adolescent inpatients. *Journal of the American Academy of Child Psychiatry, 20*, 761–776.
American Psychiatric Association. (1982). Guidelines for the psychiatric hospitalization of minors. *American Journal of Psychiatry, 139*, 971–974.
Ellis, J. W. (1974). Volunteering children: Parental commitment of minors to mental institutions. *California Law Review, 62*, 840–916.
Walding, J. K. (1990). What ever happened to *Parham* and *Institutionalized Juveniles:* Do minors have procedural rights in the civil commitment area? *Law and Psychology Review, 14*, 281–302.

V. Research

Abramovitch, R., Freedman, J. L., Thoden, K., & Nikolich, C. (1991). Children's capacity to consent to participation in psychological research: Empirical findings. *Child Development, 62*, 1100–1109.
Gaylin, W., & Macklin, R. (1982). *Who speaks for the child: The problems of proxy consent*. New York: Hastings Center.
Langer, D. H. (1984). Medical research involving children: Some legal and ethical issues. *Baylor Law Review, 36*, 1–39.
Langer, D. H. (1985). Children's legal rights as research subjects. *Journal of the American Academy of Child Psychiatry, 24*, 653–662.
Levine, R. J. (1986). *Ethics and regulation of clinical research* (2nd ed.). New Haven: Yale University Press.
National Commission for the Protection of Human Subjects of Biomedical and Behavioral Research. (1977). *The Belmont Report: Ethical principles and guidelines for the protection of human subjects of research*. (Publication No. 03 77–004). Washington, DC: Department of Health, Education, and Welfare.
Stanley, B., & Sieber, J. (Eds.). (1992). *Social research on children and adolescents: Ethical issues*. Newbury Park, CA: Sage.

VI. Child Abuse and Sexual Abuse

A. *Cases*

Groff v. State, 390 So.2d 361 (Fla.App. 1980).
People v. McKean, 418 N.E.2d 1130 (Ill.App. 1981).
Commonwealth v. Collett, 439 N.E.2d 1223 (Sup.Jud.Ct.Mass. 1982).
Goldade v. State of Wyoming, 674 P.2d 721 (Sup.Ct.Wyo. 1983).
People v. Stritzinger, 194 Cal.Rptr. 431 (1983).
Weber v. Stony Brook Hospital, 456 N.E.2d 1186 (N.Y.Ct.App. 1983).
People v. Battaglia, 203 Cal.Rptr. 370 (App. 1984).

State ex rel. D.M. v. Hoester, 681 S.W.2d 449 (Sup.Ct.Mo. 1984).
State v. R.H., 683 P.2d 269 (Alaska App. 1984).
State of Minnesota v. Andring, 342 N.W.2d 128 (Sup.Ct.Minn. 1984).
Meador v. State of Nevada, 711 P.2d 852 (Sup.Ct.Nev. 1985).
State v. Munyon, 726 P.2d 1333 (Kan. 1986).
Gross v. Myers, 748 P.2d 459 (Sup.Ct.Mont. 1987).
Krikorian v. Barry, 242 Cal.Rptr. 312 (App. 1987).
Robinson v. Commonwealth of Massachusetts, 503 N.E.2d 31 (Sup.Jud.Ct.Mass. 1987).
Rubinstein v. Baron, 529 A.2d 1061 (N.J.Super. 1987).
Taylor v. Ledbetter, 818 F.2d 791 (11th Cir. 1987).
People v. John B., 237 Cal.Rptr. 659 (App. 1987).
Commonwealth v. Moore, 548 A.2d 1250 (Pa.Super. 1988).
Montoya by Montoya v. Bebensee, 761 P.2d 285 (Colo.App. 1988).
People v. Bass, 529 N.Y.S.2d 961 (Sup.Ct. 1988).
State of Florida Department of Human and Rehabilitative Services v. Yamuni, 529 So.2d 258 (Fla. 1988).
DeShaney v. Winnebago County Department of Social Services, 109 S.Ct. 998 (1989).
Jensen v. South Carolina Department of Social Services, 377 S.E.2d 102 (S.C.App. 1989).
Shurn v. Monteleone, 769 S.W.2d 188 (Mo.App. 1989).
State v. Sypult, 800 S.W.2d 402 (Sup.Ct.Ark. 1990).
Commonwealth v. Moyer, 595 A.2d 1177 (Pa.Super. 1991).
Newmark v. Williams, 588 A.2d 1108 (Del.Sup.Ct. 1991). [Christian Science parents may refuse cancer chemotherapy for their child]
People v. Bowman, 812 P.2d 725 (Colo.App. 1991).
Roe v. Superior Court, 280 Cal.Rptr.380 (App. 1991).
Walstad v. State, 818 P.2d 695 (Alaska App. 1991).
Annotation: Validity, construction, and application of statute limiting physician–patient privilege in judicial proceedings relating to child abuse or neglect. 44 A.L.R.4th 649.
Annotation: Abused or neglected children: Tort liability of public authority for failure to remove parentally abused or neglected children from parents' custody. 60 A.L.R.4th 942.

B. *Articles and Books*

American Academy of Child and Adolescent Psychiatry. (1980). Guidelines for the clinical evaluation of child and adolescent sexual abuse. *American Academy of Child and Adolescent Psychiatry, 27*, 655–657.
American Medical Association. (1985). AMA diagnostic and treatment guidelines concerning child abuse and neglect. *Journal of the American Medical Association, 254*, 796–800.
Benedek, E. P., & Schetky, D. H. (1987). Problems in validating allegations of sexual abuse: 1, Factors affecting perception and recall of events. *Journal of the American Academy of Child and Adolescent Psychiatry, 26*, 912–915.
Benedek, E. P., & Schetky, D. H. (1987). Problems in validating allegations of sexual abuse: 2, Clinical evaluation. *Journal of the American Academy of Child and Adolescent Psychiatry, 26*, 916–921.
Berlin, F. S., Malin, H. M., & Dean, S. (1991). Effects of statutes requiring psychiatrists to report suspected sexual abuse of children. *American Journal of Psychiatry, 148*, 449–453.
Besharov, D. J. (1987). Reporting out-of-home maltreatment: Penalties and protections. *Child Welfare, 66*, 399–408.
Besharov, D. J. (1988). *Protecting children from abuse and neglect: Policy and practice*. Springfield, IL: Thomas.
Brosig, C. L., & Kalichman, S. C. (1992). Clinicians' reporting of suspected child abuse: A review of the empirical literature. *Clinical Psychology Review, 12*, 155–168.
Browne, A., & Finkelhor, D. (1986). Impact of child sexual abuse: A review of the research. *Psychological Bulletin, 99*, 66–77.
Coleman, P. (1986). Creating therapist-incest offender exception to mandatory child abuse reporting statutes—When psychiatrist knows best. *University of Cincinnati Law Review, 54*, 1113–1152.
Cunningham, C. D. (1984). Vanishing exception to the psychotherapist-patient privilege: The child abuse reporting act. *Pacific Law Journal, 16*, 335–352.
Eckenrode, J., Munsch, J., Powers, J., & Doris, J. (1988). The nature and substantiation of official sexual abuse reports. *Child Abuse and Neglect, 12*, 311–319.
Everson, M. D., & Boat, B. W. (1989). False allegations of sexual abuse by children and adolescents. *Journal of the American Academy of Child and Adolescent Psychiatry, 28*, 230–235.

Faller, K. C. (1984). Is the child victim of sexual abuse telling the truth? *Child Abuse and Neglect, 8*, 473–481.
Finkelhor, D. (1984). *Child abuse: New theory and research*. New York: Free Press.
Green, A. H. (1986). True and false allegations of sexual abuse in child custody disputes. *Journal of the American Academy of Child Psychiatry, 25*, 449–456.
Holder, W., & Hayes, K. (1984). *Malpractice and liability in child protective services*. Longmont, CL: Bookmakers Guild.
Hurley, M. M. (1985). Duties in conflict: Must psychotherapists report child abuse inflicted by clients and confided in therapy? *San Diego Law Review, 22*, 645–668.
Kalichman, S. C., Craig, M. E., & Follingstad, D. R. (1989). Factors influencing the reporting of father–child sexual abuse: Study of licensed practicing psychologists. *Professional Psychology: Research and Practice, 20*, 84–89.
Maddock, J. W. (1988). Child reporting and testimony in incest cases: Comments on the construction and reconstruction of reality. *Behavioral Sciences and the Law, 6*, 201–220.
Mantell, D. M. (1988). Clarifying erroneous child sexual abuse allegations. *American Journal of Orthopsychiatry, 58*, 618–621.
McDonald, A. E., & Reece, R. M. (1979). Child abuse: Problems of reporting. *Pediatric Clinics of North America, 26*, 785–791.
Melton, G. B., & Limber, S. (1989). Psychologists' involvement in cases of child maltreatment. *American Psychologist, 44*, 1225–1233.
Meriwether, M. H. (1986). Child abuse reporting laws: Time for a change. *Family Law Quarterly, 20*, 141–171.
Miller, R. D., & Weinstock, R. (1987). Conflict of interest between therapist-patient confidentiality and the duty to report sexual abuse of children. *Behavioral Sciences and the Law, 5*, 161–174.
Morris, J. L., Johnson, C. F., & Clasen, M. (1985). To report or not to report: Physicians' attitudes toward discipline and child abuse. *American Journal of Diseases of Children, 139*, 194–197.
Newberger, E. H. (1983). The helping hand strikes again—Unintended consequences of child abuse reporting. *Journal of Clinical Child Psychology, 12*, 307–311.
Quinn, K. M. (1988). The credibility of children's allegations of sexual abuse. *Behavioral Sciences and the Law, 6*, 181–199.
Quinn, K. M., White, S., & Santilli, G. (1989). Influences of an interviewer's behaviors in child sexual abuse investigations. *Bulletin of the American Academy of Psychiatry and the Law, 17*, 45–52.
Racusin, R. J., & Felsman, J. K. (1986). Reporting child abuse: The ethical obligation to inform parents. *Journal of the American Academy of Child Psychiatry, 25*, 485–489.
Religious confidentiality and the reporting of child abuse: A statutory and constitutional analysis. (1987). *Columbia Journal of Law and Social Problems, 21*, 1–53.
Schetky, D. H., & Green, A. H. (Eds.). (1988). *Child sexual abuse*. New York: Brunner/Mazel.
Smith, S. R., & Meyer, R. G. (1984). Child abuse reporting laws and psychotherapy: A time for reconsideration. *International Journal of Law and Psychiatry, 7*, 351–366.
Watson, H., & Levine, M. (1989). Psychotherapy and mandated reporting of child abuse. *American Journal of Orthopsychiatry, 59*, 246–256.
Weisberg, R., & Wald, M. (1984). Confidentiality laws and state efforts to protect abused or neglected children: The need for statutory reform. *Family Law Quarterly, 18*, 143–212.
White, S., & Quinn, K. M. (1988). Investigatory independence in child sexual abuse evaluations: Conceptual considerations. *Bulletin of the American Academy of Psychiatry and the Law, 16*, 269–278.
Widom, C. S. (1989). Child abuse, neglect and adult behavior. *American Journal of Orthopsychiatry, 59*, 355–367.
Widom, C. S. (1989). Does violence beget violence? A critical examination of the literature. *Psychological Bulletin, 106*, 3–28.
Yates, A., & Musty, T. (1988). Preschool children's erroneous allegations of sexual molestation. *American Journal of Psychiatry, 145*, 989–992.
Zellman, G. L. (1990). Child abuse reporting and failure to report among mandated reporters: Prevalence, incidence, and reasons. *Journal of Interpersonal Violence, 5*, 3–22.
Zellman, G. L., & Bell, R. M. (1990). *The role of professional background, case characteristics, and protective agency response in mandated child abuse reporting*. Santa Monica, CA: Rand Corporation.

VII. Child Custody

Ash, P., & Guyer, M. (1984). Court implementation of mental health professionals' recommendations in contested child custody and visitation cases. *Bulletin of the American Academy of Psychiatry and the Law, 12*, 137–147.

Ash, P., & Guyer, M. (1986). The functions of psychiatric evaluation in contested child custody and visitation cases. *Journal of the American Academy of Child Psychiatry, 25,* 554–561.
Barnum, R. (1987). Understanding controversies in visitation. *Journal of American Academy of Child and Adolescent Psychiatry, 26,* 788–792.
Benedek, E. P., & Schetky, D. H. (1985). Custody and visitation. *Psychiatric Clinics of North America, 5,* 857–873.
Berkman, C. F. (1984). Psychodynamic and family issues in post-divorce child custody. *Journal of the American Academy of Child Psychiatry, 23,* 708–712.
Bernet, W. (1983). The therapist's role in child custody disputes. *Journal of the American Academy of Child Psychiatry, 22,* 180–183.
Bolocofsky, D. N. (1989). Use and abuse of mental health experts in child custody determinations. *Behavioral Sciences and the Law, 7,* 197–213.
Derdeyn, A. P. (1976). Child custody contests in historical perspective. *American Journal of Psychiatry, 133,* 1369–1376.
Emery, R. E., & Wyer, M. M. (1987). Divorce mediation. *American Psychologist, 42,* 472–480.
Foster, H. H. (1983). Child custody and divorce: A lawyer's view. *Journal of the American Academy of Child Psychiatry, 22,* 392–398.
Goldstein, J., & Freud, A. (1979). *Before the best interests of the child.* New York: Free Press.
Goldstein, J., Freud, A., & Solnit, A. (1973). *Beyond the best interests of the child.* New York: Free Press.
Goldzband, M. G. (1988). *Custody cases and expert witnesses: A manual for attorneys* (2nd ed.). Clifton, NJ: Prentice-Hall Law & Business.
Group for the Advancement of Psychiatry. (1981). *Divorce, child custody and the family.* San Francisco: Jossey-Bass.
Haller, L. H. (1981). Before the judge: The child-custody evaluation. *Adolescent Psychiatry, 9,* 142–164.
Hayman, R. L. (1990). Presumptions of justice: Law, politics, and the mentally retarded parent. *Harvard Law Review, 103,* 1201–1271.
Jacobs, J. W. (1986). Divorce and child custody resolution: Conflicting legal and psychological paradigms. *American Journal of Psychiatry, 143,* 192–197.
Racusin, R. J., Albertini, R., Wishik, H. R., Schnurr, P., & Mayberry, J. (1989). Factors associated with joint custody awards. *Journal of American Academy of Child and Adolescent Psychiatry, 28,* 164–170.
Santilli, L. E., & Roberts, M. C. (1990). Custody decisions in Alabama before and after the abolition of the Tender Years Doctrine. *Law and Human Behavior, 14,* 123–137.
Schoettle, U. C. (1984). Termination of parental rights: Ethical issues and role conflicts. *Journal of the American Academy of Child and Adolescent Psychiatry, 23,* 629–632.
Simons, V., & Meyer, K. G. (1986). The child custody evaluation: Issues and trends. *Behavioral Sciences and the Law, 4,* 137–156.
Volkmar, F. R., Nordhaus, B., Provence, S., Leckman, J. F., Berkman, M., & Solnit, A. J. (1990). A custody and placement evaluation of an infant with a psychotic, mentally retarded mother. *Journal of the American Academy of Child and Adolescent Psychiatry, 29,* 661–666.
Wallerstein, J. S. (1989). *Second chances: Men, women and children a decade after divorce.* New York: Ticknor & Fields.
Wallerstein, J. S., & Kelly, J. B. (1979). *Surviving the breakup: How children and parents cope with divorce.* New York: Basic Books.
Weiner, B. (1985). An overview of child custody laws. *Hospital and Community Psychiatry, 36,* 838–843.
Weiner, B. A., Simons, V. A., & Cavanaugh, J. (1985). The child custody dispute. In D. Schetky & E. Benedek (Eds.), *Emerging issues in child psychiatry.* New York: Brunner/Mazel.
Weithorn, L. H. (Ed.). (1987). *Psychology and child custody determinations: Knowledge, roles, and expertise.* Lincoln: University of Nebraska Press.
Wolchik, S. A., & Karoly, P. (Eds.). (1988). *Children of divorce: Empirical perspectives on adjustment.* New York: Gardner Press.

VIII. Right to an Education

A. Cases

Mills v. Board of Education, 348 F.Supp. 866 (D.D.C. 1972).
Pennsylvania Association for Retarded Children v. Commonwealth, 343 F.Supp. 279 (D.C.Pa. 1972).
New York State Association for Retarded Children v. Carey, 612 F.2nd 644 (2nd Cir. 1979).
Board of Education v. Rowley, 458 U.S. 176 (1982).

IX. Juvenile Justice and Delinquency

A. Cases

Kent v. United States, 383 U.S. 541 (1966).
In re Gault, 387 U.S. 1 (1967).
In re Winship, 397 U.S. 358 (1970).
Morales v. Turman, 364 F.Supp. 166 (D.D.C. Tex. 1973).

B. Articles and Books

Barnum, R. (1987). Clinical evaluation of juvenile delinquents facing transfer to adult court. *Journal of the American Academy of Child and Adolescent Psychiatry, 26,* 922–925.
Cornell, D. G., Benedek, E. P., & Benedek, D. M. (1987). Juvenile homicide: Prior adjustment and a proposed typology. *American Journal of Orthopsychiatry, 57,* 383–393.
Davis, G. E., & Leitenberg, H. (1987). Adolescent sex offenders. *Psychological Bulletin, 101,* 417–427.
Fagan, J. (1991). Community-based treatment for mentally disordered juvenile offenders. *Journal of Clinical Child Psychology, 20,* 42–50.
Goetting, A. (1989). Patterns of homicide among children. *Criminal Justice and Behavior, 16,* 63–80.
Grisso, T. (1981). *Juveniles' waiver of rights: Legal and psychological competence.* New York: Plenum Press.
Grisso, T., Tomkins, A., & Casey, P. (1988). Psychosocial concepts in juvenile law. *Law and Human Behavior, 12,* 403–437.
Johnson, T. C., & Berry, C. (1989). Children who molest: A treatment program. *Journal of Interpersonal Violence, 4,* 185–203.
Kavoussi, R. J., Kaplan, M., & Becker, J. V. (1988). Psychiatric diagnoses in adolescent sex offenders. *Journal of the American Academy of Child and Adolescent Psychiatry, 27,* 241–243.
Keith, C. R. (Ed.). (1984). *The aggressive adolescent: Clinical perspectives.* New York: Free Press.
Lewis, D. O. (1981). *Vulnerabilities to delinquency.* New York: SP Medical and Scientific Books.
Offer, D., Marohn, R. C., & Ostrov, E. (1979). *The psychological world of the juvenile delinquent.* New York: Basic Books.
Patterson, G. R., DeBaryshe, B. D., & Ramsey, E. (1989). A developmental perspective on antisocial behavior. *American Psychologist, 44,* 329–335.
Quay, H. C. (Ed.). (1987). *Handbook of juvenile delinquency.* New York: Wiley.
Rutter, M., & Giller, H. (1983). *Juvenile delinquency: Trends and perspectives.* New York: Guilford Press.
Saunders, E. B., & Awad, G. A. (1988). Assessment, management, and treatment planning for male adolescent sexual offenders. *American Journal of Orthopsychiatry, 58,* 571–579.
Workgroup on Psychiatric Practice in the Juvenile Court, American Psychiatric Association. (1992). *Handbook of psychiatric practice in the juvenile court.* Washington, DC: American Psychiatric Association.
Workgroup on Quality Issues, American Academy of Child and Adolescent Psychiatry. (1992). Practice parameters for the assessment and treatment of conduct disorders. *Journal of the American Academy of Child and Adolescent Psychiatry, 31,* IV-VII.
Yeager, C. A., & Lewis, D.O. (1990). Mortality in a group of formerly incarcerated juvenile delinquents. *American Journal of Psychiatry, 147,* 612–614.

11

Involvement with Litigation

I. Why Attorneys Need Expert Witnesses • II. Mental Health Issues in the Courtroom • A. Civil Commitment • B. Proceedings Related to Children • C. Guardianship and Incompetency Proceedings • D. Personal Injury Cases • E. Workers' Compensation and Disability Claims • F. Criminal Cases • **III. Why the Professional Should Serve as an Expert Witness • IV. What to Expect from the Attorney •** A. Background of the Case • B. Clarification of the Legal Issue • C. Clarification of What the Attorney Wants • D. Access to All Records • E. The Evaluator's Setting the Terms of the Evaluation • F. Fees • G. Conferences • **V. When a Case Should Be Declined • VI. Preparing Reports •** A. Preparation for Writing the Report • B. Format for the Report • C. Content of the Report • **VII. Consulting with the Attorney before Trial • VIII. Depositions • IX. Testifying at Trial •** A. Preparation • B. Testifying • C. Cross-Examination • **X. Commonly Asked Questions • XI. Bibliography**

For many mental health professionals, even the thought of becoming involved in a case which may have legal ramifications is unpleasant. Typically, clinicians do not want to deal with attorneys, particularly in an adversary setting. Generally, juggling one's schedule to meet the unpredictable demands of courtroom appearances is unappealing. The court appearance itself may be seen as highly aversive. The professional may believe that time spent on a legal case is not time well spent. Yet, involvement in a forensic matter is often involuntary.

Common examples of clinical issues which have legal implications are the need for civil commitment, the awareness of child abuse or neglect, the client's involvement in a child custody dispute, or the client's suffering psychological harm as a result of personal injury.

In addition, the mental health professional's expertise may prompt an attorney or the court to seek the professional for an opinion on a mental health issue which impacts on a case. These types of cases will often involve a complex question which may have a major impact on the life of the person being evaluated. These cases frequently afford the professional an opportunity to bring to bear his clinical training and experience. The realities of practice dictate that one may not avoid clinical-legal matters; attempting to do so may cause the professional to miss some of the most interesting cases in clinical practice.

This chapter will provide an understanding of attorneys' and courts' need to utilize mental health professionals and the types of legal cases in which they will commonly become involved. Specific advice is offered about working with attorneys, writing reports, and testifying. The chapter also reviews when a professional should not become involved in testifying in a case. It is hoped that the reader who has avoided involvement with clinical-legal cases will become more comfortable if testimony is required.

We wish to stress that this chapter is intended to make the treating clinician more comfortable should he be compelled to appear in court or to testify about his patient. Generally, we believe that clinicians should not serve as expert witnesses unless prepared to obtain the training and experience necessary to address the psychological and forensic issues which arise in a legal forum. For this reason we have not provided details of how to evaluate a litigant for specific forensic issues. Numerous books and articles have been written on serving as a forensic mental health expert and performing specific types of forensic evaluations. Specialized forensic mental health training programs in psychology and psychiatry are also available for this purpose. In contrast, we only briefly set forth the issues which may be raised in the legal context, to help the clinician better understand what the litigant, whether his patient or not, may be facing.

I. WHY ATTORNEYS NEED EXPERT WITNESSES

Many cases involve disputes which are more complicated than the word of one person against another. The fair resolution of the dispute will turn on the interpretation of the facts in the case as well as the relevant law. Expert witnesses are needed to provide the court with sufficient information to render a just decision. They are called upon when the issues being addressed are not part of the common knowledge of the average person. The role of the expert is to educate the judge and jurors by elaborating upon the facts before the court and providing an explanation for what has occurred or should have occurred. The expert may also describe why it might have happened, who is responsible for any problems, and the extent of the harm done. In some cases, one expert can address these issues, while in other circumstances, a variety of experts will be needed. The goal of the court will be to settle the dispute by assessing responsibility and trying to return the injured party to the position he was in before the injury. This will usually take the form of monetary compensation but can also require that the losing party take specific actions to benefit the injured party. These might include performing under the terms of a contract, reinstating a person to his job, or taking other steps which will return things to the prelitigation circumstances.

Experts are called upon in many types of legal cases, from contract disputes to personal injury actions. If a hotel walkway collapses and people are injured or killed, there will be a great deal of litigation. The law seeks to accurately assess responsibility and compensate the injured parties. An architect will testify about the building's design and any flaws in it. A structural engineer will testify whether the walkway was designed and constructed in a way which made it likely to withstand the weight of many people. A building contractor may be called upon to testify as to whether the construction was completed in a proper manner and met industry standards. Once fault has been determined, experts will testify as to the extent of harm done to the injured people. These experts may include physicians, who will describe the medical injuries and prognosis; mental health professionals, who describe the psychological injuries and prognosis; and actuaries, who calculate the loss of income for someone who previously had a particular occupation and can no longer work.

Despite the volume of cases before the courts, it is relatively infrequent that the issues involve the testimony of a mental health professional. Yet it is often in cases needing a mental health expert that the decision will have the most profound impact on the individual.

II. MENTAL HEALTH PROFESSIONALS IN THE COURTROOM

Mental health professionals may be called upon to testify in civil, criminal, juvenile, or family law matters. In addition, employers may turn to mental health professionals for an opinion about whether someone is psychologically appropriate for a particular job, such as law enforcement. Other issues requiring expertise may include whether a person is fit to return to his job after having taken a leave of absence due to substance abuse or a psychiatric disorder. Summarized below are some of the most common types of proceedings in which a mental health professional is needed to provide the court with information to make an informed and fair decision. This is not an exhaustive list, but one which illustrates the involvement of mental health professionals in the courtroom as expert witnesses.

A. Civil Commitment

In all states, the participation of a mental health professional, usually a physician and sometimes other professionals, is required before someone can be civilly committed. The evaluation by the professional establishes that the person meets the civil commitment standard and is in need of treatment. Civil commitment may be the only way to obtain psychiatric treatment for an unwilling person. In civil commitment proceedings, the professional will testify about the presence and type of mental illness, its impact on the person's ability to care for himself, and any potential violence to himself or others. Mental health professionals usually testify in civil commitment hearings as treating clinicians. Sometimes, however, they testify as expert witnesses on behalf of the patient who is challenging the commitment (see Chapter 3).

B. Proceedings Related to Children

Mental health professionals may be called upon when there is a question of child abuse, child neglect, or termination of parental rights. They are also likely to be called upon when there is a custody or visitation dispute. In other circumstances, the child or adolescent will have broken the law, and the professional may become involved in juvenile court proceedings.

Juvenile courts employ social workers, psychologists, and psychiatrists, who often perform court-referred evaluations. These mental health professionals will be asked to render advice on special needs for an individual child or placement in specific rehabilitation programs. In addition, the professional may be called upon to address whether a particular child should be tried as an adult. In each of these cases involving children, the goal of the court is to serve the needs of the child. Treating clinicians can also be called on to testify about these issues when they occur during the course of a treatment which began prior to the legal case. (See Chapter 10.)

C. Guardianship and Incompetency Proceedings

Proceedings to declare a person legally incompetent and to appoint a guardian occur when the person is allegedly no longer able to make or communicate decisions related to his basic needs or is unable to manage his finances. In almost every state, a health care professional is required to provide the court with documentation or testimony that the individual is lacking a particular ability. When guardianship of the estate is sought, then the professional must address whether the alleged incompetent person is able to handle financial matters. If a guardian of the person is sought, the professional should describe why the alleged incompetent cannot make or communicate personal decisions. (See Chapter 9.)

A mental health professional who testifies in incompetency proceedings usually provides a needed service to the person, although it is not treatment as such. These proceedings are typically implemented to protect the alleged incompetent's rights or his assets. If the person is declared incompetent, then a substitute decision maker will be appointed and supervised by the court. As in the case of other civil litigation, the testifying professional might be the primary therapist for the patient or an expert witness expressly and solely retained for the litigation.

D. Personal Injury Cases

When a person has been negligently injured as the result of the fault of another, part of his claim will involve recovery for his mental suffering. Most commonly, these cases arise from injuries due to automobile or other transportation accidents, negligently maintained property, medical malpractice, or faulty products. Expert testimony will be needed to describe the extent of the psychological damage. The evaluator will try to determine the impact of the injury on the plaintiff. He will also need to know the extent of the person's functioning before the accident in order to determine how much of his current psychological problems can be attributed to the accident. Since each person responds differently to an injury, a full understanding of the individual's history and personality is necessary before one concludes that the trauma is the cause of a current symptom or behavior. For example, being injured as a result of the collapse of a building may be painful for anyone, but the psychological trauma inherent in such an event is more intense and long-lasting for some people than for others.

Another type of personal injury action which will require the expert testimony of the mental health professional is when a malpractice suit is brought against a therapist. Since the therapist must be judged by the standards of his profession, a similarly credentialed clinician must establish in his court testimony the standard of clinical practice and then testify about any deviations from that standard in the particular case at bar (see Chapter 6 for further discussion).

E. Workers' Compensation and Disability Claims

In each state, specific laws provide coverage for workers for job-related injuries. In some cases, there will be a debate about the extent of the worker's injury and whether he is now partially or fully disabled. In many states, the ability to recover for work-related psychological injury is being broadened, particularly when there has been no physical injury at work but only emotional stress. Experts are necessary to determine the extent of the injury and its impact on the person's employability. Mental health professionals are needed when the issue relates to psychological injury.

Individuals may also seek to obtain disability benefits under the Social Security system. To establish such a disability based on a mental illness requires the report of a psychologist or psychiatrist. In some instances, the disability will be challenged, and the mental health professional may be called upon to testify at a determination hearing.

F. Criminal Cases

A person's mental condition can have profound implications in the criminal justice system. One's mental condition may determine whether he is charged with a crime or taken by the police to a mental health facility. It will affect the defendant's passage through the criminal justice system and whether the person is excused from criminal responsibility. If the defendant is found guilty, the fact of some mental defect or illness may affect the sentencing conditions or disposition. There are three major criminal court proceedings in which the mental health professional can testify: (l) competency to stand trial, (2) criminal responsibility, and (3) sentencing alternatives.

1. Competency to Stand Trial

The most common mental health issue which arises in the trial context is whether the defendant has the mental ability to participate in the trial process. Without the defendant's being competent, the trial will not proceed. For the mental health professional, the issue is quite narrow: At the present time, does the defendant understand the nature of the charges and proceedings against him, and does he have sufficient ability to collaborate with his attorney in his own defense? If he does, then the defendant will be considered competent to stand trial, and the trial will proceed. If the court decides that the defendant does not have this ability, then he will be adjudicated incompetent to stand trial, and the proceedings will be suspended. In the vast majority of cases where the defendant is determined to be incompetent, he is placed in the custody of the state mental health agency for treatment to render him competent.

The issue of the defendant's trial competency can be raised by the defendant, the prosecution, or the judge. Demanding competency of the defendant serves a number of purposes. First, it safeguards the accuracy of the proceedings; if the defendant is incompetent, he cannot bring to his attorney's attention all the facts which may be relevant to his case. Second, it ensures procedural fairness. This means the defendant, by having the basic capacity to exercise the rights accorded him under the law, has the right to choose and assist counsel, act as witness on his own behalf, and confront opposing witnesses. Competency requires that the defendant be aware of the facts and be capable of communicating them to his counsel. The defendant must also understand his role in the proceedings and have some grasp of the substantive and tactical options open to him or his attorney. Third, the integrity and dignity of the legal process and general respect for our judicial and law enforcement systems would be undermined by the spectacle of trying an incapacitated defendant. Fourth, achieving the objectives of punishment or sentencing, whether they be retribution, rehabilitation, or deterrence, depends on the defendant's comprehending the punishment and the reasons for its imposition.

2. *Criminal Responsibility*

The insanity defense is a legal construct that relieves a defendant of criminal responsibility for his conduct when it is determined that he meets the insanity defense standard.

Conviction of a crime requires proof of two elements: (1) the *actus rea*, or physical act, and (2) the *mens rea*, or mental state. The prosecution must prove both elements to find a person guilty of the offense. For example, if murder is defined as the wrongful killing of a person with the intent to kill or do great bodily harm, then in order to convict someone of murder, the prosecution must prove that the defendant killed the person and also had the intent to kill or harm the person.

The Anglo-American tradition of criminal law is grounded on the premise that a person is normally capable of free and rational choice between alternative acts, and that one who chooses to harm another is thus morally accountable and liable to punishment. If, however, a person, because of mental disease or defect, lacks the capacity to make rational choices or to conform his behavior to the moral and legal demands of society, he will be relieved of criminal responsibility for his actions. Although each state has its own insanity defense standard, all standards incorporate some or all of four elements: (l) presence of a mental disease at the time of the act; (2) presence of a defect of reason because of the mental disease; (3) lack of knowledge of the nature or wrongfulness of the act as a result of the mental disease; or (4) an incapacity to refrain from the act which derives from the mental disease. When a defendant raises the insanity defense, he is admitting that he committed the physical act but is trying to shift responsibility from himself to his "mental disease," which precluded him from conforming his conduct to that required by the law.

When a defendant raises the insanity defense, he must undergo a psychiatric or psychological evaluation. Under many state laws, the evaluator must be a psychiatrist. In a growing number of states, a psychologist can also serve as the evaluator of the defendant's criminal responsibility. The evaluator must try to reconstruct the defendant's mental state at the time of the crime. The issue is not the defendant's present mental state but the defendant's mental status at the time of the commission of the alleged act. In addition to obtaining a complete psychiatric and medical history, the evaluator will need much additional information in order to clearly understand the defendant's mental state at the time of the crime. This understanding will require interviews not only with the defendant but also with any witnesses to the event and others who observed the behavior of the defendant within hours or days of the crime.

Although the insanity defense is raised in fewer than 1% of the criminal cases in the United States and is successful in only a few of these, it has generated a great deal of controversy. This controversy has focused not only on the use of the defense but also on the role of the mental health professional in evaluating and testifying in these cases. The mental health professional who undertakes such an evaluation should be familiar with the legal standard in the involved jurisdiction. At a minimum, the evaluator will need to determine if there was a major mental illness at the time of the alleged offense and its effect upon the thinking and behavior of the defendant at that time. Traditionally, the courts have required that the defendant have a mental illness of psychotic proportions at the time of the offense to meet the mental illness standard for the insanity defense.

In a growing number of states, if the person is adjudicated not guilty by reason of insanity, he will be subject to special criminal commitment statutes. The professional may also be needed to testify at such a commitment hearing as to the defendant's need for treatment and his prognosis.

3. *Sentencing Alternatives*

The mental health professional may be called upon to provide the court with recommendations regarding programs for the convicted defendant. These may include mandatory counseling or treatment as a condition of probation in lieu of imprisonment. The treatment may involve drug or alcohol rehabilitation, outpatient mental health services, or living in a halfway house. The courts will consider other types of programs which are likely to protect society from further crimes by the defendant and which are likely to increase the chance of rehabilitation.

In some states, after serving part of a prison sentence, a person can be released on parole. The parole board will be able to set conditions on the release. These will involve the same types of considerations which arise for probation regarding whether a felon is amenable to counseling or treatment.

As in civil litigation, court testimony about competency to stand trial, criminal responsibility, or sentencing can be provided by a mental health professional who has had no prior contact with the defendant and who is specifically retained for the forensic examination and testimony. On the other hand, clinicians who have been treating a person who subsequently becomes involved in criminal activity also can become involved in testifying about the defendant (who is their patient), although this is less preferred.

III. WHY THE PROFESSIONAL SHOULD SERVE AS AN EXPERT WITNESS

There are many reasons from a clinical, societal, and personal perspective why mental health professionals should sometimes involve themselves in cases which raise legal issues. Such involvement may serve the needs of the patient. It will also have the benefit of enhancing the skills of the clinician, while assisting the legal system.

From an ethical, clinical, and legal perspective, the treating clinician must become involved when the patient needs to be civilly committed. In most systems of mental health care, this is the only way to compel a patient to obtain the needed treatment. In addition, involving oneself in guardianship proceedings is also likely to serve the immediate needs of a patient who is unable to make personal or financial decisions.

For the clinician concerned about children, participating in cases involving children may be the only way to bring to the court's attention the particular problems and needs of a child. The involvement of the mental health professional ensures that the court will have the broadest data base to work with and will hopefully be able to reach a decision which is likely to be the best alternative for the child given the circumstances. In these cases, the professional should always view himself as the child's advocate, no matter who has requested his services.

From a societal perspective, serving as an expert helps further the ends of justice. At the outset of a case, the expert may help to prevent a case from going to trial. The initial consultation between the attorney and the expert may lead the attorney to conclude that there is no basis for litigation. The attorney may also conclude that a quick settlement makes more sense than going through the long and costly process of a trial. Should a trial occur, the role of the expert witness is to expand the knowledge of the judge or jurors. With this knowledge and an understanding of the issues, it is more likely that the truth will be clarified and justice will prevail.

IV. WHAT TO EXPECT FROM THE ATTORNEY

Much of the success of a lawsuit depends on the facts of the case and the skill of the attorney. The attorney's skill will be revealed in the experts he chooses and how he works with them. Yet each attorney is different, and some are more skilled or experienced than others in working with mental health professionals. This means that the clinician who is considering consulting on a forensic case should clarify a number of points at the outset with the attorney so that there will not be any subsequent misunderstandings. This section will detail those points.

A. Background of the Case

The expert should expect a briefing on what the case is about. This includes being aware of the range of issues the case involves, as well as the more narrow issue that the expert must be concerned with. How did the attorney get the case? When? Were there other attorneys involved before this attorney? Who is the opposing party? What is the status of the litigation at this point? Does this look like a case which will settle out of court or go to trial? Answers to these questions will help put into perspective the expert's role and give him a better understanding of what the attorney is trying to achieve.

B. Clarification of the Legal Issue

It is important that the expert understand the narrow clinical-legal issue that he is being asked to address. It would be wise to have the attorney specify in writing the legal question or questions, and in some instances, the expert may want to request a copy of the pertinent statutes. If, after receiving the statute, the clinician is still unclear about the state of the law in the area, then the clinician should ask the attorney for clarification, which may be provided with the help of cases which have interpreted the law.

C. Clarification of What the Attorney Wants

When a clinician is contacted by an attorney to serve as an expert, he needs to know what the attorney is seeking. This can vary depending on at what stage in the litigation the expert is consulted. Early in the process, the attorney may want an expert only to review the records to determine whether there is a basis for filing a lawsuit. The attorney may also want an informal evaluation of his client. At this stage, any work by the expert will be considered part of the attorney's work product and is not discoverable by the opposing party. The attorney may want a full evaluation but may request that the results be discussed before they are committed to writing. Until the attorney knows the expert's recommendations, he will not want to invest in the cost of the expert's writing a report which is unfavorable to his client. He also may want the expert to stress certain factors when the report is written.

D. Access to All Records

If the clinician decides to proceed beyond the preliminary investigation, the attorney must provide the evaluator with access to all the needed records. This includes making the expert aware of everything the attorney has, both favorable and unfavorable to his case. The records must be provided in complete form, not summarized or edited by the attorney. Unless the evaluator is aware of the aspects of the case which are unfavorable to the retaining attorney, he can be caught off guard during cross-examination and look as though he failed to do a thorough evaluation. Though experienced trial attorneys understand this, not every attorney who seeks expert advice will be willing to share with the expert the data which could hurt his case.

E. The Evaluator's Setting the Terms of the Evaluation

At the outset, the evaluator must make clear to the attorney his expectations and limitations in agreeing to undertake the evaluation. This may include insisting on having the ability to retain other consultants if necessary. It may require multiple interviews of the plaintiff, defendant, or others, especially when the evaluee is new to the evaluator. The evaluator should be clear that he will have the freedom to do the kind of evaluation that will enable him to render an opinion that he believes he can support with a reasonable degree of professional certainty.

The attorney will be concerned about the costs of the case since funds are often limited. He therefore may require preapproval for any unexpected expenditures. At that point the attorney may want to discuss with the expert the necessity and importance of the additional expenditures. In all cases, a balance must be reached, given the cost constraints on the attorney and what the clinician believes is necessary to render an opinion with which he is comfortable.

F. Fees

At the outset, the expert should clarify his fee arrangement. The expert should remember that he is selling his time and expertise and should take fees seriously. Attorneys are familiar with the use of retainer fees prior to the beginning of work; the expert can request a fee which is adequate to cover the initial work. This is especially important when one is approached by a private defense attorney in a criminal case or by a plaintiff's attorney in a civil case. The retainer assures the expert that he will be paid for his initial services even if his opinion or consultation is unhelpful to the retaining attorney. Thus, the retainer assures the expert is compensated for his time and it enhances the objectivity of the expert's work.

There are many ways to establish a fee. Some experts set an hourly rate which is the same for all aspects of the work on a case (reviewing records, interviewing, writing reports, consulting with counsel, or testifying). Other experts set a rate which varies for the type of work. It is not uncommon to charge more for giving depositions or testifying in court because of the stressfulness of the situation and the inconvenience to the expert's scheduling. Alternatively, a certain fee could be set for a given task such as a record review. In cases where testimony is likely and the clinician will be away from the office, he may want to set a minimum half-day or whole day rate. This would also be true in cases where travel out of town is required. Experts should never set their fees based on the outcome of a case. Such contingency fees are considered unethical, and in many states, illegal. Additionally, such a fee arrangment raises questions about the expert's impartiality and motives. The expert is to be compensated for his time and knowledge, and the outcome of the case should not be his concern.

Whatever the fee arrangement, it should be confirmed in writing. The attorney should sign a letter stating that he agrees to the arrangement, or he should send a separate letter setting forth his agreement with the fee arrangement. This provides a contract between the evaluator and the attorney. In the event of nonpayment, the correspondence provides the legal documentation to pursue collection of fees.

It is also important for the expert to periodically bill the attorney and make sure the bills are paid in a timely manner. Once payments fall behind, no further work should be done on the case. The attorney should be advised of any unexpected expenditures, and his approval should be obtained before these are undertaken. The expert should make it clear to the attorney that the agreement is for payment from him and not his client. This is especially important when the evaluator is the therapist; here, the attorney may claim that it is the patient's responsibility to pay for the evaluation and court testimony.

G. Conferences

If the case goes to a deposition or to trial, the attorney must meet with the expert to review his testimony. At the outset, the clinician should expect the attorney to set aside sufficient time for him to go through the questions he will ask at trial and those which he anticipates will be raised on cross-examination. This meeting should occur several days before the scheduled testimony and may take more time than is expected, especially if the attorney and the expert have not previously worked together. Although reviewing the testimony of a witness is a cardinal rule of good trial practice, some attorneys are so involved in the demands of their work that this review may be neglected. Even the testimony of the experienced expert witness should be reviewed so no one is surprised by the questions asked or the answers given.

V. WHEN A CASE SHOULD BE DECLINED

Sometimes a mental health professional will be approached by an attorney to consider accepting a forensic matter but the professional should decline the case. For many reasons, the authors believe that those with specific forensic training and experience are in the best position to accept such referrals. Besides lack of forensic experience, another reason for declining a case is that the clinician has no training, experience, or knowledge in an area. Perhaps the clinician had some knowledge of the topic but has not practiced in that area for many years. Or perhaps the clinician has never seen a case with the particular diagnosis in question. When the clinician is not competent or experienced in the area, the case should not be accepted. There is always another expert to be found, perhaps even one recommended by the clinician. A clinician does himself, his profession, the attorney, the attorney's client, and the court system a disservice by accepting a case for which he is unqualified.

The clinician should also decline cases in which the person who is involved in the litigation is his patient. It is important to clarify for the patient that the clinician is serving as a treatment provider and not as an expert witness. Taking on the dual role of being both is likely to interfere with the treatment relationship and to undermine the clinician's effectiveness, especially if the outcome of the legal proceedings does not go as the patient expects.

Related to this are cases in which the therapist formerly treated the litigant but the treatment has been terminated and the litigant or his attorney requests the therapist's testimony. Here, the therapist may be less reluctant to testify since there is no longer a clinical relationship which could be compromised by the court testimony. On the other hand, the therapist may not have the information relevant to the legal issue in question because it was not an issue during the treatment. In these situations, the former therapist needs to specifically indicate the areas and limitations of any possible testimony before agreeing to testify.

The clinician should also decline a case when there is an apparent conflict of interest. Sometimes the conflict will be obvious, when one of the parties is a close friend or relative. In other instances, the conflict may be less apparent, such as cases involving a former teacher, student, or colleague. The clinician may even be consulted about a case where the other side has already contacted him. It is advisable when entering the case as a forensic expert, and not the treating therapist, to have no personal knowledge of any of the litigating parties.

Finally, the clinician should not accept a case when he is uncomfortable in dealing with attorneys or testifying in court. In cases in which fear of involvement with the legal system is too anxiety-provoking, the fees generated by the case are not worth the anxiety. In addition, an anxious witness will be a poor witness and will thus do a disservice to everyone.

VI. PREPARING REPORTS

When the mental health professional is called upon for an opinion related to legal issues, he must be prepared to set forth his views in writing. Written reports will typically be required when the expert has been appointed by the court or has been agreed to by both sides. However, when the expert has been retained by one side, the attorney may decide he wishes only a brief written report or only an oral report. In these cases, the attorney will provide the guidelines as to the points to be brought out in the report. In this section, we describe how to write a report which will be read by both sides and may be admitted into evidence. Our goal is to help the clinician communicate effectively in the legal context.

A. Preparation for Writing the Report

Writing a good forensic report requires a great deal of thought and organization. Before writing the report, the evaluator must understand the legal issue being addressed and the applicable legal standard. A misunderstanding on this point could invalidate the entire report. All the data related to the case should be reviewed. As the evaluator prepares to reach his conclusion, he should review the steps he took to come to his recommendation. Finally, he must be able to explain how he reached his conclusion.

A helpful way to write a good report is to work from an outline. The evaluator can begin by restating the legal issue, then listing the materials reviewed and the interviews undertaken. The report should state the conclusion and make a list of the points that favor it and also those which are not relevant. An outline provides an easy way to obtain an overview of the points which should be included and where they should be included. A well-developed outline will lead to a well-written report (see Table 11.1).

B. Format for the Report

The report should be organized in a way which is simple to read and easy to understand (see Table 11.2).

Table 11.1. Writing the Forensic Report

1. Know the legal question and the applicable legal standard.
2. Before writing the report, review all the records and other materials used during the evaluation.
3. Prepare an outline prior to writing the report.
4. Define psychiatric terminology.
5. Avoid ultimate issue conclusions.
6. Support the opinion with specific data from the case.
7. Avoid including extraneous material or conclusions.

Table 11.2. Forensic Report Format

1. Introduction: Summarize the issue to be addressed and briefly state the conclusion.
2. Basis of the evaluation: List the documents reviewed and the interviews and testing conducted, including telephone interviews.
3. Presenting problem: Give a statement about and description of the presenting forensic issue.
4. History: Describe the relevant history of the evaluee.
5. Mental status examination: Include the evaluee's informed consent to the evaluation.
6. Psychiatric diagnosis: Specify and describe the symptoms.
7. Conclusions and recommendations regarding the forensic issues and any necessary interventions.

1. Introduction

The introduction provides a statement of the issues addressed as well as a brief statement of the conclusion, for example:

> This 45-year-old single white male, presently charged with attempted murder, was referred for an evaluation of competency to stand trial by Ms. Susan Smith, Assistant State's Attorney. In my opinion, to a reasonable degree of psychiatric certainty, Mr. Jones understands the charges against him and is able to assist his attorney in his own defense.

2. Basis of the Evaluation

The section on the basis of the evaluation lists the materials which the evaluator reviewed as part of the evaluation. There should also be a list of all interviews conducted and the date and amount of time spent on each interview. Telephone interviews should also be included. If there have been numerous interviews or materials reviewed, the length of the list will strengthen the weight given to the evaluator's conclusion.

3. Presenting Problem

Information about the presenting forensic problem should be reported here, including that obtained from official records and documents and, in many cases, that obtained from the interviewee.

4. History

The history describes the relevant background of the person being evaluated. Subsections are often useful to organize the history. For example, the use of subsections entitled "Psychiatric History," "Drug and Alcohol History," and "Family History" permit the reader to rapidly find relevant information. When the report relates to a criminal issue, the defendant's criminal history may also be included because of its relevance.

5. *Mental Status Examination*

The mental status examination should include a review of the person's behavioral, emotional, and cognitive status through detailed examples rather than conclusions. For example, describing a person as having "poor hygiene" is less effective than stating, "The individual presented with clothes which were torn and soiled and with a strong body odor and dirty fingernails." Particular emphasis should be given to observations relevant to the examination. For example, if an elderly man referred for competency to stand trial cannot remember the evaluator at the second appointment, this finding is highly significant. This section should also note that the interviewee was informed of the nature, purpose, and nonconfidentiality of the evaluation process and should record his understanding of this information.

6. *Diagnosis*

When the evaluator has reached a formal psychiatric diagnosis, then the diagnosis or diagnoses should be recorded next. The evaluator should first indicate the diagnostic system used to make the diagnosis (e.g., the revised third edition of the American Psychiatric Association's Diagnostic and Statistical Manual of Mental Disorders, or DSM-III-R). The evaluator should then indicate what was the basis for making the diagnosis in the particular case and should identify the relevant symptoms. Diagnostic terms should be explained as necessary to ensure that the nonclinician reader will understand their meaning. Any relevant diagnoses which were excluded should also be noted or discussed.

7. *Conclusion and Recommendations*

In the final section, the conclusion will be restated and discussed in full. In some instances, it will be worth mentioning why another conclusion was rejected. In a custody dispute in which the recommendation is for the mother, for example, it may be advisable to state that "joint custody was inappropriate because of the high degree of conflict between the parents and their inability to speak to each other, even on issues related to their child."

This section also contains any treatment recommendations. Although these may or may not be requested as part of the forensic evaluation, a therapist has an ethical obligation to bring to the attorney's attention the treatment needs of his client. For example, an evaluation may reveal a seriously depressed person with intermittent suicidal ideas who is not currently in any form of treatment. In such a case, the forensic evaluator should make a clinical assessment of the need for immediate treatment and communicate this recommendation directly to the individual being evaluated and his attorney. The recommendation should also be noted in writing in the final forensic report.

C. Content of the Report

When writing a forensic report, it is important to bear in mind the purpose for which the report is written and the fact that it will be read by nonclinicians, including the person who was evaluated. Thus, anything contained in the report should be enlightening for the purpose of addressing the legal issue.

Utmost care must be given when using psychiatric terminology and labels. If a psychological term is used, then it should be defined. For example, "Mr. Jones has manic-depressive disorder, which means that. . . ." Psychiatric labels should be used only when they will be meaningful to the reader. For example, describing a person as "neurotic" will generally have no relevance to the case and therefore will be of no value in the report. In contrast, describing a person as a "schizophrenic" or an "alcoholic" may be meaningful, particularly when the terms are defined. For example, the evaluator might report that "Because of Mrs. Smith's schizophrenic illness, she is unable to parent effectively due to her preoccupation with her paranoid delusions and auditory hallucinations."

It is also important to omit any superfluous information or statements. For example, the gender identity of a defendant is not relevant to his competency to stand trial and should ordinarily be excluded from the report. It is important to write clearly and concisely so that the attorney who reads each line can relate the data to the conclusion. Extraneous information or comments will not only detract from the report but will subject the evaluator to rigorous cross-examination on something that may have no relevance to the conclusion.

The conclusion should address the legal question without specifically answering the ultimate legal issue. In the example of competency to stand trial, the report should avoid stating that "Mr. Jones is incompetent to stand trial." Although the evaluator's input has been requested, the competency determination is made by the court based on a number of factors. Instead, the conclusion could state, "In my opinion, Mr. Smith is unable to understand the charges against him or assist his counsel in his defense because he is presently in an episode of schizophrenia with marked paranoia which interferes with his ability to cooperate with his attorney." In a malpractice example, the expert would not want to state that the therapist was "negligent" in the way he treated the patient/plaintiff but instead could state, "After reviewing all the materials, I have concluded, to a reasonable degree of medical certainty, that Dr. Doe did not meet the standard of care expected of a psychiatrist under the circumstances presented by this case."

Attorneys sometimes request that the expert add or delete a portion of the report so that the report appears more favorable to the case. For similar reasons, they may also ask the expert to rephrase part of the report. While it is reasonable for the attorney to request a particular format or length of the report, the expert should be free to present the content of the report in whatever manner he chooses. To avoid any later misunderstandings, the expert should review his findings with the attorney prior to preparing the report. The attorney may then decide not to use the expert or his report if the expert reaches a particular conclusion or refuses to modify the report as requested.

VII. CONSULTING WITH THE ATTORNEY BEFORE TRIAL

In seeking consultation with an expert witness, the attorney is looking for someone who is qualified in the area of the litigation, is able to testify effectively about the points in favor of his case, and will educate him as he prepares the case for trial. The primary role of the expert witness is to be an educator. If the case proceeds to trial, the expert witness educates the judge or jury. If the case does not get to trial, then the expert serves only as a consultant for the attorney who hired him. This is a important role, since the expert will be actively involved in providing suggestions to the attorney about paths to follow or discard as he prepares for trial.

Once the initial evaluation has been completed, the evaluator should discuss his findings with the attorney. If the issues are simple and the attorney is likely to be familiar with the type of case involved, a telephone consultation will be sufficient. However, in more complex cases a personal meeting is invaluable. It forces the attorney to set aside ample time to hear all the points the clinician wishes to make. By the end of the meeting, the attorney should have a good idea of what, if anything, he wishes the expert to do next, including whether he wants a written report and what its format should be.

The expert must understand that a primary function of his role is to educate the attorney so he can effectively pursue his case. Experienced trial attorneys will make this clear by specifically asking the expert for advice on problems with their case and what literature they should read. Inexperienced attorneys may neglect to do this. It is then incumbent upon the expert to thoroughly review with the attorney the points he should bring out which favor his client. Even more important, the expert must fully inform the attorney of the weaknesses or potential flaws in his position.

As part of the educative function, the expert should refer the attorney to or provide him with the pertinent literature in the area. The attorney must be made aware of the research, articles, and books which support as well as disagree with the position he is taking. At the time of the trial, the attorney should be sufficiently knowledgeable on the narrow issues so that he could be viewed as a "mini-expert" on the topic. This is critical if the attorney is to make a good presentation in court.

Another way the expert will assist the attorney is advising him about the experts who have been retained by the other side. What are their credentials? What is their reputation in the community? Is their theory of the case plausible? If not, why not?

The expert should be able to anticipate the kinds of questions he may be asked on cross-examination as well as the types of questions the attorney should ask any opposing experts.

VIII. DEPOSITIONS

An oral deposition consists of questions asked of a witness under oath by an attorney, with the opportunity for the opposing party to cross-examine the witness. This is a method of pretrial discovery. The purpose of discovery is to obtain a good understanding of the strength of the case of the opposing side. As a result of discovery, most cases are settled.

The oral deposition serves a number of purposes. First, it provides the attorney with the ability to appraise the opposition and their witnesses. It will reveal not only the strengths and weaknesses of the opposition's case but also the status of their experts. An expert may have excellent credentials on paper, but if he is arrogant and condescending when testifying, the jury will not find him as credible as another expert witness who speaks well, maintains eye contact with the jury, and relates well to them. The oral deposition will also serve to clarify some of the disputed facts and may narrow the issues in controversy. Since the deposition is taken under oath, it can be used to challenge or impeach the witness later, if at trial he makes a statement which is contrary to the one he made at his deposition.

For the attorney, preparation for a deposition is critical and should be done with the same care as if preparing for a trial. It should not be viewed as a "fishing expedition," but as a means to anticipate what the response of the witness would be should the case go to trial. The attorney should be well prepared with carefully designed questions. The deposition is one of the most important factors in determining whether a case will settle before trial.

The expert should meet with the attorney before the deposition to discuss again his findings and to review what to expect during the deposition. This not only helps in making the expert feel more comfortable because he knows what to expect, it also provides practice in answering questions and teaches him the format the answers should take.

The oral deposition will usually be conducted in an attorney's office. Present will be the opposing side, which has requested the deposition, and the attorney for the side utilizing the expert. A court reporter will take down the proceedings word for word, which will then be transcribed. The deposition may cover anything relevant to the subject matter of the suit, including the evidence at the trial and what may lead to evidence. The deposition may not invade the areas of privilege.

The attorney who has retained the expert may, during the course of the deposition, object to questions. This will be only for the record since there will be no judge present to rule on the objection. Generally, the witness will be advised to answer the question anyway. However, there will be some issues on which the attorney who has retained the expert will instruct him not to respond pending a ruling by a judge. At the end of the deposition, the witness will be asked if he wishes to review and sign the transcript. This should typically be done. It permits the witness to verify that his answers accurately reflect what he wished to convey. If they are incorrect, he can provide the necessary corrections to the deposition transcript.

An evidence deposition, as contrasted to a discovery deposition, is taken for the purpose of being admitted as part of the trial record when the witness will be unavailable at trial. The law of each jurisdiction specifies the circumstances in which such a deposition is appropriate. There may be times when a discovery deposition becomes an evidence deposition. This is most likely to occur when a witness has become gravely ill or died between the time of the deposition and the trial. In those circumstances, the discovery deposition will be admitted into the trial if relevant to the proceedings.

At the time of the meeting with the attorney, the expert should be sure the fee arrangements are settled. The expert should be paid in full for his work to this point, and there should be clarification of the fee arrangements for preparing for and giving the deposition. When one is called as an expert witness to give a deposition, the costs are generally borne by the side that has retained the professional as their expert, rather than by the side taking the deposition. This is a stated rule in most jurisdictions. If, however, the witness is being deposed as a result of having been the treating therapist, the side calling the witness must bear the expense. This could be limited to some minimal statutory amount to cover travel expenses. However, if the testimony of the therapist turns out to be valuable, the attorney will want to fully compensate the therapist for his time, to ensure having a cooperative witness when the case goes to trial.

A major strategy for attorneys taking discovery depositions is to attempt to "freeze" the opposing experts' testimony. This strategy is to limit the experts' testimony at trial to that given during the deposition. Experts should thoroughly explain their reasoning when answering questions at a deposition. If the expert does not recall all the factors, this should be stated during the deposition, so that it can be reviewed during trial.

IX. TESTIFYING AT TRIAL

The trial is the culmination of the work the parties have done on the case. As a result of the pretrial discovery process, the vast majority of cases are settled before trial. These include not only the meritless cases but also those where it is clear that one side violated the rights of the opposing party. Those cases which go to trial are generally the ones in which the facts and law of the case are closely matched. Therefore, who will win may turn on fine distinctions, and often the expert witnesses will be expected to convey those distinctions to the judge or jury.

It is important for the expert witness to bear in mind that generally he is one of many witnesses in a case. Usually the expert will be testifying about part of the case and will represent only a small part of the larger picture. The success or failure of the case depends not on the expert witness but on the facts of the case and how each attorney presents them.

A. Preparation

Before entering the courtroom, the expert should be fully prepared for his testimony. In many instances, the evaluation of the parties to the litigation and the consultation with the attorney may have occurred many months or even years before the trial. The expert should review in his mind the nature of the case and where he fits into the general trial strategy of the attorney. When he meets with the attorney before trial, he may want to discuss these topics. Having an overview of the case will provide the expert with a better perspective of where his testimony fits into the overall presentation.

The evaluator should carefully review his notes, any documents used during the course of the evaluation, his report, and his deposition transcript. He may want to abstract the transcript if he thinks there are matters on which the opposing side will challenge him on cross-examination. If the evaluator relied on other consultants, a telephone call to verify an understanding of their report is a good idea. The expert will also have had the opportunity to review the reports or read the depositions of the opposing experts. These should be reviewed carefully, with the expectation that questions will be asked about why the evaluator came to a different conclusion.

The expert should insist that the attorney review the expert's testimony in advance of the trial. The evaluator's curriculum vitae should be updated, and he should point out any accomplishments which should be emphasized in court. This should also be the opportunity, if it has not been done earlier, to reiterate fee arrangements for pretrial preparation and trial time. The bill up to this point should be paid in full, and advance payment for services at trial should be received. This not only ensures that if the attorney loses the case, the evaluator will have been paid, but it also protects the expert witness and the attorney should a question be asked about whether the evaluator's fee depends on his client's winning the case. The implication of such a question is that the expert is a "hired gun," there only to help the attorney win the case. By being able to respond, "I was compensated for the professional time spent on this matter, and my fee did not depend upon the outcome of the case," makes the expert appear impartial. In some cases the expert may want to elaborate further, stating, "I insist on payment before trial, so I don't have to worry about being compensated for my time, and I can freely answer any questions posed to me without concern about payment."

B. Testifying

Court testimony is the culmination of the expert's work on the case. To be effective, the expert should view himself as an educator and consider the judge or jury his students. The expert will explain the complexities of the subject area as it relates to the case. The listeners should be viewed as being on par with high school students. Their attention must be obtained early and retained throughout the direct and cross-examination testimony. They should not be expected to remember more than the most important points, and they should not be exposed to areas which are not germane to the topic before the court. In part, the ability to be a good educator will depend on the questions asked by the attorneys. It is hoped that during pretrial preparation, the expert provided the attorney a list of questions to be asked. Even if not asked questions in the ideal form, the expert can respond in a way which will make his point. There are a number of points to remember when testifying (see Table 11.3).

1. *Appearance and Presentation*

The initial impression of the expert witness is formed by the judge or jury as soon as he takes the stand. It is important for the expert to make a good first impression, even before anything is said. The expert needs to be dressed neatly and conservatively, perhaps in a business suit. This will establish him as a professional. If he appears unkempt, he will seem disorganized. The expert should turn to face the jury and look directly at them when testifying. Eye contact will help to establish the expert's trustworthiness with the jury. If questioned by the judge, the expert should turn and respond directly to him.

Table 11.3. Giving Direct Testimony

1. Dress neatly and conservatively.
2. Be thoroughly prepared.
3. Have a pretrial conference.
4. Look at the jury or judge when testifying.
5. Speak simply and define any technical terms.
6. Take time answering questions, and qualify any answers if necessary.
7. Speak confidently but with humility and dignity.
8. Admit the limitation of knowledge or certainty.
9. Testify to reasonable certainty; do not speculate.
10. Avoid using *always* or *never*.
11. Advocate for the expert opinion, not the litigants.

2. *Being Prepared*

The expert should have thoroughly reviewed his notes, all available records, and other relevant documents prior to his appearance in court. Because much litigation is "on and off," the expert will probably not have the material fresh in his mind if the consultation was performed months or even years before. The expert should expect that the attorneys will be familiar with the details of the case, and his credibility with the jury or judge may be reduced if he appears unfamiliar with even part of the case.

3. *Talking in Simple Terms*

It is important for the expert to speak in a manner which is understandable to the average person. The expert will only confuse and offend jurors if he uses unfamiliar language. Whenever psychiatric terminology is used, the expert should define it, for example, "My evaluation revealed Mrs. Hill to be a schizophrenic. This means that she . . ." The expert then describes the symptoms which led to the conclusion that she was schizophrenic.

4. *Qualifying Answers*

The expert should not hesitate to think about the question and take whatever time is needed to respond. Answers should be qualified in any way the expert thinks is necessary to fully inform the court. For example, to the question "Do you believe that Ryan's best interests would be served by being in the custody of his mother?" the response might be "Yes, provided that Mrs. O'Brien obtains family counseling and continues to encourage frequent visitation with Ryan's father."

5. *Admitting the Limitations of Knowledge*

Although there are few things that are certain in this world, many would argue that there is a great deal of uncertainty in dealing with issues related to the mind. It is important for the expert to admit these limitations. This not only dispels the "crystal ball" myth of mental health professionals but also can provide the expert with an opportunity to increase his credibility with the court. If asked on cross-examination, "Doctor, isn't it true that psychiatrists cannot predict violence better than other people?" the expert could respond, "Mental health professionals have not been found to have unique expertise in predicting long-term violence. However, newer studies have indicated our ability to make meaningful predictions about violence in the short-term (e.g., 48–72 hours) decisions which may be encountered in emergency settings, such as in this case."

In addition to admitting the limits of knowledge in the expert's specialty, he may also want to indicate the limits of his knowledge in the specific case. For example, in an insanity defense case, the expert may be asked, "Isn't it true that you did not see the defendant at the time of the murder and therefore do not know whether he was psychotic at that time?" The expert's response could be, "In an ideal world, I would have been able to observe the defendant at the time of the crime and then been able to give the most accurate clinical description of his behavior. However, I had to reconstruct his mental state based on interviews with him, other witnesses, and reviewing his history and the other material involved in the case. Having done all that, I have concluded to a reasonable degree of psychiatric certainty that at the time of the murder, the defendant was mentally ill."

There also may be times when the expert does not have access to all the information he desired for a complete evaluation. He should acknowledge that his conclusion is based on the information he had available. He might want to elaborate by adding that he was unable to obtain an interview with the defendant's mother because of his attorney's prohibition, and that such an interview might have given him additional important information.

6. *Not Being Limited to Yes or No Answers*

When responding to a question, the expert should remember that he is there as an educator. The expert should not give simple yes or no answers when an elaboration is necessary to explain what he means. Fact witnesses can be limited in testimony to a yes or no answer, but experts, who are in court to testify to their expert opinions, should not be. If the attorney objects to the expert's elaborations, the expert can turn to the judge and ask, "May I elaborate?" It is important that the expert give an answer he believes fully responds to the question. If the judge instructs the witness to respond with the short answers that the cross-examiner demands, then the expert will have an opportunity on redirect examination to fully explain his earlier responses.

7. *Not Answering More Than Is Necessary*

The attorney will ask questions to bring out the points in which he is interested. He will not want to repeat the entire case for the judge or jury. The expert's testimony will highlight certain narrow issues, and his responses should be limited to the questions asked. The expert should elaborate to the point of giving an answer which accurately describes his views, without including facts or issues which have not been raised.

8. *Avoiding Advocacy*

The expert should remember that he is in court to educate. It is the attorney's job to advocate the case for his client. It is the role of the attorney, rather than the expert, to be partial and to try to win the case for the client. By appearing partial and trying to win the case for the client, the expert will lose credibility and diminish his worth to the client. On the other hand, the expert may defend or advocate for his own expert opinions about the matter once he has formulated them.

It is also important for the expert to remember that the courtroom is the working territory of the attorney, not the expert. The expert should not try to play attorney or give legal opinions about any matter. The expert should also avoid responding to the attorney's jokes or sarcastic comments. It is important for the expert to appear competent, well informed, and intelligent, but he should never appear to be impudent.

9. Knowing the Literature

The expert should be familiar with the literature in the field which supports and opposes the position he has taken. On cross-examination, the expert will be confronted with opposing literature. He should be prepared to acknowledge the article and then state why he disagrees with it. Such literature may be outdated, the theory may not be generally accepted, or the article may be counter to the expert's clinical experience. Given the volumes of scientific papers published each year, it will often be possible to locate an article on almost any topic which takes a different position from that of the expert. The expert should not become disconcerted because there is some literature which takes a contrary view.

10. Admission about Fees

The expert should not be embarrassed to admit the amount that he has been paid for the services rendered on the case. Many attorneys prefer to ask about the fee arrangements on direct examination, rather than have the opposing side ask on cross-examination. If asked, "Doctor, how much were you paid for your opinion in this case?" the expert could respond by stating, "I was not paid for my opinion in this case but was paid my normal consultation fee of (describe fee arrangements) for the time I spent on this matter."

C. Cross-Examination

One purpose of cross-examination is to clarify answers to questions raised during the direct examination. (See Table 11.4.) In practice, the opposing attorney will use cross-examination to elicit the weaknesses in his opponent's case and, if possible, will utilize the expert witness to make a few points that will favor his position. In many jurisdictions, the attorney is limited in cross-examination to questions related to information that was brought out on direct examination. If the opposing attorney attempts to bring up new issues on cross-examination, the other attorney will properly object to the questions as being "beyond the scope of the direct examination." At the end of the cross-examination, the other attorney will have an opportunity to further clarify the witness's answers during redirect examination. During cross-examination, the expert witness must bear in mind the opposing attorney's role. He is there to win the case for his client in as effective a manner as possible. This means

Table 11.4. Giving Cross-Examination Testimony

1. Accept that the opposing attorney's job is to win his case, even if it is at the expense of making the witness look inadequate, incompetent, or biased.
2. Maintain composure despite a hostile cross-examiner.
3. Respond in a dignified manner without argument.
4. Do not answer any questions without fully understanding them.
5. Admit limitations, lack of knowledge, or disagreement with other experts.
6. Answer only the question asked; do not give more information than is necessary.
7. Do not be limited to a yes or no answer.
8. Admit the fee arrangements if asked.

the attorney will not be concerned about the sensitivity of the expert witness. The opposing attorney will try to strengthen his case by attempting to impeach the credentials or testimony of the opposing side's expert witness. This is not a reflection of the opposing attorney's feelings about the expert or what level of respect he may have for the expert's views. The expert should not take offensive behavior by the cross-examiner personally. This is just part of the opposing attorney's job to represent his client. The expert should bear in mind his role as an educator and should bring to cross-examination the calmness and control one expects from a well-respected teacher.

It is also important for the expert to remember that most issues are not clear-cut. An experienced trial attorney can make something which is apparently impressive appear otherwise, and something which seems unimpressive look good. For example, when questioning the credentials of the world's leading expert on schizophrenia, the opposing attorney may ask on cross-examination, "Doctor, from all the articles and books you have published on schizophrenia, and your frequent worldwide lectures, how do you find time for a routine clinical practice?" This gives the impression that the expert is an academic who does not deal with real people. In contrast, the same attorney who is using an expert who has never published anything will ask on direct examination, "Doctor, how much of your time is devoted to clinical practice?" The response will be "All my professional time is spent seeing patients and consulting on cases." The attorney will then ask his expert, "Doctor, have you ever published a professional article?" The doctor will respond with "I have been so busy taking care of my patients that I have not had time to write any articles, and in addition, I didn't believe I had anything new to add to the literature." Not only does this answer make the expert witness appear concerned about his patients, but his humility may appeal to the jury.

It is as important for the expert to admit his limitations on cross-examination as it is on direct examination. When asked, the expert should admit the possibility of error or uncertainty. The expert should avoid using the terms *always* or *never*. The expert should point out why he is confident of what he has said, but also what limitations there are on either his knowledge or the general state of knowledge in the field. The expert should emphasize that he has evaluated a person at one point in time and cannot predict the future.

X. COMMONLY ASKED QUESTIONS

1. *What is the difference between a fact witness and an expert witness?*

A fact witness is one who has direct knowledge about the issues in dispute. The fact witness can answer questions only about what he observed. In contrast, an expert witness is called upon to offer an opinion related to an issue in the case which would not be within the knowledge of the average person. An expert witness is not limited in testimony to the facts of a case.

2. *If a client or former client raises an issue about his mental condition as a claim or defense, can his therapy records be discovered?*

Yes. If someone makes a claim based on his mental condition, he will be asked about any previous psychological treatment. Once it is revealed, the opposing attorney will attempt to discover the records. In a personal injury action, the opposing attorney may attempt to show that any claims for psychological pain or suffering are inappropriate because the person was in treatment before the injury, and those psychological problems were preexisting.

When records are subpoenaed for these purposes, the attorney representing the client will attempt to quash the subpoena based on the records' being irrelevant to the litigation.

3. *If a former client makes a claim based on psychological suffering, can the therapist be called to testify?*

Yes, the former therapist can be subpoenaed to give a deposition or testify at trial. If the information is helpful to one side, that side will call the therapist to the stand. In those circumstances, the therapist will be testifying as a fact witness. However, the therapist may be qualified as an expert witness to answer certain questions based on his knowledge of the former client and his experience in the field. To preserve the therapeutic relationship, it is preferable for the therapist to avoid testifying at deposition or trial, and to leave this to outside evaluators trained and experienced in forensic work.

4. *What is a subpoena?*

A subpoena is a demand, under the authority of the court, that a person present himself to participate in a legal proceeding, to give a deposition or to testify.

5. *What is a subpoena duces tecum?*

It is an order to produce certain documents.

6. *How should one respond to a subpoena or a subpoena duces tecum?*

The expert or therapist should immediately notify the client or former client that he has been subpoenaed. If the client does not wish the professional to release records or testify, then the client's attorney should move to quash the subpoena. If the subpoena is not quashed, it must be honored, and the professional must appear in court, produce the records, or present a motion to quash based on the information being privileged. (See Chapter 7 for further discussion.)

If the subpoena requests the professional's appearance at an inconvenient time, he should contact the attorney who issued the subpoena and arrange a more convenient time. In many jurisdictions, a court order must be obtained to subpoena a physician for a deposition.

If the professional has questions about what to do, he should contact his attorney, given the circumstances of the case.

7. *When a mental health professional serves as an expert, what assurance is there of being fully compensated?*

The expert must protect himself. This begins by fully explaining to the attorney the fee policy and then obtaining a written letter from the attorney agreeing to this arrangement. In addition, a retainer should be paid to make sure the initial work is covered. The expert should periodically bill the attorney and, if payment is not forthcoming, delay any further work. Payment should also be obtained in advance of a deposition or trial.

8. *If the attorney does not wish a written report, but the evaluation reveals the person to be in need of immediate treatment, what should be done?*

The attorney should be immediately notified by telephone of his client's need for treatment. It may also be reasonable to speak to the client or his family about obtaining treatment. If possible, the evaluator should not become the treatment provider and certainly cannot serve as the therapist as well as the evaluator for the court. Should he become the treatment provider, then a new expert witness is needed for the evaluation phase.

9. *Does a mental health professional retained to conduct a forensic evaluation have any obligations to the person being evaluated?*

Yes. First, the evaluator should explain the nonconfidential nature of the interview to the person. Second, the evaluator has an obligation to bring to the individual's or his attorney's attention any immediate treatment needs of the person. Suicide or homicide intentions, for example, should be brought to the attorney's attention.

10. *What is the purpose of a discovery deposition?*

A discovery deposition is for the purpose of the opponent's learning what the expert witness for the other side will testify to. The expert will be asked questions by the opposing attorney, with the attorney who has retained him being present, and with a court reporter recording the testimony. Once all the discovery is completed in the case, including taking the depositions of the expected witnesses, the attorneys will know the strengths and weaknesses of the case and will be in a position to determine whether to settle the case and for what amount.

11. *Can a mental health expert who is retained by one party to a legal case but does not testify in the case be later compelled to testify by the opposing party?*

This is a complex legal and ethical matter with different rules in different jurisdictions. If contacted or subpoenaed by the opposing side, the expert should contact the retaining attorney to inform him of this event. The attorney may then approve or disapprove of the expert's contact with the opposition. The attorney may also attempt to quash the subpoena, but this might be unsuccessful. Courts may have the authority to compel the expert to testify over the objections of the retaining attorney. If the expert refuses to testify, despite the order of the court, he risks fines or imprisonment for contempt of court.

12. *If a patient who is in long-term outpatient therapy asks the therapist to testify in a current legal matter, should the therapist do so?*

In most such cases, the therapist should inform the patient or his attorney that it is strongly preferable to retain another mental health professional to conduct an evaluation and testify in court, rather than have the current therapist testify on behalf of the patient. Any involvement in the case, especially testimony, by the therapist may jeopardize the therapeutic relationship with the patient either by inappropriately gratifying the patient, by disclosing information which was previously intended to be kept within the therapy, or by the therapist's disputing the patient's views of his legal problem. Also, testimony by the therapist may not be as objective as that provided by an outside expert. Even with an outside expert who can address the forensic or legal issues involved in the case, however, it may still be necessary for the patient's attorney to call the therapist to court, but the therapist's testimony might be restricted to the patient's diagnosis and treatment, thus avoiding the forensic or legal issues involved in the case and reducing the chance that the therapeutic relationship will be compromised.

XI. BIBLIOGRAPHY

A. Cases

Bartlett v. Weimer, 268 F.2d 860 (7th Cir. 1959).
Ake v. Oklahoma, 105 S.Ct. 1087 (1985).
Lundgren v. Eustermann, 370 N.W.2d 877 (Minn.Sup.Ct. 1985).
Michigan v. Tyson, 377 N.W.2d 738 (Mich.Sup.Ct. 1985).
Brewington v. Texas, 702 S.W.2d 312 (Tex.App. 1986).
State of Iowa v. Chancy, 391 N.W.2d 231 (Iowa Sup.Ct. 1986).
Sutphin v. Platt, 720 S.W.2d 455 (Tenn.Sup.Ct. 1986).
Trower v. Jones, 500 N.E.2d 1134 (Ill.App. 1986).
Bell v. Hart, 516 So.2d 562 (Ala.Sup.Ct. 1987).
Cogdell v. Brown, 531 A.2d 1379 (N.J.Super. 1987).
Polo by Shipley v. Gotchel, 542 A.2d 947 (N.J. 1987).
Cross v. Lakeview Center, 529 So.2d 307 (Fla.App. 1988).
DiMaggio v. Makover, 536 A.2d 595 (Conn.App. 1988).
Ex Parte Morris v. Craddock, 530 So.2d 785 (Ala.Sup.Ct. 1988).
Florida Bar v. Harris, 531 So.2d 151 (Fla.Sup.Ct. 1988).
Tolisano v. Texon, 533 N.Y.S.2d 874 (A.D. 1988).
Plitt v. Griggs, 585 So.2d 1317 (Ala.Sup.Ct. 1991).
Annotation: Right of accused in criminal prosecution to presence of counsel at court-appointed or approved psychiatric examination, 3 A.L.R.4th 910.
Annotation: Physician's negligence in conducting or reporting physical examination as rendering him liable to third person relying thereon, 24 A.L.R.4th 1310.
Annotation: Propriety of cross-examining expert witness regarding his status as "professional witness," 39 A.L.R.4th 742.
Annotation: Right of independent expert to refuse to testify as to expert opinion, 50 A.L.R.4th 680.
Annotation: Compelling testimony of opponent's expert in state court, 66 A.L.R.4th 213.
Annotation: Attorney's personal liability for expenses incurred in relation to services for client, 66 A.L.R.4th 256.

B. Articles and Books

American Bar Association. (1989). *American Bar Association Criminal Justice Mental Health Standards.* Washington, DC: Author.
Appelbaum, P. S. (1987). In the wake of *Ake*: The ethics of expert testimony in an advocate's world. *Bulletin of the American Academy of Psychiatry and the Law, 15,* 15–25.
Black, B. (1988). Evolving legal standards for the admissibility of scientific evidence. *Science, 239,* 1508–1512.
Brennan, T. P., Gedrich, A. E., Jacoby, S. E., Tardy, M. J., & Tyson, K. B. (1986). Forensic social work: Practice and vision. *Social Casework, 67,* 340–350.
Brodsky, S. L. (1991). *Testifying in court: Guidelines and maxims for the expert witness.* Washington, DC: American Psychological Association.
Curran, W. J., McGarry, A. L., & Shah, S. A. (Eds.). (1986). *Forensic psychiatry and psychology: Perspectives and standards for interdisciplinary practice.* Philadelphia: F. A. Davis.
Diamond, B. L. (1983). The psychiatrist as expert witness. *Psychiatric Clinics of North America, 6,* 597–609.
Ennis, B. J., & Litwack, T. R. (1974). Psychiatry and the presumption of expertise: Flipping coins in the courtroom. *California Law Review, 62,* 693–752.
Faust, D., & Ziskin, J. (1988). The expert witness in psychology and psychiatry. *Science, 241,* 1–35.

Goldstein, R. L. (1988). Consequences of surveillance of the forensic psychiatric examination: An Overview. *American Journal of Psychiatry, 145,* 1243–1247.
Gothard, S. (1989). Power in the court: The social worker as an expert witness. *Social Work, 34,* 65–67.
Grisso, T. (1987). The economic and scientific future of forensic psychological assessment. *American Psychologist, 42,* 831–839.
Grisso, T. (1987). Psychological assessments for legal decisions. In D. Weisstub (Ed.), *Law and mental health,* Vol. 3, pp. 125–257. New York: Pergamon Press.
Heilbrun, K. (1992). The role of psychological testing in forensic assessment. *Law and Human Behavior, 16,* 257–272.
Hoffman, B. F. (1986). How to write a psychiatric report for litigation following a personal injury. *American Journal of Psychiatry, 143,* 164–169.
Holleman, W. L., & Holleman, M. C. (1988). School and work release evaluations. *Journal of American Medical Association, 260,* 3629–3634.
Kunn, C. M. (1984). The expert witness in medical malpractice litigation. *Annals of Internal Medicine, 100,* 139–143.
Melton, G. B., Petrila, J., Poythress, N. G., & Slobogin, C. (1987). *Psychological evaluations for the courts: A handbook for mental health professionals and lawyers.* New York: Guilford Press.
Rachlin, S., & Schwartz, H. I. (1988). The presence of counsel at forensic psychiatric examinations. *Journal of Forensic Sciences, 33,* 1008–1014.
Rogers, R. (1986). *Conducting insanity evaluations.* New York: Van Nostrand Reinhold.
Rogers, R. (Ed.). (1988). *Clinical assessment of malingering and deception.* New York: Guilford Press.
Saks, M. J. (1990). Expert witnesses, nonexpert witnesses, and nonwitness experts. *Law and Human Behavior, 14,* 291–313.
Shuman, D. W. (Ed.). (1986). *Psychiatric and psychological evidence.* New York: McGraw-Hill.
Slovenko, R. (1987). The lawyer and the forensic expert: Boundaries of ethical practice. *Behavioral Sciences and the Law, 5,* 119–147.
Smith, S. R. (1989). Mental health expert witnesses: Of science and crystal balls. *Behavioral Sciences and the Law, 7,* 145–180.
Wasyliw, O. E., Cavanaugh, J. L., Jr., & Rogers, R. (1985). Beyond the scientific limits of expert testimony. *Bulletin of the American Academy of Psychiatry and the Law, 13,* 147–158.
Ziskin, J., & Faust, D. (1988). *Coping with psychiatric and psychological testimony* (4th ed.). Marina Del Ray, CA: Law & Psychology Press.

Glossary of Legal Terms

Accused Person charged with a crime, the defendant.

Acquit To be found not guilty of a criminal charge.

Actus rea The physical act that has been declared a crime.

Adjudication The determination of a controversy and pronouncement of judgment.

Adjudicatory hearing Juvenile court proceeding determining a youth's guilt or innocence.

Adversary Opponent in legal controversy.

Adversary proceeding Hearing or trial involving a controversy between two or more opposing parties.

Adverse party The opposing party in a lawsuit.

Advocacy The act of taking up a legal cause; the act of persuasion.

Affidavit A written statement made under oath before an officer of the court or a notary public.

Affirm To approve or confirm. If an appellate court affirms the decision of the lower court, it means it agrees that the lower court's judgment was correct.

A fortiori A term of logic that denotes an argument to the effect that because one ascertained fact exists, therefore another, which is included in it or analogous to it, and which is less important, unusual, or surprising, must also exist.

Age of majority The age at which a person is considered an adult, generally 18 years of age in the United States.

Allegation A statement in a pleading that the party expects to prove.

Amicus curiae "Friend of the court." This kind of brief is submitted by one who is not a party to the lawsuit, to give the court additional information. The court first decides if it will accept an *amicus curiae* brief. The brief argues the interests of a group, not a party to the lawsuit, which will be affected by the court's decision.

Answer The formal response by the defendant to the allegations made in the plaintiff's complaint.

Appeal A request for a higher court to review the decision of the lower court. The appellate court is limited to determining whether the lower court erred in its interpretation of the law or reached a conclusion which was contrary to the evidence presented at trial.

Appearance The required coming to court of either the plaintiff or the defendant.

Appellant The party to a lawsuit who appeals the decision to a higher court.

Appellee The party who prevailed in the lower court against the appellant and is arguing against setting aside the lower court's verdict.

Arraignment An initial step in the criminal process in which the defendant is formally charged with an offense; is given a copy of the complaint, the indictment, the information, or other accusatory instrument; and is informed of his constitutional rights. At that time the defendant can make a plea.

Bail A monetary amount or other security given to secure the release of a defendant until the time of trial. The bail is set in an amount which is likely to ensure his appearance at trial. Bail will be forfeited if the defendant does not appear.

Bailiff A court attendant.

Bench trial A trial held without a jury. This term is usually used in the context of a criminal trial.

Bindover hearing A hearing in juvenile court to determine if the juvenile will be tried as a juvenile or an adult.

Brief A written argument in which the lawyer states the facts of the case and the questions of law involved and provides supporting legal documentation of why the law should be interpreted in a way which is favorable to his client.

Burden of proof The weight of evidence required for the plaintiff to win his case.

Charge In criminal law, a description of the offense.

Circumstantial evidence Indirect evidence. This is evidence which is secondary. From it something can be inferred.

Citation Reference to a legal authority, such as a statute or case.

Cite To make reference to a legal authority.

Civil action An action to protect a private right or to compel a civil remedy in a dispute between private parties.

Civil law The branch of law that is concerned with noncriminal matters.

Civil liability A liability to actions seeking private remedies or the enforcement of personal rights.

Civil procedure The rules of court on adjudicating civil matters.

Claim The assertion of a right to money or property.

Class action A suit brought by one or more members of a large group of persons on behalf of all members of that group.

Commitment Order by a court requiring a person be confined in a facility for the mentally disabled.

Common law System of jurisprudence which originated in England and was later adopted in the United States. This system is based on judicial precedent (court decisions) rather than legislative enactments (statutes) and is therefore derived from principles rather than rules. When there are no statutes on a subject, the court will refer to the common law for guidance in reaching its decision.

Common law marriage A marriage created by cohabitation and an agreement to marry, but without a marriage ceremony as required by law. Only a limited number of states recognize common law marriages and in those instances the persons must have cohabited for a number of years, typically more than seven.

Comparative negligence A demonstration that the plaintiff may have been partly at fault for the harm which occurred to him. In comparative negligence cases, a determination is made as to what percentage of harm was caused by each party, and damages are awarded based on the contribution to the injury.

Competent Capable of understanding or of acting reasonably within a particular legal context.

Complainant Party who files the lawsuit.

Complaint The first legal document filed in a case, which sets forth the plaintiff's facts on which his claim is based.

Conclusion of fact A conclusion as to a factual matter, reached solely through the use of facts and natural reasoning rather than through rules of law. Conclusions of fact are within the province of the jury.

Conclusion of law A conclusion as to a legal issue, which is reached by the judge, who applies the rules of law.

Consent decree Recorded agreement of the parties as to the form of the judgment.

Conservator Court-appointed guardian of the property of a person who has been declared incompetent.

Constitution The written instrument which has been agreed to by the people of a state or a country, which sets forth the authority of government.

Constitutional rights Individual liberties granted by the state and federal constitutions and protected from governmental interference.

Contempt A determination that someone is to be held in contempt of court means they have disobeyed an order of the court. This could result in a fine or imprisonment.

Contingency fee A fee arrangement in which the attorney is paid a certain amount contingent upon the successful outcome of the case.

Continuance The postponement of the matter until a subsequent court date.

Contributory negligence The plaintiff's contribution to the harm which has occurred to him. By having contributed to his own injury through negligence, the plaintiff may be barred from recovering money for his damages in some states.

Convict To find one guilty of a crime.

Count A distinct claim by the plaintiff which is part of his complaint. A complaint will often contain many counts.

Counterclaim A response by the defendant which asserts claims against the plaintiff.

Cross-examination Questioning of a witness, by a lawyer other than the one who called the witness to the stand, concerning matters about which the witness testified to during the direct examination.

Damages Monetary compensation which is awarded to one who has been injured by the actions of another.

Decree The decision rendered by the court.

Defamation Injuring a person's reputation by false and malicious statements.

Defendant In a criminal case, the person charged with a crime. In a civil action, the party who is being sued.

Defense Response to plaintiff's claims in the form of a denial, answer, or plea.

Deponent Person who gives a deposition.

Depose To take a deposition from a person, or to give a deposition.

Deposition A method of pretrial discovery that consists of a stenographically transcribed statement of a witness under oath, in response to an attorney's questions, with the opportunity for the opposing party or his attorney to be present and cross-examine.

Dictum A statement in a judicial opinion not necessary for the decision of the case. The *dictum* differs from the holding of the case in that it does not establish a rule binding on the courts in subsequent cases.

Directed verdict A verdict returned by the jury at the direction of the trial judge, by whose direction the jury is bound. In civil proceedings, a directed verdict can be granted to either side, if the opposing party fails to sufficiently establish its case. In criminal cases, there may only be a directed verdict of acquittal, not of conviction.

Direct examination The questioning of the witness by the attorney who has called the witness on his client's behalf.

Discovery A pretrial process for learning information about the opposing party's case.

Dismiss To terminate a case or some part of it, such as a particular count in a complaint.

Dispositional hearing A juvenile court proceeding which determines the services to be imposed on the juvenile.

Docket List of cases on the court's calendar.

Due care The degree of care a person of ordinary prudence would use in a given set of circumstances.

Due process of law The principle that the government may not deprive a person of life, liberty, or property without following certain rules and procedures.

Duty Legal obligation by one person to another.

Emancipated minor Someone under the age of 18 who has been declared by a court to be independent, and who is thus able to make all the decisions an adult can.

En banc A decision by the full court. Many appellate courts sit in divisions of three or more judges from among a large number on the full court.

Estoppel A restraint. One can be estopped from using a certain argument because it will lead to an unjust result.

Ex parte An *ex parte* proceeding is one brought on behalf of one party without the expectation of an adverse party. An *ex parte* communication is one in which one side speaks with the judge without the opposing counsel present. This is considered improper.

Expert witness A witness having special knowledge, skill, or experience in the subject about which he is to testify. An expert can give an opinion as a result of his special knowledge.

Extenuating circumstances Unusual factors tending to contribute to the consummation of an illegal act. These are factors over which the actor had little or no control and thus would work against his being held responsible for the criminal act.

Fact finder The person or group responsible for determining the facts in the case. In a jury trial, it is the jury. In a bench trial, the judge is the finder of fact and the trier of law.

Fault The person who is responsible for the wrongdoing or harm.

Felony A serious crime that is punishable by imprisonment in a penitentiary or by death.

Fiduciary One who has a legal duty to act for the benefit of another.

Finding A decision of a court.

Foreseeability A concept used to limit a person's liability to the certain consequences forseeable from his negligent behavior.

Good cause Substantial or legally sufficient reason for doing something.

Good faith An honest intention to fulfill one's obligations.

Good samaritan doctrine A doctrine that provides immunity from liability for the negligent actions of persons who come to the aid of an injured person.

Grand jury A group of 23 persons who determine whether the facts and accusations presented by the prosector warrant the indictment and eventual trial of the accused.

Guardian A person who is legally responsible for the care of another. This could be a person appointed to serve as the guardian of a child, or one who is to serve as the guardian of an incompetent adult.

Habeas corpus The writ of *habeas corpus* is used to challenge someone's confinement in a state mental hospital or a correctional facility.

Hearsay Evidence proceeding not from the personal knowledge of the witness but from the mere repetition of what he has heard others say.

Holding A ruling of the court.

Hung jury A jury which cannot reconcile their differences and reach a verdict by the degree of agreement necessary. (In most criminal cases, a verdict requires unanimous agreement.)

Immaterial Not relevant to the case, insignificant.

Impeach To question the truthfulness of the testimony of the witness by means of evidence that the witness is unworthy of belief.

In camera In the judge's chambers.

Indemnify To insure against or to compensate for loss or damage.

Indictment A formal written accusation drawn up and submitted under oath to a grand jury by the prosecuting attorney, charging one or more persons with a crime.

Information An accusation against a person for a criminal offense without an indictment by a grand jury.

Injunction A judicial remedy to restrain a particular activity. It is a preventive measure to guard against future injuries.

In loco parentis "In the place of a parent," a person or agency which has assumed the obligations of a parent.

In re "In the matter of." This is a title used for cases involving one individual, such as in civil commitment or probate proceedings. This title may also be used in juvenile proceedings.

Insufficient evidence A decision by a judge that the amount of evidence presented by the prosecutor in a criminal trial was insufficient to provide the minimum evidence necessary to prove guilt.

Intent State of mind wherein the person knows or desires the consequences of his act.

Inter alia "Among other things."

Interrogatories A pretrial discovery tool in which written questions are served on the opposing party, who must respond in writing, under oath.

Issue A point of law or fact disputed by the parties.

Joint custody Child custodial arrangement when the parents are divorced in which both parents continue to be legally responsible for making decisions regarding the child. They also will share the physical custody of the child.

Judgment The decision by the court.

Jurisdiction The geographic or political entity governed by a particular legal system or body of laws; also means the power to hear and determine a case. If a court has jurisdiction, then it can hear the case.

Jury A group of people chosen to decide the facts at issue in a trial. A petit jury is a trial jury in a civil or criminal case.

Juvenile delinquent A minor who has committed an offense ordinarily punishable by criminal process, but who is under the age set by statute to be tried as an adult.

Leading question A question asked of a witness at trial, which may be improper because it suggests to the witness the answer he is to give or prompts him to give an answer which is not from his memory.

Legal custody The parent who has the right to make decisions for the child, including those related to education, medical care, and religious upbringing. In an intact family both parents have this right and responsibility.

Legal duty That which the law requires someone to do.

Liable Responsible for.

Libel A tort which consists of a false, malicious, unprivileged publication aimed at defaming a living person.

Malfeasance The doing of a wrongful or unlawful act.

Malpractice A professional's negligent or unskillful performance of his professional duties as determined by a judge or jury.

Material Necessary or relevant to a given matter.

Mediation Use of a neutral third party to try to settle disputes between two other parties by helping them reach agreement.

Mens rea "The guilty mind."

Mental anguish A compensable injury covering all types of mental pain, including grief, distress, anxiety, and fright.

Misdemeanor A class of crimes in which the penalty is either a fine or time spent in a jail, rather than a prison. The possible sentence will be less than a year.

Misfeasance The wrongful or injurious performance of an act that might have been lawfully done.

Mistrial A trial that has been terminated before the jury has returned a verdict because of some extraordinary circumstance (e.g., the death of a necessary juror or the attorney) or because of some fundamental prejudicial error to the defendant which cannot be cured by appropriate instructions to the jury. A mistrial will also occur when there is a hung jury. When there has been a mistrial, a new trial can be scheduled, since no judgment was rendered during the first trial.

Motion A request to the court for an order in favor of the party making the motion.

Negligence Failure to exercise the degree of care a reasonable person would exercise under the same circumstances.

Non compos mentis "Not of sound mind."

Nonsuit A judgment rendered against a plaintiff who fails to proceed to trial or fails to prove his case.

Not guilty In a criminal case, a plea of innocence. When a person is found not guilty, then he is considered innocent.

Notice Informing a person that there is a legal proceeding against him and the specifics of the suit.

Opinion The reasoning for the court's ruling. A concurring opinion is one which agrees with the result but expresses different reasoning. A dissenting opinion is one written by the minority, which disagrees with the decision of the majority.

Order A direction by the court on a matter before it. If the order disposes of the case, it is a final order.

Overrule To deny an objection or motion made. When an objection is overruled, then the witness can answer the question. This could also mean the decision of a court to overturn or void another decision or the decision of the lower court in the same case.

Parens patriae The role of the state as guardian of persons under legal disability.

Per curiam An opinion by the court which is not authored.

Petition The formal documents which are filed with the court, stating the basis for a cause of action and requesting relief.

Petitioner The person who files the petition with the court.

Plaintiff The one who initially files the lawsuit.

Plea Response by the defendant to the allegations of the plaintiff.

Pleading Statement, in logical and legal form, of the facts that constitute the plaintiff's cause of action and the defendant's grounds of defense. Pleadings are either allegations by parties affirming or denying certain matters of fact, or other statements in support or derogation of certain principles of law, which are intended to describe to the court the real matter in dispute.

Plenary guardian A guardian with full or unqualified powers.

Police power Inherent power of state government, often in part delegated to local governmental bodies, to impose upon private rights those restrictions that are reasonably related to the promotion and maintenance of the health, safety, morals, and general welfare of the public. For example, building codes, fire codes, and rules about the equipment needed in hospitals are all part of the state's police power.

Power of attorney A written document by which one person appoints another as his agent and confers upon him the authority to perform certain specified acts. A durable power of attorney continues to provide another person the authority to act, even though the principal is now incapable of acting.

Prayer for relief Request in the petition or complaint which sets forth the specific relief the plaintiff is requesting.

Precedent Previously decided case law recognized as authority for the disposition of future cases.

Prima facie Something that does not need further support to establish its existence. It is clear on its face.

***Prima facie* case** A case sufficient on its facts, which are free from obvious defects.

Privileged communication Those conversations between certain groups which are protected when one seeks to have them divulged in a litigation setting. Many states have statutes regarding attorney–client privilege, therapist–patient privilege, and religious leader–penitent privilege, for example.

Pro bono (publico) Applied when an attorney accepts a case "for the public good" and does not charge a fee.

Pro forma "For the sake of form."

Pro se "For himself," when a person represents himself in a lawsuit.

Prosecution The act of pursuing a lawsuit; generally used to refer to the state initiating a criminal action.

Prosecutor Attorney for a governmental agency who conducts the prosecution of persons charged with crimes.

Proximate cause That which, in a natural and continuous sequence, unbroken by any intervening cause, produces the injury, and without which the injury would not have occurred.

Punitive damages Compensation in excess of the actual damages which is designed to punish the wrongdoer for his or her acts.

Quash To annul or vacate. To quash a subpoena is to make it void.

Question of fact Disputed factual question which is left for the jury to decide, unless the trial is being conducted without a jury, and then the judge decides. Whether or not something occurred is a question of fact.

Question of law Disputed legal contention which is left for the judge to decide. The legal significance of an event is a question of law.

Quid pro quo "Something for something." For example, the *quid pro quo* of civil commitment exchanges a loss of liberty for treatment.

Reasonable doubt The degree of certainty required of a juror before he can make a legally valid determination of the guilt of a criminal defendant. The juror must be convinced beyond a reasonable doubt that the defendant is guilty before convicting him.

Reasonable person A phrase used to denote hypothetically how an ordinary person would act in similar circumstances.

Record The history of the suit from beginning to end, including all the filings with the court, as well as the transcript of the trial proceedings and the court's decision.

Recovery The amount of the judgment; also, the amount actually collected as a result of the judgment.

Release A written document by which some claim, right, or interest is given up to the person against whom the claim, right, or interest could have been enforced.

Relief The award of the court. This could include monetary damages, as well as requiring some specific act, such as giving a person his job back or forcing the losing party to go through with the contract.

Res ispa loquitur "The thing speaks for itself." This is a rule of evidence in which negligence may be inferred from the facts of the case and no expert testimony is necessary to establish negligence, for example, when a surgeon removes the wrong arm.

Res judicata "Something already decided." This reflects a rule in which the final judgment of a court is binding on the parties in any subsequent litigation involving the same cause of action.

Respondeat superior "Let the master reply." This is a theory in which the employer is held responsible for the actions of his employees or others under his control.

Respondent Person responding to a legal action.

Sequester To hold the jury or a witness incommunicado in a place specified by the court so they/he cannot communicate with the public or other witnesses about the case.

Service Providing the opposing side with a copy of the documents filed with the court.

Settlement A compromise between the parties before the case has been decided. A settlement is a resolution of the matter.

Sine qua non An indispensable thing or condition.

Slander The speaking of base and defamatory words tending to injure a person's reputation.

Standing The legal right to challenge the conduct of another in a legal forum. One must have standing to be able to bring a lawsuit.

Stare decisis Rule by which the courts follow the precedents of earlier decisions which addressed similar legal questions.

Statute An act of the legislature; a law.

Statute of limitations A law which sets a certain amount of time in which someone may take legal action to enforce his rights. If the time has passed, then a person is barred by the statute of limitations from seeking to enforce his rights. There are also statutes of limitations which set the time frame in which the state must prosecute someone.

Stay A halt in the judicial proceedings which will stop things until another event occurs.

Stipulation An agreement by the parties related to some matter before the court.

Strict liability The holding of someone liable without a showing of fault.

Sua sponte Without being prompted. If a person makes a statement *sua sponte*, it means the statement was made without the person's being asked about it.

Subpoena A writ issued under the authority of the court to compel the appearance of a witness at a judicial proceeding. This is usually a routine form and is not issued from a direct order of the court. Disobedience of the subpoena (not appearing) may be punished by holding someone in contempt of court.

Subpoena duces tecum An order to produce documents.

Summary judgment The court will grant a motion for summary judgment to either party if it determines that there is no factual dispute.

Summons A mandate requiring a defendant to appear in court. Judgment can be entered against the defendant if he does not appear to answer the issues raised in the suit. An initial appearance is accomplished by filing an "answer" to the suit.

Sustain To approve. When an objection to a question is sustained, then the witness shall not answer the question, because the judge agrees with the basis for the objection.

Testacy The condition of leaving a valid will.

Testator One who writes a will.

Testimony Statement made by a witness under oath.

Tort A private or civil wrong resulting from a breach of a legal duty which exists as a result of society's expectations regarding interpersonal conduct.

Tortfeasor One who is guilty of a tort.

Trial court The court of original jurisdiction which hears the case. Testimony is taken in the trial court.

Verdict The opinion rendered by a jury, or by a judge if there is no jury, on the questions before it.

Vicarious liability A liability that is imputed to one person for the actions of another, where the law contemplates that the other should be held responsible for the wrong in fact committed by someone else.

Voir dire The preliminary examination the court may make of one presented as a witness or juror.

Waiver The intentional and voluntary surrender of some known right.

Waiver hearing A hearing in juvenile court to determine if a juvenile will be tried as an adult.

Warrant An order issued by a court to a law enforcement office to arrest someone.

Will A person's written statement of how he wishes his property to be distributed after his death.

Willful Intentional, as in a willful act.

Witness One who gives evidence before a court under oath.

Work product Work done by an attorney in the course of representing his client which is not discoverable.

Wrongful act An act which will infringe on the rights of another and damage him.

Wrongful death statute A statute which permits administrators of estates to sue for the wrongful death of someone and seek damages as a result.

ABOUT THE AUTHORS

BARBARA A. WEINER, J.D. is an attorney who specializes in health law, with offices in Highland Park, Illinois. Her clients include hospitals, community mental health agencies, and individual health care providers. She is the coauthor of the award-winning *Mentally Disabled and the Law* (3rd edition), and has written more than 25 articles and book chapters in the mental health law field. Ms. Weiner frequently speaks to groups of mental health professionals and is an Assistant Professor in the Department of Psychiatry and Behavioral Sciences, Northwestern University Medical School. This book grows out of Ms. Weiner's past experiences as the Executive Director of a grant-in-aid agency which specialized in addressing the interface issues between law and the behavioral sciences.

ROBERT M. WETTSTEIN, M.D. is an academic psychiatrist with subspecialty training and experience in law and psychiatry. He is Co-Director of the Law and Psychiatry Program at the Western Psychiatric Institute and Clinic, and is on the full-time faculty of the Department of Psychiatry at the University of Pittsburgh. In that capacity, he teaches and consults with other mental health professionals about clinical-legal issues. In addition, he has been a consultant to legal professionals regarding both policy issues and specific litigation. He has published in several areas of psychiatric and law, including psychiatric malpractice, criminal responsibility, violence, and suicide. Dr. Wettstein is Editor of the interdisciplinary journal *Behavioral Sciences and the Law.*

Index

Abandonment, as malpractice lawsuit basis, 164–165
Abortion
  parental consent and notification requirements for, 318–320
  women's right to, 218, 319
Acquired immunodeficiency syndrome (AIDS), 221
Actus rea, 354
Ad litem guardianship, 283
Administrative agencies, published regulations of, 20
Administrative decisions, by governmental agencies, 5
Admission, to psychiatric hospitals, 43–47. *See also* Civil commitment; Voluntary admission
  on emergency basis, 45–46, 63–64
Adolescents
  civil commitment of, 339
  competency of
    clinical, 274, 275–276, 317
    legal, 274
  confidentiality right of, 219, 226–227
  contraceptive use by, 340
  as mature minors, 311–312
  as parents, 338
  prenatal care for, 340
  as runaways, 339–340
  as sex offenders, 340
  treatment decision-making involvement, 317–318, 338–339
Adoption, family assessment for, 168
Adult-protective services, 294
Advance directives
  for impaired decision making, 296–299
  for psychiatric treatment, 302–303
Adversarial system, 23–24
Advocacy
  of attorney, 85–86, 369
  of expert witness, 369
Agencies, legal liability of, 173–174
Age of majority, 310–311
Akron Center for Reproductive Health v. *Ohio*, 320
Alcohol abuse counseling, for minors, 320–321
Alcoholism treatment records, confidentiality of, 219–221
American Psychiatric Association
  duty to protect third parties model statute, 248, 262–263
  electroconvulsive therapy guidelines, 157, 166
  restraints and seclusion use task force report, 136
Americans with Disabilities Act, 207
Amicus curiae, 9
Amicus curiae brief, 9
Answer, by defendant, 14
Appeal, right to, 16
Appellate courts
  decisions, published sources of, 5, 18–19
  federal, 6, 7–9, 17, 18, 19. *See also* United States Supreme Court
  review process of, 7–8, 24
  state, 11, 18–19
"As needed" order, for psychotropic medication administration, 139

Attorney, 23–39
  advocacy role, 85–86, 369
  circumstances for contacting, 31–33
  conflict of interest of, 31, 34
  expert witness's interaction with, 356–359
    conferences, 358–359
    fees, 358, 365, 366–367, 370, 372
    pretrial consultation, 363–364
    setting terms of evaluation, 357
    witness's access to records, 357, 369
  fees, 25, 35–37, 153
  hiring of, 33–35
  impact on mental health system, 37–38
  in malpractice lawsuits, 189
    case analysis, 152–154
    clinician's relationship with, 183–184
  points of involvement, 26–30
  referral of clients by, 31
  referral of clients to, 34
  representation of children, 30
  representation of the family, 28–29
  representation of mentally disabled patients, 26–28, 30–31, 85–86
    advocacy role, 85–86, 369
    at civil commitment hearings, 56
    visitation rights during, 84
  representation of the state, 28
  representation of the treatment facility, 29
  representation of the treatment provider, 29–30
  responsibilities to client, 25
Attorney-client privilege, 25–26
Attorney in fact, 298
Aversive behavior modification, 136–137

Baby Jane Doe case, 316, 340
Behavioral assessment, 278–279
Behavior modification, legal regulation of, 136–137
"Beyond a reasonable doubt" standard, 15–16
Bill of Rights, 3–4
Bills, passage of, 4–5
Bind over, of juvenile offenders, 337–338
Board of Education v. *Rowley*, 335
Brief, *amicus curiae*, 9
Burch v. Zinermon, 44

Carey v. *Population Services International*, 319
Case citations, 17–19
Case law, 5
  as common law basis, 2
  law reporters of, 17
Causation
  attorney's analysis of, 153–154
Causation (*cont.*)
  as negligence claim requirement, 151–152
  tests for, 152
Certiorari, writ of, 9
Child abuse and neglect
  assessment of, 168, 327–328
  definition, 326–327
  diagnostic and treatment guidelines for, 327
  interventions for, 328–329
  investigation of, 168, 327–328
  reporting of, 226, 326–329
    for adult clients, 340–341
    breach of confidentiality in, 205
    failure to, 171–172
    good-faith liability protection for, 172
Child abuse and neglect cases
  breach of confidentiality in, 33
  testimonial privilege and, 212
Child custody, 329–334, 340
  best interests of the child standard, 214, 330–332, 339
  confidentiality issues, 334
  expert testimony for, 351–352, 356
  family assessment for, 168
  joint custody, 331, 332–333
  least detrimental alternative in, 339
  legal custody, 331
  modification of custody, 331
  noncustodial parent's rights, 341
  patient-litigant exception in, 214–215
  physical custody, 331
  types of, 331
Child-related proceedings, expert testimony at, 351–352, 356
Children
  arrest of, 336. *See also* Juvenile justice system
  definition, 309
  developmental stages of, 309–310
  disabled
    access to education, 334–336
    termination of care for, 316, 340
  inappropriate hospital discharge of, 339
  legal representation for, 30
  legal rights of, 309–347
    in abuse and neglect, 326–329
    competency, 274, 275–276, 310–312
    confidentiality of records, 324–325
    disabled, access to education, 334–336
    disabled, access to medical treatment, 315–316, 340
    and juvenile justice system, 336–338
    medical treatment access, 311, 314–318
    medical treatment decision-making, 317–138

Children (*cont.*)
legal rights of (*cont.*)
outpatient counseling access, 320–322
parens patriae and, 310
during psychiatric hospitalization, 322–324
reproductive rights, 317, 318–320
research participation, 325–326
as witness, 312–314
mentally retarded, sterilization of, 320
sterilization of, 317, 320
voluntary admission of, 44
Child welfare workers, child abuse and neglect involvement, 328–329
Circuit court, 10, 11
Circuit Court of Appeals, 7–8, 18
Circumstantial proof, *res ipsa loquitur* doctrine of, 154, 155
Citation, legal system of, 16–22
case citations, 17–19
regulatory citations, 20
Shepard's, 21–22
statutory citations, 19–20
Civil cases, 13
Civil commitment, 37, 41–79
application for, 26–27, 54
breach of confidentiality during, 53, 204–205
duration of, 60–62
duty to protect third parties and, 244–245
financial responsibility for, 62
by guardian, 300
hearings for, 55–59
expert testimony, 58–59, 64, 351
mental health professional's refusal to testify, 64
mental health professional's testimony, 58–59, 64, 351
patient's attendance at, 64–65
patient's rights during, 55–58, 85
prosecutor's role, 58
testimonial privilege and, 211, 212
historical background, 41–43
of incompetent persons, 86–87, 275, 300–301
initiation of, 53–54
least-restrictive-alternative in, 88–89
legal criteria of, 47–53
danger to others, 47, 48, 49–51
danger to self, 51–52
inability to care for self, 52
mental illness, 48–49
medical evidence for, 46–47
of minors, 322–323
outpatient, 59–60
parens patriae basis, 47, 55
patients' discharge following, 60–62, 99
Civil commitment (*cont.*)
recommitment and, 61–62
states' standards for, 65–75
as threat by therapist, 64
of voluntarily-admitted patients, 45, 63
wrongful, 63
Civil law system, 2
Civilly-committed patients
discharge of, 60–62, 99
habeas corpus action by, 61
rights of
habilitation, 114–115
selection of own therapist, 140
treatment, 111–112
Civil rights lawsuits, 172–173
Class action lawsuits, 10
impact on mental health system, 38
"Clear and convincing evidence" standard, 15
Clergy
access to hospitalized patients, 84
testimonial privilege of, 210
Code of ethics, breach of, 217–218
Code of Federal Regulations (CFR), 5, 20
Co-guardians, 290
Colleagues
impaired, 191
sexual misconduct by, 228
College students, as emancipated minors, 311
Common law, 2
for therapist-patient communications, 218
as treatment refusal basis, 128–129
Communication
as hospitalized patients' right, 82–85, 98–99
conjugal visits, 84
mail rights, 82–83, 98–99
telephone access, 84–85
visitation rights, 83–84, 99, 100
privileged, 210–217
exceptions to, 212–217
malpractice implications, 181
Community, rights of disabled persons in, 27
Community-based treatment
least-restrictive-alternative basis, 89
Competency, 273. *See also* Incompetency; Incompetency declaration; Incompetent persons
of children, 274, 275–276, 310–312
clinical, 87, 116–117, 119, 274, 275–281
criminal, 275
definition, 310
evaluations of, 276–280
historical background, 274
legal, 116, 274–275
restoration to, 293

Competency (*cont.*)
standards of, 280–281
types of, 274–276
Competency to stand trial proceedings, expert testimony at, 353–354
Confidentiality, 201–235
breach of, 203–210
civil commitment-related, 53, 204–205
client advisement about, 206–207, 226–227
following client's death, 227
by disclosure to investigative agencies, 20, 208, 228–229, 244, 245, 246, 248
Fax machines and, 229
as lawsuit basis, 171
legally-justified, 204–206
legally-mandated, 33
malpractice and, 203
with patient's family, 209
social factors affecting, 208–210
in child abuse and neglect cases, 329
in child custody cases, 34
definition of confidential material, 203
disclosure of records and, 222–225
of drug abuse and alcoholism treatment records, 219–221
duty to protect third parties and, 239, 242
in family therapy, 226
importance of, 201–203
of minor's health care records, 219, 224, 324–325
nonstatutory protection of, 217–219
privileged communications and, 210–217
waivers of, 207–208
Congress
constitutional empowerment of, 3
publication of laws enacted by, 19–20
statutory law enactment by, 4–5
Conjugal visits, of hospitalized patients, 84
Conservator, 287–288
Constitution, U.S., 2–4, 19, 110, 125, 310, 336
Constitutional law, 3–4
Consultants, legal liability of, 175
Consultation
malpractice liability and, 182, 189
negligent release and, 255
for potentially violent clients, 246–247, 255
by social workers, 168
for unorthodox therapy, 164
Continuity of care, 182–183
Contraception, 218, 318–39
Contract law, 2
Corporations, legal representation of, 31
Co-therapist, legal liability of, 175
Counterclaim, by defendant, 14
Court of Appeals
Circuit Court of, 7–8, 18
of state court systems, 11
Court system, 5–12
federal court system, 6–9
Circuit Court of Appeals, 7–8, 18
federal district courts, 6–7
Supreme Court. *See* United States Supreme Court
juvenile justice system, 11–12, 336–338, 351–352
state court system, 9–11
Craig v. *Maryland*, 313
Criminal behavior, by clients, reporting of, 228–229, 260
Criminal cases, 12–13
defense, client's records for, 371–372
expert testimony at, 353–355
competency to stand trial proceedings, 353–354
criminal responsibility proceedings, 354–355
sentencing alternatives recommendations, 355
rights of mentally-disabled persons during, 27–28
Cross-examination, 15, 370–371
Cruel-and-unusual punishment, as treatment refusal basis, 110
Cruzan v. *Director, Missouri Department of Health*, 296–297
Custodial relationships, 238

Damages
award of, 158
determination of, 153, 157–158, 168
proof of, 151
Danforth v. *Planned Parenthood of Central Missouri*, 319
Dangerousness, as civil commitment basis, 47, 48, 49–52. *See also* Duty to protect third parties
recent overt act requirement, 49
Decisionally incapacitated persons. *See also* Guardian(s); Guardianship
adult-protective services for, 294
advance directives for, 296–299
elder abuse reporting for, 294–295
public guardians for, 295–296
representative payees for, 93–95, 99–100, 293–294
surrogate consent law for, 299
Decision-making capacity, 275–276
evaluation of, 276–280

Decision-making capacity (*cont.*)
incompetency declarations and, 281
standards of, 280–281
Defendants
answer by, 14
counterclaim by, 14
in criminal cases, 12–13
notice of, 13
rights of, 13–14, 15
Deinstitutionalization, 90
Depositions, 364–366
discovery, 364–366, 373
evidence, 365
subpoena for, 32
Diagnosis, failure to, as malpractice lawsuit basis, 160–161
Diagnostic procedures, refusal of, 138
Disability claims
breach of confidentiality in, 216
expert testimony for, 353
patient-litigant exception in, 216
Disabled children
access to education, 334–336
access to medical treatment, 315–316, 340
termination of care for, 316, 340
Disabled persons. *See also* Incompetency; Incompetency declaration; Incompetent persons
definition, 282
Discharge
of civilly commited patients, 60–62, 99
court review for, 254
negligent. *See* Negligent release
of noncompliant patients, 188
of voluntarily admitted patients, 45, 61
Discharge planning, negligent release implications, 253–254. *See also* Negligent release lawsuits
Discovery, right of, 13–14
Divorce
child custody and, 329–334, 340
joint custody, 331, 332–333
legal custody, 331
modification of custody, 331
noncustodial parent's rights, 341
physical custody, 331
vistitation/access, 331
of incompetent persons, 286
Dix, Dorothea Lynde, 42
Donaldson v. *O'Connor*, 111, 112
Driving ability impairment
of incompetent persons, 286
reporting of, 206
Drug abuse treatment records, confidentiality of, 219–221
Drug abuse, negligent release implications, 251
Due Process clause, 3–4
Duty
breach of, 152–153
of health care provider, 151
as negligence claim element, 152
Duty to protect third parties, 237–272. *See also* Negligent release lawsuits
breach of confidentiality for, 205
with HIV-infected clients, 227
legal immunity statutes for, 247–248
methods of discharging, 243–245
assessment of violence potential, 243
notification of police, 244, 245, 246, 248
notification of potential victims, 244–245, 248, 258–260
risk management and implementation, 243–245
statutes, 247–248
American Psychiatric Association's model for, 248, 262–263
legal immunity, 247–248

Eanes v. *United States*, 252
Eastern Lunatic Asylum, Kentucky, 42
Education, disabled children's access to, 334–336
Education for All Handicapped Children Act, 334–335
Educational record, parents' right of review of, 324
Elder abuse, reporting of, 206, 294–295
Elderly persons
adult-protective services for, 294
functional status assessment of, 279
Electroconvulsive therapy
competency to consent to, 276
guardian's consent for, 289
legal regulation of, 133–134, 140
as malpractice lawsuit basis, 166–167
for minors, 321, 323
Emancipated minors, 311
Emergency admission, 45–46, 63–64
Emergency care, children's access to, 314–315
Emergency situations
breach of confidentiality during, 204
detention of clients during, 189
psychotropic medication administration during, 132, 138
restraints and seclusion use during, 135–136
right to refuse medication during, 127–128, 129–130

Employer
release of client's records to, 171
responsibility for employees' actions, 174
Employment
confidentiality waivers for, 207–208
of patients, 91–92, 99–100
Epileptic patients, 256
Equal Protection Clause, 4
Estate, of incompetent persons, 284, 285
guardianship for, 287–288
Ethics, professional code of, breach of, 217–218
Evidence
attorney-client privilege of, 25–26
for civil commitment, 54, 58
standard of proof for, 15–16
Examination, 15
cross-examination, 15, 370–371
Expert witness, 349–375
advocacy by, 369
appearance of, 367
attorney's interaction with, 356–359
access to records, 357, 369
briefing about case, 356
clarification of legal issue, 356–357
clarification of witness's role, 357
conferences, 358–359
fees, 358, 365, 366–367, 370, 372
pretrial consultation, 363–364
setting terms of the evaluation, 357
benefits of serving as, 355–356
in child-related proceedings, 351–352, 356
in civil commitment proceedings, 58–59, 351
comparison with fact witness, 371
in criminal cases, 353–355
declining to serve as, 359
depositions, 364–366, 373
fees, 365, 366, 370
in forensic cases, 359
"freeze" of testimony of, 365–366
in negligence cases, 152
opposing party's use of, 373
in personal injury cases, 352
psychiatric terminology use by, 362–263, 368
qualification of answers by, 368
report preparation by, 360–363
content of report, 362–363
format of report, 360–362
preparation for writing, 360
role of, 350–351
selection of, 155–156
testimony on behalf of patient, 359, 372, 373–374
trial testimony by, 366–371
cross-examination, 370–371
preparation for, 366–367
in worker's compensation and disability claims, 353

Fact witness
comparison with expert witness, 371
testimony by, 369, 372
Family, of mentally-disabled persons
breach of confidentiality with, 209
civil commitment proceedings by, 28
financial responsibility of, 62
legal representation of, 28–29
treatment plan involvement, 88
Family law, 3
Family planning, by minors, 319
Family therapy, confidentiality of, 222
Fax machines, confidentiality implications, 229
Federal court system, 6–9
Circuit of Appeals, 7–8, 18
federal district courts, 6–7, 17
Supreme Court. *See* United States Supreme Court
Federal District Courts, 6–7
citations of decisions, 17
Federal government, constitutional law and, 3–4
Federal laws
interaction with state laws, 2
publication of, 19–20
Federal Register, 5
Federal Reporter System, 18
Federal Supplement, 17, 18
Fees
of attorney, 25, 35–37, 153
of expert witness, 358, 365, 366–367, 370, 372
of therapist, 182
Financial responsibility and rights
of hospitalized patients, 92–95
of incompetent persons, 284, 285
guardian's responsibility for, 287–288, 291, 301, 302
Forensic cases, expert witnesses, 359
Forensic evaluation, evaluator's obligations in, 373
Forensic report, 360–363
content, 362–363
format, 360–363
preparation for writing of, 360
Foster care, 318
Functional status assessment inventories, 278–279

Gault, In re, 322, 336
Good-faith actions and reports. *See also* Immunity
for child abuse reporting, 172

Good-faith actions and reports (*cont.*)
for civil commitment, 63
for elder abuse, 295
for negligent release, 252
Governmental immunity, 175–176
Group therapy, confidentiality of, 222
Guardian(s)
appointment of, 287–292
authority of, 287–290
civil commitment by, 300
as co-guardians, 287, 290
of estate, 287–288, 291
health care provider's consultation with, 286
incapacitated, 293
limited, 289–290
of the person, 288–289
plenary, 289
public, 295–296
selection of, 287
surrogate decision-making by, 290–292
in best interests of third party or family, 291–292
in best interests of ward, 290
for financial decisions, 287–288, 291
as prudent person/administrator, 291
as substituted judgment, 291
in treatment setting, 117, 286, 292- 293
temporary, 281, 289
Guardian *ad litem*, 283
Guardianship
for authorization of treatment, 117
incompetency declaration and, 281
right to refuse medication and, 130
Guardianship Individual Functional Assessment Tool, 279
Guns, violent patients' access to, 254

Habeas corpus action, by civilly commited patients, 61
Habilitation, right to, 114–115
Halderman v. *Pennhurst*, 114–115
Hamman v. *County of Maricopa*, 241
Hammurabi, Code of, 1–2
Handicapped infants/children, medical care of, 315–316
termination of, 316, 340
Harper v. *Washington*, 126
Health Care Quality Improvement Act of 1989, 190
Health insurance claims
appeals of, 258
fraudulent, 161
for mental illness, 207–208
Health insurance coverage
confidentiality waivers and, 207–208
periodic patient review and, 91
Hearings
adjudicatory, for juvenile delinquency, 336
for civil commitment, 55–59
expert testimony, 351
mental health professional's testimony, 58–59, 64, 351
patient's attendance at, 64–65
patient's rights during, 55–58, 85
prosecutor's role, 58
refusal to testify at, 64
testimonial privilege and, 211, 212
dispositional, for juvenile delinquency, 336
Hearsay, at civil commitment hearings, 56–57
Hicks v. *United States*, 250
Hippocratic Oath, 211, 217
H.L. v. *Matheson*, 319
Hodgson v. *Minnesota*, 320
Homicide, client's confession of, 260
Homicide ideation, reporting of, 259
Homicide potential, evaluation of, 182, 259
Hospital(s). *See also* Treatment facilities
legal liability of, 173–174
Hospitalization
competency to consent to, 276. *See also* Competency; Voluntarily committed patients
health care coverage of, periodic review and, 91
Hospitalized patients. *See also* Civilly commited patients; Voluntarily admitted patients
rights of, 81–108
access to attorney, 85–86
communication, 82–85, 98–99
employment, 91–92, 99–100
humane care and treatment, 87–88
knowledge of rights, 100
least restrictive alternative, 88–90, 99
periodic review, 90–91, 99
personal possessions, 97–98
presumption of competency, 86–87
religious freedom, 98
right to manage funds, 92–95
right to refuse research participation, 95–97, 100
states' statutes for, 81, 100–104
voting rights, 98
Wyatt v. *Stickney* decision for, 81–82, 87, 89, 111, 114
Humane care, of hospitalized patients, 87–88
Human experimentation. *See* Research participation

Human immunodeficiency virus-infected clients
breach of confidentiality with, 221, 227, 261–262
duty-to-protect-third-parties and, 261–262
Human immunodeficiency virus testing, release of results, 221

Immunity
for civil commitment, 63
for duty to protect third parties compliance, 247–248
for elder abuse reporting, 295
governmental, 175–176
for impaired driver reporting, 257
for living will compliance, 297
from negligent release lawsuits, 252–253
In camera inspection, of patient's records, 225
Incapacitated person. *See also* Incompetency; Incompetency declaration; Incompetent persons
definition, 282
Incompetency, definition, 282
Incompetency declaration, 86–87, 116
adjudication proceedings for, 282–284
expert testimony, 352
initiation of, 282
mental health professional's role in, 281, 283–284, 352
reasons for, 274–275
clinician's recommendation for, 281
as to estate, 284, 285
guardianship for, 287–288
legal effects of, 273, 281
of minors, 273
as to person, 284, 285–286
guardianship for, 170, 288–289
rights affected by, 284–286
Incompetent persons
civil commitment of, 86–87, 275, 300–301
protective devices for, 293–299
adult-protective services, 294
advance directives, 296–299
elder abuse reporting, 294–295
public guardians, 295–296
representative payees, 93–95, 99–100, 293–294
Index to Legal Periodicals, 21
Individualized Education Program, 334–335
Infants, handicapped, medical care of, 315–316
termination of, 316, 340
Information disclosure, for informed consent, 118
Informed assent, for research participation, 325, 326
Informed consent, 115–119
for competency evaluation, 276
competency to consent to treatment and, 116–117
for duty to protect third parties victim notification, 245
for electroconvulsive therapy, 166
failure to provide, 169–171
information necessary for, 118
for malpractice prevention, 182
for psychosurgery, 137
for psychotropic medication administration, 139
for research participation, 96, 97
substituted, 292–293, 299
therapist's responsibility for, 140, 187
voluntariness of, 117–118
In re Gault, 322
In re Winship, 336
Insanity defense, expert testimony for, 354–355
Institutional policies, clinician's familiarity with, 183
Institutional Review Board, for human research participation, 96, 325–326
Insurance. *See also* Health insurance
for malpractice, 176–177
notification of carrier in lawsuit, 183
sexual misconduct lawsuits and, 163
Insurance companies, confidentiality waivers and, 208
Involuntary hospitalization. *See* Civil commitment
Iowa v. *Coy*, 313

J.L. and R.L. v. *Parham*, 322–323
Job discrimination, mental illness-related, 171, 207–208
Judiciary
federal, 6
of state court system, 10
U.S. Supreme Court, 9
Jury trial, 15, 57
Juvenile delinquency, 336–338
Juvenile justice system, 11–12, 336–338
court-referred evaluations for, 351–352

Kaimowitz v. *Department of Mental Health (Michigan)*, 96, 137

Law enforcement agencies
confidential records release to, 20, 227
notification of
about client's criminal behavior, 228–229, 260
as duty to protect third parties, 244, 245, 246, 248

Law review articles, 20–21
Lawsuits
civil cases, 13
criminal cases, 12–13
defense, client's records for, 371–372
expert testimony at, 353–355
rights of mentally disabled persons in, 27–28
filing procedures for, 12–16
rights of parties during a trial, 14–16
rights of parties involved in litigation, 13–14
right to appeal, 16
Law Week, 18
Least-restrictive-alternative, 88–90, 99
restraints and seclusion as, 135–136
Legal aid organizations, class action lawsuits by, 27
Legal aid programs, for mentally ill patients, 85–86
Legal system
citation system, 16–22
court system, 5–12
federal, 6–9, 18. *See also* United States Supreme Court
juvenile justice, 11–12, 336–337, 351–352
state, 9–11
Liability, of incompetent persons, 286
Liability, professional, 149–200
breach of confidentiality-related, 171
civil rights violations-related, 172–173
duty to protect third parties-related, 171. *See also* Duty to protect third parties
effect on patient care, 149
failure to report child abuse-related, 171–172
of hospitals and treatment facilities, 173–174
lack of informed consent-related, 169–171. *See also* Informed consent
malpractice. *See* Malpractice
for negligent release. *See* Negligent release lawsuits
problems in proving, 168–169
record keeping and, 177–181
of state employees, 175–176
of supervisory personnel, 174–175
third-party. *See also* Duty to protect third parties; Negligent release lawsuits
for managed care, 257–258
for motor vehicle accidents, 256–257
sexual activity with a patient-related, 161–163
of social workers, 158, 161, 162, 167–168
suicide and attempted suicide-related, 158–160
Liberty interest
as medication refusal basis, 124, 125–128
restraints and seclusion as impingement on, 134–135
License suspension, for incompetency, 286
Licensure
malpractice insurance requirements for, 177
sexual misconduct reporting requirement for, 162
Living will, 117, 297–299

Mail rights, of hospitalized patients, 82–83, 98–99
Majority, age of, 310–311
Malpractice, 150–168
areas of liability, 158–168
abandonment, 164–165
breach of confidentiality, 203
electroconvulsive therapy, 166–167
failure to diagnose, 160–161
improper psychotherapy, 163–164
negligent administration of medication, 165–166
negligent release, 161
negligent psychological evaluation, 167
sexual activity with patient, 161–163
social worker negligence, 158, 161, 162, 167–168
suicide and attempted suicide, 158–160
attorney's analysis of, 152–154
definition, 150
elements of
breach of duty, 151
causation, 151–152
duty, 151
proof of damages, 151
managed care and, 258
negligence basis of, 150–152
reporting of, 187
to National Practitioner Data Bank, 190
standard of care violation and, 155–157
statute of limitations of, 152
Malpractice insurance, 176–177
notification of carrier in lawsuit, 183
premiums, 149, 150, 158
sexual misconduct lawsuits and, 163
Malpractice lawsuits, 10
breach of confidentiality in, 216
coping with, 185–186
expert testimony in, 155–156, 352
incidence of, 158
legal representation in, 29–30, 32–33
patient-litigant exception in, 214, 216
prevention of, 181–183
response to, 183–185, 183–185
separate counsel in, 184
standard of care and, 240
Malpractice stress syndrome, 185–186
Managed care, 257–258

Maryland v. *Craig*, 313
Matheson v. *H.L.*, 319
Mature minor, 311–312
Medicaid
fraud statute, 218
patient self-determination requirement, 296
sterilization requirement, 320
Medical care. *See* Treatment
Medicare, 296
Medication. *See also* Psychotropic medication
negligent administration of, 161, 165–166
nonphysician therapist's monitoring of, 189
refusal of, constitutional basis of, 110
standard of care for, 157
Mens rea, 354
Mental health agencies
legal liability of, 173–174
legal representation of, 29
Mental health care. *See* Treatment
Mental health examination. *See* Psychiatric examination
minors' access to, 321–322
Mental hospitals. *See* Psychiatric hospitals
Mental illness, as defined by state statutes, 48–49, 65–75
Mentally disabled persons, legal representation of, 26–28
general legal rights, 27
special representation needs
in civil commitment proceedings, 26
in criminal proceedings, 27–28
for institutional rights, 27
problems of, 30–31
Minors. *See also* Adolescents; Children
confidentiality right of, 219
disclosure of records of, 224, 324–325
emancipated, 311
legal incompetency of, 273
mature, 311–312
treatment access by, 321–322
treatment statutes regarding, 312
Misdiagnosis, as malpractice suit cause, 160–161
Motor vehicle accidents. *See also* Driving ability impairment
professional liability for, 256–257, 261

National Commission for the Protection of Human Subjects of Biomedical and Behavior Research, 95
National Institutes of Health, 3
National Practitioner Data Bank, 190, 191
National Reporter System, 18–19
Negligence
definition, 150
elements of
breach of duty, 152–153
causation, 153–154
damages, 153
duty, 152
statute of limitations, 152
as malpractice basis, 150–152
proof of, 154–158
standard of care violation, 155–157
Negligent release lawsuits, 161, 237–238, 249–256
immunity from, 252–253
Noncompliance, discharge from care and, 188
Non compos mentis laws, 42
Notice, of defendants, 13
Nurse
inadequately-trained, 174
malpractice suits against, 158

O'Connor v. *Donaldson*, 111, 112
Ohio v. *Akron Center for Reproductive Health*, 320
Okin v. *Rogers*, 127–128
Organ transplantation, guardian's consent for, 289
Outpatient(s)
civil commitment of, 59–60
danger caused by. *See* Duty to protect third parties; Negligent release
Outpatient treatment
minors' access to, 320–322
patient's suicide during, 159

Parens patriae, 28, 47, 55, 111–112, 284, 310, 315
Parental consent
for abortion, 318–320
for contraceptive information, 318–319
for research participation, 326
for treatment, 311–312, 314–315, 316–317
for treatment records release, 226–227
Parental notification
children's right to confidentiality and, 219
for substance abuse counseling, 321
Parham v. *J.L. and R.L.*, 322–323
Parole, 355
Patient-litigant exception, to testimonial privilege, 213–217
Patient Self-Determination Act, 296–297
Peer review, in managed care, 258
Pensions, representative payee for, 293
Peonage, institutional, 92
Periodic review, of hospitalized patients, 90–91

Personal injury lawsuits, 150
breach of confidentiality in, 214, 215–216, 228
expert testimony in, 352
motor vehicle accident-related, 256–257
patient-litigant testimonial privilege exception in, 214, 215–216
Personal possessions, of hospitalized patients, 97–98
Physical abuse. *See also* Child abuse and neglect
by therapist, 164
Physical examination
inadequate, 256
malpractice implications, 160–161
pre-empolyment, 207
Physician-patient privilege statutes, 211
Plaintiff, definition, 13
Planned Parenthood of Central Missouri v. *Danforth*, 319
Police
notification of
about client's criminal behavior, 228–229
as duty to protect third parties, 244, 245, 246, 248
negligent release and, 250
release of client's records to, 20, 227
Police power, of the states, 47
Power of attorney, 298–299, 302
Precedent, definition, 2
Pregnancy
adolescent, 340
implications of treatment on, 190
Prenatal care, for adolescent mothers, 340
Press, access to mental health facilities by, 84
Privacy, right to, 4, 218–219
of hospitalized patients, 87, 88
of minors, 318–319, 321
as treatment refusal basis, 110, 124, 125–128
Privileged communication, 210–217
exceptions to, 212–217
Process notes, of trainees, 227
Professional guidelines, use in malpractice suits, 156–157
Proof, circumstantial, 154, 155
Property damage, duty to protect third parties from, 242, 260–262
Prosecutor
in civil commitment hearings, 58
in criminal cases, 12
Psychiatric examination
for civil commitment, 57
court-ordered, 213
of insanity defense defendants, 354–355
periodic, of hospitalized patients, 90–91
Psychiatric hospitals. *See also* Treatment facilities
admission status to, 43–47
civil commitment. *See* Civil commitment
emergency, 45–46, 63–64
informed, 45
observational, 46
voluntary. *See* Voluntarily admitted patients; Voluntary admission
historical background, 42
Psychiatrists
malpractice suits against, 158
sexual activity with clients, 161
Psychological tests, negligent evaluation of, 167
Psychologist(s)
malpractice suits against, 158
sexual activity with clients, 161
Psychologist-patient privilege statutes, 211–212
Psychosurgery
experimental, 96
guardian's consent for, 289
legal regulation of, 137–138
of minors, 321
Psychotherapist-patient privilege statutes, 211–212
Psychotherapy, improper, 163–164
Psychotic persons, voluntary hospital admission of, 44
Psychotropic medication
competency to consent to, 276
guardian's consent for, 130, 289
informed consent for, 139
lack of, 169
for minors, 321
negligent administration of, 161, 165–166
patient's refusal of, 87, 90, 120–133
clinical aspects of, 130–132
common law basis of, 128–129
constitutional basis of, 124–128
courts' denial of, 129, 130, 133
in emergency situations, 133
as freedom of religion, 124, 125, 128
guardian's overriding of, 130
least restrictive alternative and, 90
major cases regarding, 120, 121–124
by voluntarily admitted patients, 138–139
side effects
driver impairment, 256, 257
malpractice implications, 165–166
tardive dyskinesia/dystonia, 139, 165–166
Publication, of patients' records, 224–225
Public law, 3

Quid pro quo theory, 112

Rational relationship test, 111–112
Recent overt act requirement, 49
Records, 177–181
  contents of, 178–181
  for criminal responsibility defense, 371–372
  disclosure of, 222–225
    authorization form for, 229–230
    obligation to patient in, 224
    in publications, 224–225
    records of minors, 224, 324–325
    statutory access by others, 223
  expert witness's access to, 357
  functions of, 177–178
  informed consent documentation in, 170–171
  length of retention of, 190–191
  official, 178
  patient's access to, 181, 223
  personal notes as, 178
  of potentially violent clients, 247
  publication of, 224–225
  subpoena of, 32, 372
Redirect examination, 15
Referral
  abandonment and, 165
  for alternative treatment, 164, 170
  for driving evaluation, 257
  following ineffective treatment, 164
  malpractice prevention and, 182
Regulatory citations, 20
Regulatory law, 5
Release. *See* Discharge
  negligent. *See* Negligent release lawsuits
Religion, free exercise of, 210
  by hospitalized patients, 98
  as medication refusal basis, 124, 125, 128
  as treatment refusal basis, 98, 301
Reporters, of legal citations, 17
  federal court decisions, 17–18
  Mental and Physical Disability Law Reporter, 21
  state court decisions, 18–19
Reporting, mandatory
  of child abuse, 226, 326–329
    for adult clients, 340–341
    breach of confidentiality in, 205
    failure to, 171–172
    good-faith liability protection for, 172
  of client's criminal behavior, 228–229
  of elder abuse, 294–295
  of impaired drivers, 257
  of sexually transmitted disease, 205–206, 319
  of therapist's sexual activity with clients, 228
Reports, of expert witnessses, 360–363
  content of, 362–363
  format of, 360–362
  preparation for writing of, 360
Representative payee, 93–95, 99–100, 292, 293–294
Reproductive rights, of children, 317, 318–320
Research participation
  by children, 325–326
  competency to consent to, 276
  duty to protect third parties and, 259–260
  patients' right to refuse, 95–97, 100
Res ipsa loquitur doctrine, 154, 155
Respondeat superior doctrine, 174
Restraint
  historical background, 41–42
  legal regulation of, 134–136
R.L. and J.L. v. *Parham*, 322–323
Rogers v. *Okin*, 127–128
Romeo v. *Youngberg*, 115, 126, 134–135
Rouse v. *Cameron*, 111
Rowley v. *Board of Education*, 335
Rules
  administrtive decisions and, 5
  of evidence, 24
  law and, 1
  of procedure, 24

Schools, release of treatment records to, 226–227
Searches, of patients, 97–98
Seclusion, legal regulation of, 134–136
Secret Service, 208
Self-incrimination, during civil commitment process, 53
Self-mutilation, as civil commitment basis, 51
Sentencing alternatives, expert witness's recommendations for, 355
Sex offenders, juvenile, 337–338, 340
Sexual abuse, of children, 327, 328
Sexual activity, with clients, 161–163, 169
  reporting of, 228
  by supervisee, 191
Sexually transmitted disease, reporting of, 205–206, 319
Sexually transmitted disease counseling, for minors, 319
Shepard's citation system, 21–22
Social contacts, therapist-client, 209–210
Social Security benefits, representative payee for, 93, 94, 293
Social workers
  malpractice suits against, 158, 162, 167–168
  sexual activity with clients, 161, 162
Special education, for handicapped children, 334–335
Specialists, practice standards of, 150

Standard of care
expert testimony regarding, 352
"locality rule" of, 188–189
in malpractice lawsuits, 240
right to treatment and, 13
violations of, 155–156
Standard of proof, 15–16
State court system, 9–11
publication of decisions of, 18–19
State employees, lawsuits against, 175–176
Statute(s)
citations of, 20, 22
for psychologist-patient privilege, 211–212
Shepard's citation system of, 22
Statute of limitations
for incompetent persons, 286
for malpractice actions, 152
Statutory immunity, 175–176
Statutory law, 4–5
Sterilization
guardian's consent for, 289
of minors, 317, 320
Subpoena
definition, 372
for deposition, 32
of records, 32, 372
response to, 372
testimonial privilege and, 212
for testimony, 32, 212
therapist's response to, 225, 227–228
Subpoena duces tecum, 372
Substance abuse
by colleagues, 191
Substance abuse treatment
confidentiality of, 227
for employees, 207
for minors, 320–321
Substance-abusing clients, duty to protect third parties from, 261
Suicidal clients
civil commitment of, 51
clinical assessment of, 51–52
malpractice implications, 158–160, 182
records of, 178, 179–180
Suicide, by clients
as malpractice lawsuit basis, 33, 154, 158–160, 188
meeting with patient's family following, 188
treatment facilities' liability for, 173
Superior court, 10, 11
Supervisory personnel
lawsuits against, 174–175
legal responsibilities, 191
Supreme Court
federal. *See* United States Supreme Court
state, 10, 11
Supreme Court Reporter, 18

Tarasoff v. *Regents of the University of California*, 237, 239–240, 242, 243–245, 250
Tardive dyskinesia and dystonia, medication-related, 139, 165–166
Teaching conferences, patient's consent for participation in, 225
Telephone contact, therapist-client, documentation of, 180
Telephone rights, of hospitalized patients, 84–85, 99
Testamentary capacity, 285
evaluation of, 301
Testimonial privilege, 210–217
exceptions to, 212–217
marital, 210
physician-patient, 211
priest-penitent, 210
psychotherapist-patient, 211–212
Testimony. *See also* Expert witness
pretrial, in malpractice lawsuits, 185
subpoena for, 32, 212
Therapist
availability of, 165
qualifications of, 170
Therapist-client
social contact, 209–210
telephone contact, documentation of, 180
Therapist-client privilege statutes, 211–212
Third parties, protection of
from driving-impaired clients, 256–257, 261
negligent release and. *See* Negligent release lawsuits
from outpatients. *See* Duty to protect third parties
Tort, unintentional, 150
Tort law, 2–3
Trainees
process notes of, 227
supervision of, 170, 174
Transference
malpractice and, 162, 169
medication refusal and, 131
therapist-client sexual activity and, 162
Treatment
adolescents' decision-making about, 317–318, 338–339
alternative modalities of, 170
children's access to, 311, 314–318
emergency care, 314–315
handicapped infants, 315–316, 340

Treatment (*cont.*)
  children's access to (*cont.*)
    nonparental consent for, 318
    parental consent for, 316–317
    treatment decision-making and, 317–318
  competency to consent to, 87, 116–117, 119, 274, 275–281
  cost of, responsbility for, 62
  humane, 87–88
  informed consent for. *See* Informed consent
  institutionalized persons' right to, 110–113
    case law basis of, 111–112
    clinical implications, 112–113
  least-restrictive-alternative of, 88–90, 99
  minors' access to, 321–322
  patient's refusal of. *See* Treatment refusal
  of potentially violent clients, 244, 245
  termination of
    as abandonment, 164–165
    for disabled infants/children, 316, 340
    family's request for, 301–302
    living wills and, 117, 297–299
Treatment facilities
  as humane environment, 87–88
  legal liability of, 173–174
  legal representation of, 29
  voluntary admissions decision of, 45
Treatment plan, 88
Treatment provider, legal representation of, 29–30
Treatment refusal, 119–120
  by adolescents, 338–339
  advance directives for, 296–297
  attorney's role in, 31
  competency and, 276
  constitutional basis of, 110
  for handicapped infants, 315–316
  informed consent and, 118–119
  in involuntary hospitalization, 87
  least-restrictive-alternative basis, 89
  by minors, 323
  religious beliefs-based, 98
    for children, 315
  by surgical patients, 118–119
Trial court, 6, 9–10, 11
  federal, 6–7

United States Code (U.S.C.), 19–20
  Child Abuse Amendments, 315–316
United States Code Annotated, 19–20
United States Law Week, 18
United States Reporter, 18
United States Supreme Court, 2, 9, 18, 114–115, 125–128, 134–135
University of California Regents v. *Tarasoff*, 237, 239–240, 242, 243–245, 250
Utilization review, in managed care, 258

Verbal abuse, by therapist, 164
Veterans Administration
  benefits, representative payees for, 93, 293
  negligent release lawsuits against, 250
Videotaping, of children
  for abuse assessment, 328
  of testimony, 313–314
Violence potential, assessment and prediction of, 49–51, 63
  duty to protect third parties implications, 243
  negligent release implications, 253, 254–255
Violent patients
  access to guns, 254
  civil commitment of, 63
  civil/criminal charges against, 140
  outpatients as. *See* Duty to protect third parties
  restraint and seclusion of, 134–136
Visitation rights, of hospitalized patients, 83–84, 99
  suicide implications, 160
Voluntarily admitted patients
  adolescents as, 323
  discharge of, 45, 61
  involuntary detention of, 63, 261
  psychotropic medication refusal by, 138–139
  restraint and seclusion of, 135
Voluntary admission, 44–45, 57–58
  incompetency adjudication following, 300–301
  patient's competency to consent to, 64
  states' mental health codes for, 44
Voluntariness, of consent to treatment, 117–118
Voting rights
  age of majority for, 310
  of hospitalized patients, 98
  of incompetent persons, 286

Waiver
  of confidentiality by client, 207–208
  for juvenile offenders, 337–338
Westlaw, 22
West Publishing Company, 18, 20
Wills
  contests of, breach of confidentiality in, 217
  of incompetent persons, 285, 301
  living, 117, 297–299
  testamentary capacity and, 301
Winship, In re, 336

Witnesses, 14
  children as, 312–314
  at civil commitment hearings, 56–57
  court-ordered examination of, 213
  expert, *See* Expert witness
Worker's compensation claims, 216, 353

Wyatt v. *Stickney*, 81–82, 87, 89, 111, 114
  citation of, 17

Youngberg v. *Romeo*, 115, 126, 134–135

Zinermon v. *Burch*, 44

www.ingramcontent.com/pod-product-compliance
Ingram Content Group UK Ltd.
Pitfield, Milton Keynes, MK11 3LW, UK
UKHW020131290926
15471UKWH00003B/418
9781489916556